Contents

Preface

This concise review of microbiology and immunology is intended for medical and graduate students studying for the United States Medical Licensing Examination (USMLE) as well as other examinations. The fourth edition remains a succinct description of the most important concepts of the microbial world and the ways in which the host–parasite relationships are affected. This book is not meant to be a substitute for a major microbiology text but rather to be a review of information that has been learned in didactic courses.

Organization

The book is divided into seven chapters covering major topics of microbiology and immunology. Within each chapter, the important signs, symptoms, and etiology of diseases are described along with mechanisms of preventing infection and means of identifying and diagnosing the causative agent.

The text is presented in a tightly outlined format that facilitates rapid review of important information. Numerous tables with clinical correlations are inserted.

Each chapter is followed by review questions and answers and explanations that reflect the style and content of USMLE. A Comprehensive Examination at the end of the book serves as a practice exam and self-assessment tool to help students diagnose their weaknesses prior to reviewing microbiology and immunology.

Features of the fourth edition

- Updated and current information in all chapters
- Many new questions and explanations reflecting USMLE changes
- Numerous tables, including an alphabetized index of the distinguishing characteristics of the bacterial pathogens
- A comprehensive examination

Arthur G. Johnson, PhD
Richard J. Ziegler, PhD
Omelan A. Lukasewycz, PhD
Louise B. Hawley, PhD

Acknowledgments

The authors are grateful for the excellent organizational and secretarial skills of Ms. Sally Herstad, who aided the preparation of this edition.

1

General Properties of Microorganisms

I. The Microbial World

A. Microorganisms

—belong to the Protista biologic kingdom.

—include some eukaryotes and prokaryotes, viruses, viroids, and prions.

—are classified according to their structure, chemical composition, and biosynthetic and genetic organization.

B. Eukaryotic cells

—contain organelles and a nucleus bounded by a nuclear membrane.

—contain complex phospholipids, sphingolipids, histones, and sterols.

—lack a cell wall (plant cells and fungi have a cell wall).

—have multiple diploid chromosomes and nucleosomes.

—have relatively long-lived mRNA formed from the processing of precursor mRNA, which contains exons and introns.

—have 80S ribosomes and uncoupled transcription and translation.

1. Protozoa (kingdom Protista)

—are classified into seven phyla; three of these phyla (Sarcomastigophora, Apicomplexa, Ciliophora) contain medically important species that are human parasites.

2. Fungi (kingdom Fungi)

—are **eukaryotic** cells with a complex carbohydrate cell wall.

—have **ergosterol** as the dominant membrane sterol.

—may be **monomorphic,** existing as single-celled **yeast** or multicellular, filamentous **mold.**

—may be **dimorphic,** existing as **yeasts or molds, depending on temperature and nutrition.**

1

—may have both asexual and sexual reproduction capabilities. (Deuteromycetes, or Fungi Imperfecti, have no known sexual stages.)

C. Prokaryotic cells

—have no organelles, no membrane-enclosed nucleus, and no histones; in rare cases, they contain complex phospholipids, sphingolipids, and sterols.

—have 70S ribosomes.

—have a cell wall composed of peptidoglycan-containing muramic acid.

—are haploid with a single chromosome.

—have short-lived, unprocessed mRNA.

—have coupled transcription and translation.

1. Typical bacteria

—**have normal peptidoglycan.**

—may be normal flora or may be pathogenic in humans.

—do not have a sexual growth cycle; however, some can produce asexual spores.

2. Mycoplasmas

—are the smallest and simplest of the bacteria that are self-replicating.

—lack a cell wall.

—are the only prokaryotes that contain sterols.

3. Rickettsia organisms

—are **obligate intracellular bacteria** that are incapable of self-replication.

—depend on the host cell for adenosine triphosphate (ATP) production.

4. Chlamydiae

—are bacteria-like **obligate intracellular pathogens** with a complex growth cycle involving intracellular and extracellular forms.

—depend on the host cell for ATP production.

D. Viruses

—are not cells and are not visible with the light microscope.

—are **obligate intracellular parasites.**

—contain no organelles or biosynthetic machinery, except for a few enzymes.

—contain either RNA or DNA as genetic material.

—are called **bacteriophages** (or **phages**) if they have a bacterial host.

E. Viroids

—are not cells and are not visible with the light microscope.

—are **obligate intracellular parasites.**

—are single-stranded, covalently closed, circular RNA molecules that exist as base-paired, rod-like structures.

—cause plant diseases but have not been proved to cause human disease, although the RNA of the hepatitis D virus is viroid-like.

F. Prions

—are infectious particles associated with subacute, progressive, degenerative diseases of the central nervous system (e.g., Creutzfeldt-Jakob disease).

—copurify with a specific glycoprotein (PrP) that has a molecular weight of 27–30 kDa.

—are resistant to nucleases but are inactivated by proteases and other agents that inactivate proteins.

—are altered conformations of a normal cellular protein that can autocatalytically form more copies of itself.

II. Bacterial Structure (Table 1-1)

A. Bacterial shape

—can usually be determined with appropriate staining and a light microscope.

—is usually **round** (coccus), **rod-like** (bacillus), or **spiral** with most species; cocci and bacilli often grow in doublets (diplococci) or chains (streptococci). Cocci that grow in clusters are called staphylococci.

—may be **pleomorphic** with some species, such as *Bacteroides*.

—is used, along with other properties, to identify bacteria.

—is determined by the mechanism of cell wall assembly.

—may be altered by antibiotics that affect cell wall biosynthesis (e.g., penicillin).

B. Bacterial nucleus

—is not surrounded by a nuclear membrane, nor does it contain a mitotic apparatus.

—is generally called a **nucleoid or nuclear body.**

—consists of polyamine and magnesium ions bound to negatively charged, circular, supercoiled, double-stranded DNA; small amounts of RNA; RNA polymerase; and other proteins.

C. Bacterial cytoplasm

—contains ribosomes and various types of nutritional storage granules.

—contains no organelles.

D. Bacterial ribosomes

—have a sedimentation coefficient of 70S and are composed of 30S and 50S subunits containing 16S, and 23S and 5S RNA, respectively.

—are the sites of action of many antibiotics that inhibit protein biosynthesis.

Table 1-1. Components of Microbial Cells

Structure	Composition	Cell Type					
		Fungi	Gram-Positive Bacteria	Gram-Negative Bacteria	Myco-plasmas	Chlamydia*	Rickettsia*
Envelope capsule	Polysaccharide or polypeptide	–	+ or –	+ or –	–	–	–
Wall							
Chitin	Poly-N-acetylglucosamine	+	–	–	–	–	–
Peptidoglycan	Poly-N-acetylglucosamine-N acetylmuramic acid-tetrapeptide	–	+	+	–	–	+
Periplasm	Proteins and oligosaccharides	–	–	+	–	+	+
Lipoprotein	Lipoprotein	–	–	+	–	+	+
Outer membrane	Proteins, phospholipids, and lipopolysaccharide	–	–	+	–	+	+
Appendages							
Pili	Protein	–	+ or –	+ or –	–	–	–
Flagella	Protein	–	+ or –	+ or –	–	–	–
Cell membrane	Proteins and phospholipids	+ (plus ergosterol)	+	+	+	+	+
Cytosol							
Organelles	Protein, phospholipids, and nucleic acids	+	–	–	–	–	–
80S Ribosomes	Protein and RNA	+	–	–	–	–	–
70S Ribosomes	Protein and RNA	–	+	+	+	+	+
Genetic material							
Nucleus	Protein, phospholipids, and nucleic acids	+	–	–	–	–	–
Nucleoid	Protein and nucleic acids	–	+	+	+	+	+
Plasmids	DNA	+ or –	+ or –	+ or –	+ or –	+ or –	+ or –
Transposons	DNA	+	+	+	+	+	+
Spores							
Reproductive spores	All cellular components	+	–	–	–	–	–
Endospores	All cellular components plus dipicolinic acid	–	+ or –	–	–	–	–

*Obligate intracellular pathogens because they cannot synthesize ATP

—have proteins and RNAs that differ from those of their eukaryotic counterparts.

—form the basis for the selective toxicity of antibacterial protein synthesis–inhibiting agents, which affect 70S ribosomes (e.g., erythromycin) but not 80S ribosomes.

—are membrane-bound if engaged in protein biosynthesis.

E. Cell (cytoplasmic) membrane

—is a typical phospholipid bilayer.

—contains the cytochromes and enzymes involved in electron transport and oxidative phosphorylation.

—contains carrier lipids and enzymes involved in cell wall biosynthesis.

—contains enzymes involved in phospholipid synthesis and DNA replication.

—contains chemoreceptors.

—is responsible for selective permeability and active transport, which are facilitated by membrane-bound permeases, binding proteins, and various transport systems.

—is the site of action of certain antibiotics, such as polymyxin.

F. Mesosomes

—are **convoluted invaginations** of the plasma membrane.

—function in DNA replication and cell division as well as in secretion.

—are termed **septal mesosomes** if they occur at the septum (cross-wall) or **lateral mesosomes** if they are nonseptal.

G. Plasmids

—are small, circular, nonchromosomal, double-stranded DNA molecules.

—are capable of self-replication.

—are most frequently extrachromosomal, but may become integrated into bacterial DNA.

—contain genes that confer protective properties, such as antibiotic resistance, virulence factors, or their own transmissibility to other bacteria.

H. Transposons

—are small pieces of DNA that move between the DNA of bacteriophages.

—are bacteria or plasmids not capable of self-replication.

—code for antibiotic resistance enzymes, metabolic enzymes, or toxins.

—may alter expression of neighboring genes or cause mutations to genes into which they are inserted.

I. Cell envelope (Figures 1-1 and 1-2)

—is composed of the macromolecular layers that surround the bacterium.

—always includes a cell membrane and a peptidoglycan layer.

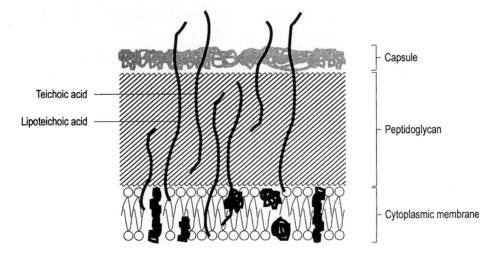

Figure 1-1. Diagrammatic representation of a gram-positive bacterial cell envelope.

—includes an outer membrane layer in gram-negative bacteria.

—may include a capsule, a glycocalyx layer, or both.

—contains antigens that frequently induce a specific antibody response.

1. Cell wall

—refers to that portion of the cell envelope that is external to the cytoplasmic membrane and internal to the capsule or glycocalyx.

—confers osmotic protection and gram-staining characteristics.

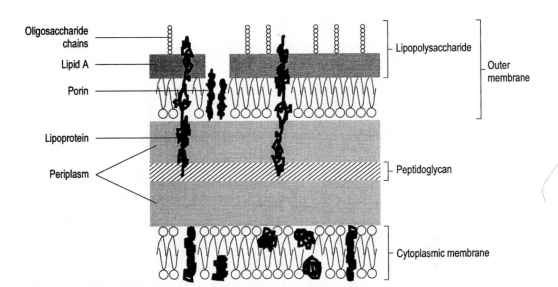

Figure 1-2. Diagrammatic representation of a gram-negative bacterial cell envelope.

—is composed of peptidoglycan, teichoic and teichuronic acids, and polysaccharides in **gram-positive bacteria.**

—is composed of peptidoglycan, lipoprotein, and an outer phospholipid membrane that contains lipopolysaccharide in **gram-negative bacteria.**

—contains **penicillin-binding proteins.**

2. Peptidoglycan

—is also called **mucopeptide** or **murein** and is unique to prokaryotes.

—is found in all bacterial cell walls, except *Mycoplasma*.

—is a **complex polymer** that consists of a **backbone,** which is composed of alternating *N*-acetylglucosamine and *N*-acetylmuramic acid and a set of identical tetrapeptide **side chains,** which are attached to the *N*-acetylmuramic acid and that are frequently linked to adjacent tetrapeptide side chains by identical peptide **cross-bridges** or by direct peptide **bonds.**

—contains the β-1,4 glycosidic bond between *N*-acetylmuramic acid and *N*-acetylglucosamine, which is cleaved by the bacteriolytic enzyme **lysozyme** (found in mucus, saliva, and tears).

—may contain **diaminopimelic acid,** an amino acid unique to prokaryotic cell walls.

—is the site of action of certain antibiotics, such as penicillin and the cephalosporins.

—comprises up to 50% of the cell wall of gram-positive bacteria but only 2%–10% of the cell wall of gram-negative bacteria.

3. Teichoic and teichuronic acids

—are **water-soluble polymers,** containing a ribitol or glycerol residue linked by phosphodiester bonds.

—are found in **gram-positive** cell walls or membranes.

—are chemically bonded to peptidoglycan (wall teichoic acid) or membrane glycolipid (lipoteichoic acid), particularly in mesosomes.

—contain important bacterial surface antigenic determinants, and lipoteichoic acid helps anchor the wall to the membrane.

—may account for 50% of the dry weight of a gram-positive cell wall.

4. Lipoprotein

—cross-links the peptidoglycan and outer membrane in **gram-negative** bacteria.

—is linked to diaminopimelic acid residues of peptidoglycan tetrapeptide side chains by a peptide bond; the lipid portion is noncovalently inserted into the outer membrane.

5. Periplasmic space

—is found in **gram-negative** cells.

—refers to the area between the cell membrane and the outer membrane.

—contains hydrated peptidoglycan, penicillin-binding proteins, hydrolytic enzymes (including β-lactamases), specific carrier molecules, and oligosaccharides.

6. **Outer membrane**

—is found in **gram-negative** cells.

—is a **phospholipid bilayer** in which the phospholipids of the outer portion are replaced by lipopolysaccharides.

—protects cells from many things, including harmful enzymes and some antibiotics, and prevents leakage of periplasmic proteins.

—contains embedded proteins, including matrix **porins** (nonspecific pores), some nonpore proteins (phospholipases and proteases), and transport proteins for small molecules.

7. **Lipopolysaccharide**

—is found in the outer leaflet of the outer membrane of **gram-negative** cells.

—consists of **lipid A,** several long-chain fatty acids attached to phosphorylated glucosamine disaccharide units, and a polysaccharide composed of a core and terminal repeating units.

—is negatively charged and noncovalently cross-bridged by divalent cations.

—is also called **endotoxin;** the toxicity is associated with the lipid A.

—contains major surface antigenic determinants, including **O antigen** found in the polysaccharide component.

8. **Bayer's junction**

—is found in **gram-negative** cells.

—is the region of the wall where the inner leaflet of the outer membrane is contiguous with the outer leaflet of the cell membrane.

J. **External layers**

1. **Capsule**

—is a well-defined structure of polysaccharide surrounding a bacterial cell and is external to the cell wall. The one exception to the polysaccharide structure is the poly-D-glutamic acid capsule of *Bacillus anthracis.*

—protects the bacteria from phagocytosis and plays a role in bacterial adherence.

2. **Glycocalyx**

—refers to a loose network of polysaccharide fibrils that surrounds some bacterial cell walls.

—is sometimes called a **slime layer.**

—is associated with adhesive properties of the bacterial cell.

—is synthesized by surface enzymes.

—contains prominent antigenic sites.

K. **Appendages**

1. **Flagella**

—are protein appendages for locomotion.

—consist of a basal body, hook, and a long filament composed of a polymerized protein called **flagellin.**

—may be located in only one area of a cell (**polar**) or over the entire bacterial cell surface (**peritrichous**).

—contain prominent antigenic determinants.

2. Pili (fimbriae)

—are rigid surface appendages composed mainly of a protein called **pilin.**

—exist in two classes: **ordinary pili (adhesins),** involved in bacterial adherence, and **sex pili,** involved in attachment of donor and recipient bacteria in conjugation.

—are, in the case of ordinary pili, the colonization antigens or **virulence factors** associated with some bacterial species, such as *Streptococcus pyogenes* and *Neisseria gonorrhoeae.*

—may confer antiphagocytic properties, like the **M protein** of *S pyogenes.*

L. Endospores

—are formed as a survival response to certain adverse nutritional conditions, such as depletion of a certain resource.

—are metabolically **inactive bacterial cells** that are highly resistant to desiccation, heat, and various chemicals.

—possess a core that contains many cell components, a spore wall, a cortex, a coat, and an exosporium.

—contain **calcium dipicolinate,** which aids in heat resistance in the core.

—germinate under favorable nutritional conditions after an activation process that involves damage to the spore coat.

—are helpful in identifying some species of bacteria (e.g., *Bacillus* and *Clostridium*).

—are not reproductive structures.

III. Bacterial Growth

A. General characteristics—bacterial growth

—refers to an increase in bacterial cell numbers (multiplication), which results from a programmed increase in the biomass of the bacteria.

—results from bacterial reproduction due to binary fission, which may be characterized by a parameter called **generation time** (i.e., the average time required for cell numbers to double).

—may be determined by measuring **cell concentration** (turbidity measurements or cell counting) or **biomass density** (dry weight or protein determinations).

—usually occurs asynchronously (i.e., all cells do not divide at precisely the same moment).

B. Cell concentration

—may be measured by **viable cell counts** involving serial dilutions of sample followed by a determination of colony-forming units on an agar surface.

—may be determined by **particle cell counting** or **turbidimetric density measurements** (includes both viable and nonviable cells).

C. Bacterial growth curve (Figure 1-3)

—requires inoculation of bacteria from a saturated culture into fresh liquid media.

—is unique for a particular nutritional environment.

—is frequently illustrated in a plot of logarithmic number of bacteria ver-

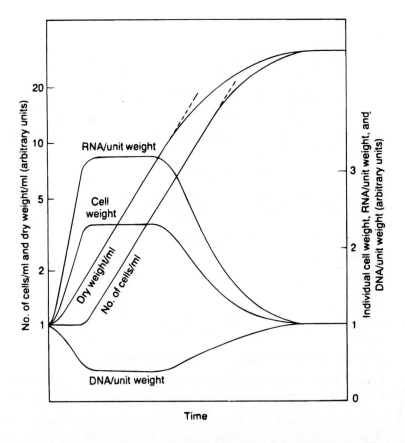

Figure 1-3. Diagram of changes in cell size and chemical composition during growth curve. The bacterial inoculum was from an early stationary-phase culture. The bacterial count and dry-weight concentration are on logarithmic scale (*left-hand ordinate*); the average bacterial dry weight and content of RNA and DNA are on arithmetic scale (*right-hand ordinate*). The initial values of all variables are taken as one unit. (Reprinted with permission from Wilson GS, Miles A, eds: *Topley and Wilson's Principles of Bacteriology, Virology and Immunity,* 6th ed, vol 1. Baltimore, Williams & Wilkins, 1975, p 125.)

sus time; the generation time is determined by observing the time necessary for the cells to double in number during the log phase of growth.

—consists of **four phases:**

1. **Lag**—metabolite-depleted cells adapt to new environment.

2. **Exponential or log**—cell biomass is synthesized at a constant rate. Cells in this stage are generally more susceptible to antibiotics.

3. **Stationary**—cells exhaust essential nutrients or accumulate toxic products.

4. **Death or decline**—cells may die due to toxic products.

D. Chemostat

—is a device that maintains a bacterial culture in a specific phase of growth or at a specific cell concentration.

—is most frequently used to maintain a bacterial culture in the exponential growth phase.

—is based on the principle that toxic products and cells are removed at the same rate as fresh nutrients are added and new cells are synthesized.

—operates best if one nutrient limits bacterial growth.

E. Synchronous growth

—refers to a situation in which all the bacteria in a culture divide at the same moment.

—may be achieved by several methods, including thymidine starvation (thymidine-requiring bacteria), alternate cycles of low and optimal incubation temperatures, spore germination, selective filtration of old (large) and young (small) cells, or "trapped cell" filtration.

IV. Bacterial Cultivation

A. General characteristics—bacterial cultivation

—refers to the propagation of bacteria.

—involves specific pH, gaseous, and temperature preferences of bacteria.

—is performed in either liquid (broth) or solid (agar) growth medium.

—requires an environment that contains:

1. A carbon source

2. A nitrogen source

3. An energy source

4. Inorganic salts

5. Growth factors

6. Electron donors and acceptors

B. Superoxide dismutase

—is an enzyme in aerobes and facultative and aerotolerant anaerobes that allows them to grow in the presence of the superoxide free radical (O_2^-).

—carries out the reaction $2O_2^- + 2H^+ \rightarrow H_2O_2 + O_2$.

—produces hydrogen peroxide (H_2O_2), which is toxic to cells but is destroyed by **catalase** or is oxidized by a peroxidase enzyme.

C. Oxygen requirements

1. Obligate aerobes

—refer to bacteria that require oxygen for growth.

—contain the enzyme **superoxide dismutase,** which protects them from the toxic O_2^-.

2. Obligate anaerobes

—are killed by the O_2^-; they grow maximally at a P_{O_2} concentration of less than 0.5%–3%.

—lack superoxide dismutase, catalase, and cytochrome *c* oxidase (enzymes that destroy toxic products of oxygen metabolism).

—require a substance other than oxygen as a hydrogen acceptor during the generation of metabolic energy.

—use fermentation pathways with distinctive metabolic products.

—outnumber aerobes 1000:1 in the gut and 100:1 in the mouth.

—comprise 99% of the total fecal flora (10^{11}/g of stool in the large bowel).

—usually cause polymicrobial infections (i.e., infections involving more than one genus or species).

—are foul smelling.

—are generally not communicable or transmissible, except as endospores, such as *Clostridium difficile.*

—generally are found proximal to mucosal surfaces; when this barrier is broken, anaerobes can escape into tissues.

—Mucosal surfaces can be disrupted by:

a. Gastrointestinal obstruction or surgery

b. Diverticulitis

c. Bronchial obstruction

d. Tumor growth

e. Ulceration of the intestinal tract by chemotherapeutic agents

3. Facultative anaerobes

—grow in the presence or absence of oxygen.

—shift from a fermentative to a respiratory metabolism in the presence of air.

—display the **Pasteur effect,** in which the energy needs of the cell are met by consuming less glucose under a respiratory metabolism than under a fermentative metabolism.

—include most pathogenic bacteria.

4. Aerotolerant anaerobes

—resemble facultative bacteria but have a fermentative metabolism both with and without an oxygen environment.

D. Nutritional requirements

1. Heterotrophs

—require preformed organic compounds (e.g., sugar, amino acids) for growth.

2. Autotrophs

—do not require preformed organic compounds for growth because they can synthesize them from inorganic compounds and carbon dioxide.

E. Growth media

1. Minimal essential growth medium

—contains only the primary precursor compounds essential for growth.

—demands that a bacterium synthesize most of the organic compounds required for its growth.

—dictates a relatively slow generation time.

2. Complex growth medium

—contains most of the organic compound building blocks (e.g., sugars, amino acids, nucleotides) necessary for growth.

—dictates a faster generation time for a bacterium relative to its generation time in minimal essential growth medium.

—is necessary for the growth of fastidious bacteria.

3. Differential growth medium

—contains a combination of nutrients and pH indicators to allow visual distinction of bacteria that grow on or in it.

—is frequently a solid medium on which colonies of particular bacterial species have a distinctive color.

4. Selective growth medium

—contains compounds that prevent the growth of some bacteria while allowing the growth of other bacteria.

—uses certain dyes or sugars, high salt concentration, or pH to achieve selectivity.

V. Bacterial Metabolism

A. General characteristics

1. Bacterial metabolism

—is the sum of **anabolic processes** (synthesis of cellular constituents requiring energy) and **catabolic processes** (breakdown of cellular constituents with concomitant release of waste products and energy-rich compounds).

—is **heterotrophic** for pathogenic bacteria.

—varies depending on the nutritional environment.

2. Bacterial transport systems

—involve membrane-associated binding or transport proteins for sugars and amino acids.

—frequently require energy to concentrate substrates inside the cell.

—are usually inducible for nutrients that are catabolized; glucose, which is constitutive, is an exception.

—frequently use phosphotransferase systems when sugars are transported.

B. Carbohydrate metabolism

1. Fermentation

—is a method by which some bacteria obtain metabolic energy.

—is characterized by a **substrate phosphorylation.**

—involves the formation of **ATP** not coupled to electron transfer.

—requires an organic electron acceptor, such as pyruvate.

—results in the synthesis of specific metabolic end products that may aid in the identification of bacterial species.

2. Respiration

—refers to the method of obtaining metabolic energy that involves an **oxidative phosphorylation.**

—involves the formation of ATP during electron transfer and the reduction of gaseous oxygen in aerobic respiration.

—involves a cell membrane electron transport chain composed of cytochrome enzymes, lipid cofactors, and coupling factors.

C. Regulation

1. Regulation of enzyme activity

—may occur because enzymes are **allosteric proteins,** susceptible to binding of effector molecules that influence their activity.

—may occur by **feedback inhibition** involving the end product.

—may involve **substrate-binding enhancement** (cooperatively) of catalytic activity.

2. Regulation of enzyme synthesis

—may involve allosteric regulatory proteins that activate (**activators**) or inhibit (**repressors**) gene transcription.

—may involve **end product feedback repression** of biosynthetic pathway enzymes.

—may involve **substrate induction** of catabolic enzymes.

—may involve **attenuation control sequences** in enzyme mRNA.

—may involve the process of **catabolite repression,** which is under positive control of the **catabolite activator protein.**

3. Pasteur effect

—occurs in **facultative bacteria.**

—is caused by oxygen blocking the fermentative capacity of the bacteria.

—means that the energy needs are met by using less glucose during aerobic growth.

VI. Cell Wall Synthesis

—involves the cytoplasmic synthesis of peptidoglycan subunits, which are translocated by a membrane lipid carrier and cross-linked to existing cell wall by enzymes associated with the plasma membrane of gram-positive bacteria or found in the periplasmic region of gram-negative bacteria.

—involves the covalent linkage of teichoic acid to *N*-acetylmuramic acid residues in gram-positive cells.

—is affected by many antibiotics, including penicillins, cephalosporins, and carbapenems.

—includes the addition of three components (lipoprotein, outer membrane, lipopolysaccharide), whose constituents or subunits are synthesized on or in the cytoplasmic membrane and assembled outside of it in gram-negative cells.

VII. Sterilization and Disinfection

A. Terminology

1. **Sterility**—total absence of viable microorganisms as assessed by no growth on any medium

2. **Bactericidal**—kills bacteria

3. **Bacteriostatic**—inhibits growth of bacteria

4. **Sterilization**—removal or killing of all microorganisms

5. **Disinfection**—removal or killing of disease-causing microorganisms

6. **Sepsis**—infection

7. **Aseptic**—without infection

8. **Antisepsis**—any procedure that inhibits the growth and multiplication of microorganisms

B. Kinetics of killing

—is affected by menstruum or medium, the concentration of organisms and antimicrobial agents, temperature, pH, and the presence of endospores.

—can be exponential (logarithmic).

—can result in a killing curve that becomes asymptotic, requiring extra considerations in killing final numbers, especially if the population is heterogeneous relative to sensitivity.

C. Methods of control include

1. **Moist heat** (autoclaving at 121°C for 15 minutes at a steam pressure of 15 pounds per square inch kills microorganisms, including endospores)

2. **Dry heat and incineration** (both methods oxidize proteins, killing bacteria)

3. **Ultraviolet radiation** (blocks DNA replication)

4. **Chemicals**

   a. **Phenol** (Figure 1-4)

      —is used as a disinfectant standard that is expressed as a phenol coefficient, which compares the rate of the minimal sterilizing con-

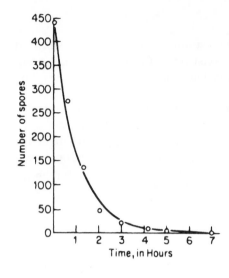

Figure 1-4. Disinfection of anthrax spores with 5% phenol at 33.3°C. The curve is drawn through a series of calculated points. The circles represent the experimental observations. (Reprinted with permission from Wilson GS, Dick HM (eds): *Topley and Wilson's Principles of Bacteriology, Virology and Immunity,* 7th ed, vol 1. Baltimore, Williams & Wilkins, 1983, p 85.)

centration of phenol to that of the test compound for a particular organism.

b. Chlorhexidine

—is a diphenyl cationic analogue that is a useful topical disinfectant.

c. Iodine

—is bactericidal in a 2% solution of aqueous alcohol containing potassium iodide.

—acts as an oxidizing agent and combines irreversibly with proteins.

—can cause hypersensitivity reactions.

d. Chlorine

—inactivates bacteria and most viruses by oxidizing free sulfhydryl groups.

e. Formaldehyde

—is used as a disinfectant in aqueous solution (37%).

f. Ethylene oxide

—is an alkylating agent that is especially useful for sterilizing heat-sensitive hospital instruments.

—requires exposure times of 4–6 hours, followed by aeration to remove absorbed gas.

g. Alcohol

—requires concentrations of 70%–95% to kill bacteria given sufficient time.

—Isopropyl alcohol (90%–95%) is the major form in use in hospitals.

VIII. Antimicrobial Chemotherapy

A. General characteristics—antimicrobial chemotherapy

—is based on the principle of selective toxicity, which implies that a compound is harmful to a microorganism but innocuous to its host.

—involves drugs that:

1. **Are antimetabolites**
2. **Inhibit cell wall biosynthesis**
3. **Inhibit protein synthesis**
4. **Inhibit nucleic acid synthesis**
5. **Alter or inhibit cell membrane permeability or transport**

   —includes both **bacteriostatic** (inhibit growth) and **bactericidal** (kill) drugs.

   —may be characterized as **broad spectrum** (effective against a wide variety of bacterial species) or **narrow spectrum** (effective against one or a few bacterial species).

   —may use synergistic combinations of bacteriostatic drugs (e.g., trimethoprim and sulfonamide).

   —incorporates both **drug–parasite** relationships (e.g., location of bacteria and drug distribution) and alterations of **host–parasite** relationships (e.g., immune response and microbial flora) to be effective.

B. **Drug antimicrobial activity**

   —is usually determined by **dilution** or **diffusion** tests.

   —is quantitated by determining the minimal inhibitory concentration.

   —may differ in vitro and in vivo.

   —is affected by pH, drug stability, microbial environment, number of microorganisms present, length of incubation with drug, and metabolic activity of microorganisms.

   —may be modified for a specific bacterium if **genetic or nongenetic drug resistance** develops.

C. **Drug resistance**

   1. **Nongenetic mechanisms of drug resistance**

      —may involve loss of specific target structures, such as cell wall by L forms of bacteria.

      —may result from metabolic inactivity of microorganisms.

   2. **Genetic mechanisms of drug resistance**

      —may result from either chromosomal or extrachromosomal (plasmid) resistance.

      —may involve a chromosomal mutation that alters the structure of the cellular target (e.g., penicillin-binding protein) of the drug or the permeability of the drug.

      —may result from the introduction of a plasmid (R factor or R plasmid) that codes for enzymes (**β-lactamase**) that degrade the drug or modify it (**acetyltransferase**), or from the introduction of proteins that pump it from the cell in an energy-dependent fashion.

   3. **R factor or R plasmid**

      —contains **insertion sequences** and **transposons**.

—may acquire additional resistance genes by plasmid fusion or from transposons.

—may consist of two plasmids, the **resistance transfer factor (RTF),** which codes for replication and transfer, and the **r or resistance determinant,** which contains genes for replication and resistance.

—can be transmitted from species to species.

—is responsible for the rapid development of multiple drug-resistant bacteria over the past 30 years.

D. Mechanisms of action (Table 1-2)

1. Antimetabolites

—include bacteriostatic (sulfonamide, trimethoprim, para-aminosalicylic acid) and bactericidal (isoniazid) drugs.

—are structural analogs of normal metabolites.

—may become bactericidal when used in combination (e.g., trimethoprim and sulfonamide).

—inhibit the action of specific enzymes.

Table 1-2. Mechanisms of Action of Antimicrobial Chemotherapy

Mechanism of Action	Agent	Site of Action	Effect
Inhibitors of cell wall biosynthesis	Cycloserine	Peptidoglycan tetrapeptide side chain	Bactericidal
	Phosphomycin	Formation of N-acetylmuramic acid	Bactericidal
	Bacitracin	Membrane carrier molecule	Bactericidal
	Penicillins	Peptidoglycan cross-linking	Bactericidal
	Cephalosporins, carbapenems	Peptidoglycan cross-linking	Bactericidal
	Vancomycin	Translocation of cell wall intermediates	Bactericidal
Inhibitors of protein biosynthesis	Streptomycin	30S ribosomal subunit	Bactericidal
	Gentamicin	30S ribosomal subunit	Bactericidal
	Tetracycline	30S ribosomal subunit	Bacteriostatic
	Spectinomycin	30S ribosomal subunit	Bacteriostatic
	Chloramphenicol	50S ribosomal subunit	Bacteriostatic
	Erythromycin	50S ribosomal subunit	Bacteriostatic
	Clindamycin	50S ribosomal subunit	Bacteriostatic
	Griseofulvin	Microtubule function	Fungistatic
Inhibitors of nucleic acid synthesis	Quinolones	DNA gyrase	Bactericidal
	Novobiocin	DNA gyrase	Bacteriostatic
	Flucytosine	Fungal thymidylate synthetase	Fungicidal
	Rifampin	DNA-dependent RNA polymerase	Bactericidal
Inhibitors of folate metabolism	Sulfonamides	Pteroic acid synthetase	Bacteriostatic
	Trimethoprim	Dihydrofolate reductase	Bacteriostatic
Inhibitor of mycolic acid synthesis	Isoniazid	Mycobacterial mycolic acid biosynthesis	Bactericidal
Alteration of cytoplasmic membrane	Polymyxins	Bacterial membrane permeability	Bactericidal
	Polyenes	Fungal membrane permeability	Fungicidal
	Azoles	Fungal ergosterol biosynthesis	Fungicidal

2. Cell wall synthesis inhibitors

—are bactericidal.

—may inhibit transpeptidation (cross-linking) of peptidoglycan (β-lactam drugs: penicillins, cephalosporins, carbapenems).

—may inhibit the synthesis of peptidoglycan (cycloserine, bacitracin, vancomycin).

—may act in the cytoplasm (cycloserine), in the membrane (bacitracin), or in the cell wall (penicillins, cephalosporins, vancomycin).

—require cell wall synthesis to be effective.

—may cause bacteria to take on aberrant shapes or become **spheroplasts.**

a. Penicillins

—inhibit the transpeptidation enzymes involved in cell wall synthesis.

—are active against both gram-positive and gram-negative bacteria.

—react with penicillin-binding proteins.

—have a β-lactam ring structure that is inactivated by β-lactamases (penicillinases), which are genetically coded in some bacterial DNA or some R plasmids.

b. Cephalosporins

—have a mechanism of action similar to that of penicillin.

—are active against both gram-positive and gram-negative bacteria.

—contain a β-lactam ring structure that is inactivated by some β-lactamases.

—are frequently used to treat patients who are allergic to penicillins.

c. Carbapenems

—have a mechanism similar to that of penicillin.

—have a β-lactam ring fused to a five-carbon ring and are resistant to β-lactamases.

3. Protein synthesis inhibitors

—include, for example, the aminoglycosides, macrolides, lincomycins, and tetracyclines.

—are frequently known as broad-spectrum antibiotics.

—require bacterial growth to be effective.

a. Aminoglycosides

—include streptomycin, neomycin, kanamycin, and gentamicin.

—are bactericidal for gram-negative bacteria and bind to the 30S ribosomal subunit.

—are not active against anaerobes or intracellular bacteria.

—may irreversibly block initiation of translation or cause mRNA misreading (or both).

—have a narrow effective concentration range before toxicity occurs, causing renal damage and eighth cranial nerve damage (hearing loss).

—may be modified (acetylation) and rendered inactive by enzymes contained in R plasmids.

b. Tetracyclines

—include tetracycline, oxytetracycline, and chlortetracycline.

—are bacteriostatic, bind to the 30S ribosomal subunit, and prevent binding of aminoacyl tRNA to the acceptor site.

—may be deposited in teeth and bones, which can cause tooth staining and structural problems in the bones of children.

—are transported out of or bound to a plasmid-derived protein in cells containing specific tetracycline R plasmids.

c. Chloramphenicol

—is bacteriostatic for gram-positive and gram-negative bacteria, *Rickettsia,* and *Chlamydia.*

—binds to the 50S ribosomal subunit and inhibits peptide-bond formation.

—may be inactivated by the enzyme chloramphenicol acetyltransferase, which is carried on an R plasmid.

—may cause anemia.

d. Griseofulvin

—is a fungistatic drug that is active against fungi with chitin in their cell walls.

—inhibits protein assembly, which interferes with cell division by blocking microtubule assembly.

e. Macrolides and lincomycins

—include erythromycin (macrolide) and lincomycin and clindamycin (lincomycins).

—are bacteriostatic.

—bind to the 23S RNA in the 50S ribosomal subunit and block translocation.

—are rendered ineffective in bacteria that have a mutation in a 50S ribosomal protein or that contain an R plasmid with specific genetic information, which results in methylation of 23S RNA and inhibition of drug binding.

4. Nucleic acid synthesis inhibitors

—can inhibit DNA (quinolones, derivatives of nalidixic acid) or RNA (rifampin) synthesis.

—are generally bactericidal and are quite toxic to mammalian cells.

—bind to strands of DNA (actinomycin and mitomycin) or inhibit replication enzymes. Nalidixic acid and its derivatives inhibit DNA gyrase activity; rifampin inhibits DNA-dependent RNA polymerase.

5. Mycolic acid synthesis inhibitor—isoniazid

—is a bactericidal drug that inhibits mycobacterial mycolic acid biosynthesis.

6. Cytoplasmic membrane inhibitors

—alter the osmotic properties of the plasma membrane (polymyxin and polyenes) or inhibit fungal membrane lipid synthesis (azoles: miconazole and ketoconazole).

—are used in the treatment of some gram-negative (polymyxin) and sterol-containing mycoplasma and fungal (polyenes: nystatin and amphotericin B) infections.

—can react with mammalian cell membranes and are therefore toxic.

—are primarily used as a topical treatment or with severe infections.

IX. Toxins

A. Definition

—Toxins are broadly defined as microbial products that damage host cells or host tissues.

B. Classification

—Toxins are generally classified into two groups: **exotoxins** and **endotoxins.**

—Table 1-3 lists the properties of each group.

C. Mechanism of action

—Many toxins possess an **A and a B polypeptide fragment.**

1. **The A (active) subunit** enters the cell and exerts its toxic effect.

2. **The B (binding) subunit** is responsible for initial attachment of the toxin to the specific target tissue.

3. **Antitoxin** interacts only with the B subunit to block its attachment; once toxin is bound, the antitoxin is ineffective.

D. Toxins composed of A and B polypeptides

1. *Corynebacterium diphtheriae*—exotoxin that inhibits protein synthesis by catalyzing transfer of the adenosine diphosphate (ADP) release moiety of nicotinamide adenine dinucleotide to tRNA elongation factor 2 (EF-2), which disrupts protein synthesis.

2. *Pseudomonas aeruginosa*—exotoxin A that also inhibits protein synthesis via the tRNA EF-2.

3. *Shigella dysenteriae*—shiga neurotoxin that inhibits synthesis via the 60S ribosomal unit by RNase action on 28S ribosomal RNA.

4. *Vibrio cholerae*—choleragen enterotoxin binds to G_{M1} ganglioside and

Table 1-3. Properties of Exotoxins and Endotoxins

Property	Exotoxin	Endotoxin
Organisms	Gram positive and gram negative	Gram negative
Composition	Proteins	Lipopolysaccharides
Released by organisms	Yes	No
Heat sensitivity	Labile	Stable
Toxoids (vaccines)	Yes	No
Neutralization by antitoxin	Yes	No
Degree of toxicity	Very potent	Less potent
Specificity for target cells	High	Low

transfers ADP-ribose to guanosine 5′-triphosphate, which stimulates adenylate cyclase to overproduce cyclic adenosine monophosphate (cyclic AMP) and induce loss of fluids and electrolytes.

5. *Escherichia coli*—heat-labile enterotoxin similar to choleragen that also stimulates adenylate cyclase to overproduce cyclic AMP and induce loss of fluids and electrolytes.

6. *Campylobacter jejuni*—an enterotoxin also similar to choleragen.

7. *Bordetella pertussis*—ADP-ribosylation of a G protein, which increases adenylate cyclase activity by preventing its inactivation.

8. *Clostridium tetani*—tetanospasm exotoxin that acts on synaptosomes; gangliosides bind the toxin and block the release of glycine, which obliterates the inhibitory reflex response of nerves, causing uncontrolled spastic impulses (hyperreflexia of skeletal muscles).

9. *Clostridium botulinum*—botulinum exotoxin that acts on myoneural junctions; cholinergic nerve fibers are paralyzed, which suppresses the release of acetylcholine, causing flaccid paralysis.

E. **Toxins composed of a single polypeptide**

1. *Clostridium perfringens*—α-toxin that is an enzyme phospholipase C; it disrupts cellular and mitochondrial membranes.

2. *E coli*—heat-stable enterotoxin that stimulates guanylate cyclase to overproduce cyclic guanosine monophosphate, which impairs chloride and sodium absorption.

3. *Salmonella*—enterotoxin that stimulates cyclic AMP.

4. *Staphylococcus aureus*—exfoliative toxin that disrupts the stratum granulosum in the epidermis.

5. *S pyogenes*—erythrogenic and pyrogenic exotoxins that act as T-cell super antigens, stimulating release of tumor necrosis factor and interleukin-1.

X. Bacteriophages

A. **General characteristics—bacteriophages**

—are bacterial viruses that are frequently called **phages.**

—are obligate intracellular parasites.

—are host-specific infectious agents for bacteria.

—are called bacteriophage virions when they are complete (genetic material and capsid) infectious particles.

—contain protein and RNA or DNA as major components.

B. **Morphologic classes of bacteriophages**

1. **Polyhedral phages**

—are usually composed of an outer polyhedral-shaped protein coat (capsid) that surrounds the nucleic acid.

—may contain a lipid bilayer between two protein capsid layers (PM-2 phage).

—have either circular double-stranded (PM-2) or single-stranded DNA (ΦX174 and M-12) or linear single-stranded RNA (MS2 and Qβ) as their genetic material, although one phage (Φ6) that has three pieces of double-stranded RNA has been described.

2. Filamentous phages

—have a filamentous protein capsid that surrounds a circular single-stranded DNA genome (f1 and M13).

—are male bacteria–specific in that infection occurs through the pili, which are only present on male bacteria.

—do not lyse their host cells during the replication process.

3. Complex phages

—have a protein polyhedral head containing linear double-stranded DNA and a protein tail and other appendages.

—include the T and lambda phages of *E coli.*

C. Genetic classes of bacteriophages

1. RNA phages

—refer to all phages with RNA as their genetic material.

—are specific for bacteria with male pili (male-specific phages).

—contain single-stranded RNA (except for Φ6) [see X B1], which can act as polycistronic mRNA.

2. DNA phages

—refer to all phages with DNA as their genetic material.

—contain nucleic acid bases that are frequently glucosylated or methylated.

—may contain some unusual nucleic acid bases, such as 5-hydroxymethyl cytosine or 5-hydroxymethyl uracil.

—are classified as **virulent** or **temperate,** depending on whether their pattern of replication is strictly lytic (virulent) or alternates between lytic and lysogenic (temperate).

D. Bacteriophage replication

—requires that the phage use the biosynthetic machinery of the host cell.

—follows a basic sequence of events, which includes adsorption; penetration; phage-specific transcription, translation, or both; assembly; and release.

—is initiated by interaction of phage receptors and specific bacterial surface receptor sites.

—involves injection of the phage genome into the host cell (filamentous phages are the exception).

—follows one of two types of patterns, **lytic** or **lysogenic,** for DNA phages.

—is usually complete in 30–60 minutes for virulent phages.

1. Lytic replication cycle

—occurs with virulent phages (*E coli* T phages) and results in **lysis of the host cell.**

—is the basis for **phage-typing** of bacteria, which can identify strains of bacteria based on their lysis by a selected set of phages.

—may be analyzed in an experimental situation using a **one-step growth curve.**

a. **One-step growth curve**

—is the result of an experimental situation in which one cycle of lytic phage replication is monitored.

—is a plot of infectious virus produced versus time after infection.

—involves the use of a **plaque assay,** which is an infectious-center assay in which counts are made of focal areas of phage-induced lysis on a lawn of bacteria.

b. **Data obtained from one-step growth curve**

(1) **Replication time**

—is the average time necessary for a phage to replicate within a specific host cell and be released from that cell.

(2) **Burst size**

—is the number of infectious phages produced from each infecting phage.

(3) **Eclipse period**

—is the time from infection to the synthesis of the first intracellular infectious virus.

2. **Lysogenic replication cycle**

a. **General characteristics—lysogenic replication**

—may occur only with temperate phages (*E coli* lambda phage).

—involves limited phage-specific protein synthesis, because of the synthesis of a phage-specific **repressor protein** that inhibits phage-specific transcription.

—includes the incorporation of **prophage** (phage DNA) into specific attachment sites in the host cell DNA.

—confers immunity to infection by phages of a type similar to the infecting phage.

—results in passage of the prophage to succeeding generations of the bacteria.

—can revert to lytic replication if the phage repressor is destroyed.

—can result in the generation of **specialized or restricted transducing phages.**

—may result in **lysogenic phage conversion.**

b. **Lysogenic phage conversion**

—refers to a change in the phenotype of the bacteria as a result of limited expression of genes in a prophage.

—occurs in *Salmonella* polysaccharides as a result of infection with the epsilon prophage.

—is the genetic mechanism by which nontoxigenic strains of *C diphtheriae* are converted to toxin-producing strains.

—results in the conversion of nontoxigenic *C botulinum* types C and D to toxin-producing strains.

Review Test

1. Which of the following toxins has phospholipase C activity?

(A) *Escherichia coli* heat-labile toxin
(B) *Clostridium tetani* exotoxin
(C) *Corynebacterium diphtheriae* exotoxin
(D) *Pseudomonas aeruginosa* exotoxin
(E) *Clostridium perfringens* α-toxin

2. What type of phage is used in phage-typing?

(A) Prophage
(B) Virulent phage
(C) Temperate phage
(D) Filamentous phage

3. Which of the following microorganisms contains RNA or DNA as a genetic material?

(A) Viruses
(B) Fungi
(C) Prions
(D) Bacteria
(E) Viroids

4. Which of the following enzymes would be most likely to affect sugar transport into bacteria?

(A) Acetyltransferase
(B) Neuraminidase
(C) Oxidase
(D) Phosphotransferase

5. Polymers of *N*-acetylglucosamine and *N*-acetylmuramic acid are found in which one of the following chemical structures?

(A) Teichoic acid
(B) Cell wall
(C) Glycocalyx
(D) Lipopolysaccharide

6. What type of phage is not inactivated by proteases?

(A) Prophage
(B) Virulent phage
(C) Temperate phage
(D) Filamentous phage

7. What type of bacteria synthesize organic compounds from inorganic compounds?

(A) Heterotrophs
(B) Obligate anaerobes
(C) Aerobes
(D) Facultative anaerobes
(E) Autotrophs

8. Which of the following microorganisms is dimorphic?

(A) Viruses
(B) Fungi
(C) Prions
(D) Bacteria
(E) Viroids

9. Which of the following bacterial structures is most involved in adherence?

(A) Capsule
(B) Lipopolysaccharide
(C) Ordinary pili
(D) O-specific side chain

10. What type of bacteria display the Pasteur effect?

(A) Heterotrophs
(B) Obligate anaerobes
(C) Aerobes
(D) Facultative anaerobes
(E) Autotrophs

11. Which of the following characteristics applies to cephalosporin antibiotics?

(A) Are bacteriostatic
(B) Inhibit protein biosynthesis
(C) Treat fungal infections
(D) Treat patients allergic to penicillin

12. Which of the following toxins acts on synaptosomes?

(A) *Escherichia coli* heat-labile toxin
(B) *Clostridium tetani* exotoxin
(C) *Corynebacterium diphtheriae* exotoxin
(D) *Pseudomonas aeruginosa* exotoxin
(E) *Clostridium perfringens* α-toxin

13. Which one of the following statements applies to bacteria that contain superoxide dismutase?

(A) Need superoxide to grow
(B) Are frequently obligate anaerobes
(C) Grow slowly in the presence of CO_2
(D) Produce hydrogen peroxide from hydrogen ion and the superoxide free radical (O_2^-)

14. Which of the following statements describes lysogenic phage conversion?

(A) The transformation of a virulent phage to a lysogenic phage
(B) A change in bacterial phenotype due to the presence of a prophage
(C) The conversion of a prophage to a temperate phage
(D) The incorporation of a prophage into the bacterial chromosome

15. Which of the following microorganisms may be inactivated by RNases with endonuclease activity?

(A) Viruses
(B) Fungi
(C) Prions
(D) Bacteria
(E) Viroids

16. Which of the following types of media would best be used to isolate bacteria capable of growth in a high-salt concentration?

(A) Minimal growth media
(B) Complex growth media
(C) Differential growth media
(D) Selective growth media

17. Which of the following characteristics applies to bacteriostatic antibiotics?

(A) Are effective when used in combination with bactericidal antibiotics to obtain a synergistic effect
(B) Include all the antimetabolites
(C) Are effective against bacteria in all phases of growth
(D) Include some broad-spectrum antibiotics

18. What type of phage is exemplified by the lambda phage?

(A) Prophage
(B) Virulent phage
(C) Temperate phage
(D) Filamentous phage

19. Which of the following statements concerning prokaryotic cells is true?

(A) They have coupled transcription and translation.
(B) They have processed mRNAs.
(C) They generally have exons and introns.
(D) They transfer secretory proteins into the Golgi apparatus before secretion.

20. What type of bacteria lack superoxide dismutase?

(A) Heterotrophs
(B) Obligate anaerobes
(C) Aerobes
(D) Facultative anaerobes
(E) Autotrophs

21. Which of the following statements applies to the regulation of enzyme activity in bacterial cells?

(A) Can be coupled to the binding of effector molecules
(B) Can be controlled by a catabolite activator protein
(C) May occur via attenuation sequences
(D) Can involve inducer molecules

22. The plasma membrane

(A) contains matrix porins.
(B) includes endotoxin.
(C) contains glycocalyx.
(D) contains the enzymes involved in bacterial oxidative phosphorylation.

23. Which of the following microorganisms has a nuclear membrane?

(A) Viruses
(B) Fungi
(C) Prions
(D) Bacteria
(E) Viroids

24. Which of the following toxins induces electrolyte loss as a result of overproduction of cyclic adenosine monophosphate?

(A) *Escherichia coli* heat-labile toxin
(B) *Clostridium tetani* exotoxin
(C) *Corynebacterium diphtheriae* exotoxin
(D) *Pseudomonas aeruginosa* exotoxin
(E) *Clostridium perfringens* α-toxin

Answers and Explanations

1–E. The phospholipase C activity of the α-toxin of *Clostridium perfringens* disrupts cellular and mitochondrial membranes.

2–B. Phage-typing is useful for identifying certain types of bacteria and depends on bacterial lysis by a selected set of virulent phages.

3–A. Viruses are the only entities that contain either RNA or DNA as genetic material. Fungi and bacteria have DNA, viroids have RNA, and the genetic material of prions is unknown.

4–D. The transport of sugar into a bacterium frequently involves the transfer of a phosphate group to the sugar molecule.

5–B. *N*-acetylglucosamine and *N*-acetylmuramic acid are polymerized to form the peptidoglycan backbone of the cell wall.

6–A. A prophage is the intracellular DNA of a phage and is, therefore, resistant to protease degradation.

7–E. Autotrophic bacteria do not require organic compounds for growth because they synthesize them from inorganic precursors.

8–B. Fungi are dimorphic; that is, they have two morphologic forms.

9–C. Ordinary pili and the glycocalyx are the two bacterial structures that are involved in adherence.

10–D. Facultative anaerobes shift from a fermentative to a respiratory metabolism in the presence of air because the energy needs of the cell are met by consuming less glucose (Pasteur effect) under respiratory metabolism.

11–D. Patients who are allergic to the various penicillins are frequently given one of the cephalosporins.

12–B. *Clostridium tetani* exotoxin acts on synaptosomes, thereby causing hyperreflexia of skeletal muscles.

13–D. Superoxide dismutase is found in aerobic and facultative anaerobic bacteria. It protects them from the toxic free radical (O_2^-) by combining it with hydrogen ion to form hydrogen peroxide, which is subsequently degraded by peroxidase.

14–B. Lysogenic phage conversion refers to a change in bacterial phenotype resulting from the presence of a lysogenic prophage of a temperate phage.

15–E. Viroids are single-stranded, covalently closed, circular RNA molecules that may be degraded by endonucleases.

16–D. A selective growth medium that contains a high-salt concentration would permit bacterial growth.

17–D. The broad-spectrum antibiotics—tetracycline, chloramphenicol, the macrolides, and the lincomycins—are bacteriostatic. They are not effective against stationary phase bacteria and do not give a synergistic effect with bactericidal drugs.

18–C. *Escherichia coli* phage lambda is a prototypic temperate bacteriophage.

19–A. Prokaryotic cells differ from eukaryotic cells in that the former have coupled transcription and translation of mRNA in the cytoplasm.

20–B. Superoxide dismutase, which is present in aerobes and facultative anaerobe organisms, protects them from the toxic O_2^- radical. This enzyme is not present in obligate anaerobes.

21–A. The biochemical activity of an enzyme may be regulated by binding of effector molecules or by biosynthetic pathway end-product feedback inhibition. Enzyme synthesis may be controlled by inducers, attenuation sequences, or catabolite activator protein.

22–D. The plasma membrane contains the enzymes involved in oxidative phosphorylation.

23–B. Fungi are eukaryotic cells and, therefore, have a distinct nuclear membrane as part of the cellular structure.

24–A. Both *Escherichia coli* heat-labile toxin and *Vibrio cholerae* choleragen stimulate the overproduction of cyclic adenosine monophosphate, resulting in fluid and electrolyte loss.

2

Bacterial Genetics

I. Organization of Genetic Information—General Concepts

A. Deoxyribonucleic acid (DNA)

—stores genetic information as a sequence of nucleotide bases (adenine, thymine, guanosine, cytosine).

—is generally double stranded, composed of complementary base pairs (A–T or G–C) joined by hydrogen bonds.

B. Ribonucleic acid (RNA)

—transcribes and translates DNA-bound genetic instructions for protein synthesis.

—is generally single stranded.

—substitutes uracil for the thymine base used by DNA; the complementary base pairs for RNA are A–U or G–C.

—is found in three types:

1. Messenger RNA (mRNA)

—is the template that carries DNA gene sequences to ribosomes, the site of protein synthesis.

2. Ribosomal RNA (rRNA)

—is a structural component of ribosomes.

—acts as a substrate for protein synthesis.

3. Transfer RNA (tRNA)

—carries specific amino acids to the triplet-encoded, mRNA-borne message that translates the message into the amino acid structure of proteins.

II. Comparison of Prokaryotic and Eukaryotic Genomes

A. Eukaryotic genomes

1. Structure

a. Except in some fungi, eukaryotes are **diploid** with two homologous copies of each chromosome.

    b. Virtually all genetic information is contained in two or more linear chromosomes located in a membrane-bound nucleus.

    c. Unlike prokaryotes and viruses, eukaryotic genomes contain **introns** (DNA sequences not translated into gene products) and redundant genetic information.

    d. Certain eukaryotic organelles (mitochondria, chloroplasts) contain a self-replicating, circular, double-stranded DNA molecule (**plasmid**) relating to their intracellular function.

2. Replication

    —begins at several points along the linear DNA molecule.

    —is regulated by specific gene inducer or repressor substances.

    —involves a specialized structure, the **spindle,** that pulls newly formed chromosomes into separate nuclei during mitosis.

B. Prokaryotic genomes

  1. Structure

    a. Most prokaryotes are **haploid** (single chromosome).

    b. Genes essential for bacterial growth are carried on a **single, circular chromosome** encoding generally several thousand genes; they are not enclosed in a membrane-circumscribed nucleus.

    c. Many bacteria contain additional, specialized genes on smaller **extrachromosomal plasmids.** Prokaryotic plasmids exist in transmissible and nontransmissible forms and may be integrated into the bacterial chromosome.

    d. Specialized information may also be carried on **transposons,** moveable genetic elements that cannot self-replicate. Transposons contain **insertion sequences** and can transfer their information by inserting themselves into other loci in the same or other genetic elements (e.g., plasmids, chromosomes, viral DNA).

  2. Replication

    a. Replicons

      —is a general term for double-stranded DNA circles (chromosomes, plasmids) capable of self-replication. Plasmid replication is independent of chromosome replication.

      —replicate bidirectionally (5′ PO_4 to 3′ OH) from a fixed origin.

      (1) The replicon attaches to a projection of the cell membrane (**mesosome**), which acts as the replication origin site, and one of the DNA strands is broken.

      (2) The 5′ end of the broken strand attaches to a new membrane site.

      (3) Elongation of the cell membrane via localized membrane synthesis pulls the broken strand through the mesosomal attachment site, where replication takes place.

      (4) Replication is completed, and the free ends of the new replicon are joined.

    b. Transposons

      —are replicated, along with the code of the host, after insertion into a replicon.

C. Viral genomes

1. Structure

a. Genetic information may be coded as DNA or RNA and in double-stranded or single-stranded form.

b. The viral genome may contain exotic bases.

2. Replication

—takes place only after successful infection of an appropriate host.

—proceeds when the injected viral genome subverts normal replicative processes of the host, producing new virus particles.

3. Bacteriophage types

—may be discerned by their mode of propagation.

a. Lytic phages quickly produce many copies of themselves as they kill the host.

b. Temperate phages can lie seemingly dormant in the host (**prophage** state), timing replication of prophage genetic material to replication of the host cell. Various activation signals trigger the prophage to enter a lytic cycle, resulting in host death and the release of new phages.

III. Gene Transfer Between Organisms

—maintains genetic variability in microbes through the **exchange and recombination** of allelic forms of genes.

—is most efficient between cells of the same species.

—may also occur as the crossing over of homologous chromosomes or by nonhomologous means (e.g., movement of plasmids or transposons, insertion of viral genes).

—can result in the acquisition of new characteristics (e.g., antigens, toxins, antibiotic resistance).

—occurs via three mechanisms: conjugation, transduction, and transformation (Figure 2-1).

A. Conjugation

—is a one-way transfer of genetic material (usually plasmids) from donor to recipient by means of physical contact.

—typically involves three types of plasmids:

1. F⁺ cell

—possesses a fertility (F) plasmid, mediating the creation of a sex pilus necessary for conjugal transfer of the F plasmid to the recipient.

—can integrate into chromosomal DNA, creating **high-frequency recombination** donors from which chromosomal DNA is readily transferred.

2. R factors

—contain genes conferring **drug resistance.** Frequently, the resistance genes are carried on transposons.

—express resistance phenotype through natural selection.

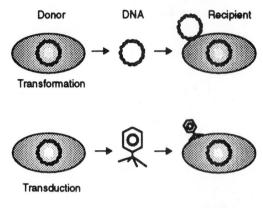

Donor   DNA   Recipient

Transformation

Transduction

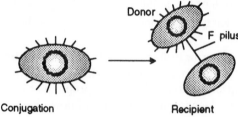

Donor

F pilus

Conjugation   Recipient

Figure 2-1. Three major mechanisms of genetic transfer in bacteria. In **transformation,** naked DNA is taken up directly by the recipient cell. During **transduction,** host DNA is transferred attached to viral DNA via bacteriophage. In **conjugation,** donor DNA is transferred via a conjugative plasmid (F pilus) to a recipient cell by physical contact. (Adapted with permission from Atlas RM: *Microbiology: Fundamentals and Application,* 2nd ed. New York, Macmillan, 1988, p 215.)

   3. **F′ and R′ plasmids**

      —are recombinant **fertility or resistance plasmids** in which limited regions of chromosomal DNA can be replicated and transferred by conjugation independently of the chromosome.

  B. Transduction (Figure 2-2)

    —is **phage-mediated transfer** of host DNA sequences.

    —can be performed by temperate phages and, under special conditions, by lytic phages.

    —occurs in two forms:

    1. In **generalized transduction,** the phage randomly packages host DNA in a bacteriophage coat and may transfer any gene. The transducing particle contains only host DNA.

    2. In **specialized transduction,** the lysogenic phage favors the transfer of host DNA segments near the site of prophage integration. Specialized transducing phages contain both viral and host genes.

  C. Transformation (Figure 2-3)

    —is the **direct uptake** and recombination of naked DNA fragments through the cell wall by competent bacteria. Natural occurrence of this process is uncommon.

    —is sometimes mediated by surface **competence factors** (DNA receptor enzymes) produced only at a specific point in the bacterial growth cycle.

    —can sometimes be forced by treatment with calcium chloride and temperature shock.

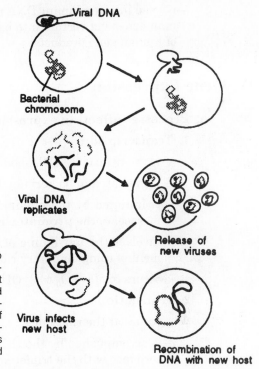

Figure 2-2. Transduction of genes from one bacterium to another. Viral DNA enters the bacterial cell after attachment of bacteriophage. As it replicates, fragments of host DNA are incorporated into the viral DNA. Newly formed virus leaves the infected cell with new, altered DNA, infects a new host bacterium, and recombines with DNA of the latter cell, thereby transducing genes from one bacterium to another. (Adapted with permission from Atlas RM: *Microbiology: Fundamentals and Application,* 2nd ed. New York, Macmillan, 1988, p 215.)

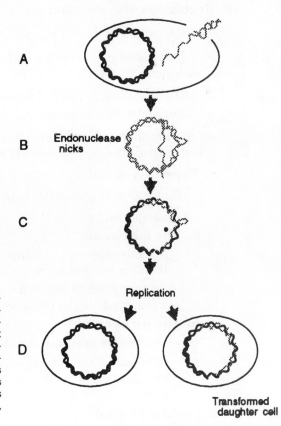

Figure 2-3. Sequential steps during bacterial transformation. (*A*) Double-stranded DNA enters the bacterial cell, where an exonuclease converts the transforming DNA into a single strand. (*B*) A heteroduplex forms when transforming DNA pairs with complementary host DNA. (*C*) A ligase completes the integration of transforming DNA. (*D*) One daughter cell is a mutant, like the recipient cell, and one other is transformed. (Adapted with permission from Atlas RM: *Microbiology: Fundamentals and Application,* 2nd ed. New York, Macmillan, 1988, p 216.)

—is used in recombinant DNA research and commercially to introduce human genes via vectors into bacteria for rapid and large-scale production of human gene products.

IV. Gene Expression

A. Processes affecting expression

1. Transcription

—is the transfer of DNA-bound protein synthesis instructions to mRNA.

—is mediated in bacteria by **RNA polymerase.**

—is initiated by the binding of **sigma factor,** a subunit of RNA polymerase, to the **promoter region** of the DNA molecule.

—involves the unwinding of a short sequence of DNA bases and alignment of complementary ribonucleotide bases onto the DNA template.

—occurs in a 5′ PO_4 to 3′ OH direction.

2. Translation

—occurs at the ribosomes.

—is accomplished by the tRNA-mediated linkage of amino acids, in accordance with the triplet-encoded mRNA transcript.

—is the assembly of polypeptide chains from the mRNA transcript.

B. Regulation of expression

—occurs primarily during transcription.

—is determined partly by the ability of the DNA promoter region to bind with sigma factor.

—can be facilitated or blocked by regulator proteins binding to operator sequences near the promoter.

—typically affects an **operon,** a group of genes under the control of one operator controlled by the action of regulatory proteins.

1. Negative control

—is inhibition of transcription by the binding of a repressor protein.

—is exemplified by:

a. The *lac* operon

—controls expression of three structural genes for **lactose metabolism** via a repressor protein.

—Transcription is induced by the presence of lactose (allolactose), which binds to the repressor protein and frees the *lac* operator.

b. The *trp* operon

—controls **tryptophan synthesis.**

—Synthesis of tryptophan is halted by the binding of a repressor protein (tryptophan complex) to the *trp* operator when excess tryptophan is available.

2. Positive control

—is the initiation of transcription in response to the binding of an activator protein.

   a. Expression of the *ara* operon proceeds only when arabinose binds to a special protein, forming an activator compound necessary for the transcription of the *ara* operon.

   b. Cyclic adenosine monophosphate (cyclic AMP) binding protein, when bound to a specific DNA sequence near the promoter, enhances the expression of many genes associated with fermentation. Cyclic AMP enhances RNA polymerase activity.

V. Mutation

—occurs approximately once for any gene in every 1 million cells.

—is an induced or spontaneous heritable alteration of the DNA sequence.

—introduces variability into the gene pool and changes in the phenotype.

—may be caused by various mutagens, including ultraviolet light, acridine dyes, base analogues, and nitrous acid.

A. Mutation types

1. Nucleotide substitutions

—arise from mutagenic activity or the mispairing of complementary bases during DNA replication.

—often do not significantly disrupt the function of gene products.

2. Frameshift mutations

—result from the insertion or deletion of one or two base pairs, disrupting the phase of the triplet-encoded DNA message.

3. Deletions

—are usually large excisions of DNA, dramatically altering the sequence of coded proteins.

—may also result in frameshift mutations.

4. Insertions

—change genes and their products by integration of new DNA via transposons.

B. Results of mutation

1. Missense mutations

—result in the substitution of one amino acid for another.

—may be without phenotypic effect (silent mutation).

2. Nonsense mutations

—terminate protein synthesis and result in truncated gene products.

—usually result in inactive protein products.

C. Reversions

—Function lost to mutation may be regained in two ways:

1. Genotypic (true) reversion

—is restoration at the site of DNA alteration.

2. **Phenotypic (suppression) reversion**

—is restoration of an activity lost to mutation, often by a mutation at a second site (**suppressor mutation**).

Review Test

1. Bacterial antibiotic resistance is frequently conveyed by

(A) a temperate bacteriophage.
(B) an R factor plasmid.
(C) a replicon.
(D) a lytic bacteriophage.
(E) an intron.

2. The expression of the *lac* operon

(A) must be initiated by the binding of an inducer protein.
(B) involves the release of allolactose from a repressor protein.
(C) does not involve the expression of structural genes.
(D) necessitates the finding of RNA polymerase followed by transcription.

3. Which of the following requires cell–cell contact?

(A) Transformation
(B) Conjugation
(C) Transduction
(D) Transcription
(E) Recombination
(F) Translation

4. Which of the following is mediated by a bacteriophage that carries host-cell DNA?

(A) Transformation
(B) Conjugation
(C) Transduction
(D) Transcription
(E) Recombination
(F) Translation

5. Which of the following involves exchange of allelic forms of genes?

(A) Transformation
(B) Conjugation
(C) Transduction
(D) Transcription
(E) Recombination
(F) Translation

6. Which of the following involves synthesis of RNA from a DNA template?

(A) Transformation
(B) Conjugation
(C) Transduction
(D) Transcription
(E) Recombination
(F) Translation

7. Which of the following creates high-frequency recombination donors?

(A) Transformation
(B) Conjugation
(C) Transduction
(D) Transcription
(E) Recombination
(F) Translation

Answers and Explanations

1–B. R factor (resistance) plasmids contain genes for proteins that degrade antibiotics or alter antibiotic transport, thus conferring antibiotic resistance. They also carry transfer genes, which facilitate their intercellular transfer to other genomes.

2–D. The transcription of the *lac* operon is under negative control. Initiation depends on the binding of allolactose to a repressor protein. This reaction prevents the repressor from binding to the operator region, thus allowing RNA polymerase to bind and transcription to proceed.

3–B. Conjugation involves the transfer of genetic information from a donor to a recipient cell during physical contact.

4–C. Bacteriophages containing portions of host-cell DNA can introduce this genetic material into new host cells via the process of transduction.

5–E. DNA or genetic recombination is the general term used to describe the exchange of allelic forms of genes in bacteria or eukaryotic cells.

6–D. The synthesis of mRNA from DNA by DNA-dependent RNA polymerase is called transcription.

7–E. High-frequency recombination donors, which result from the integration of a fertility (F) factor into chromosomal DNA, are created by recombination.

3

Bacteriology

This chapter uses a systems-based approach. Each medically important pathogen is described in greatest detail in association with the major organ system that it is most noted to affect. If other organs are infected with the same organism, the disease is highlighted and a cross-reference to the bacterial description is provided.

Taxonomic relationships of the various genera of medically important bacteria are currently determined using molecular techniques and numerical taxonomy. By contrast, clinical identification of a pathogen is determined by a variety of methods, often by demonstrating the presence of specific enzyme activities. An overview of some of the most important laboratory tests distinguishing the major genera is shown in Figures 3-1 and 3-2.

Current laboratory methods are rapidly changing. In this review book, critical standard culture media and identification methods are presented along with the newer methods because many of the older methods will continue to be used by some laboratories and will appear on national examinations.

UPPER RESPIRATORY TRACT INFECTIONS

I. *Streptococcus pyogenes* (Group A)

A. General characteristics—*Streptococcus pyogenes*

—occurs as single, paired, or chained gram-positive cocci, depending on the environment.

—is a facultative anaerobe.

—attaches to epithelial surfaces via the lipoteichoic acid portion of fimbriae (pili).

—**causes multiple clinical conditions.**

B. Classification—*Streptococcus pyogenes*

—is classified as **group A** of the 21 Lancefield groups of streptococci. Each group is distinguished serologically by slight differences in specific **cell wall carbohydrates.**

—contains group A–specific carbohydrate and several antigenic proteins (**M, T, and R antigens**) in the cell wall.

39

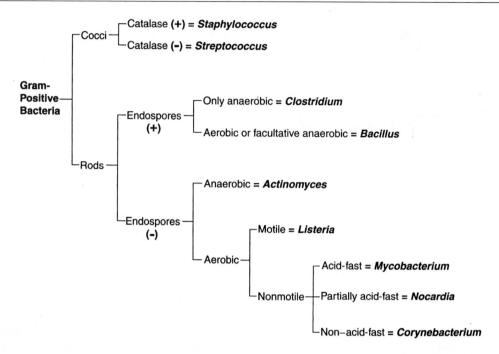

Figure 3-1. Flow chart for differentiating gram-positive bacterial genera. (Reproduced with permission from Hawley LB: *High-Yield Microbiology and Infectious Diseases.* Philadelphia, Lippincott Williams & Wilkins, 2000, p 43.)

—is subdivided into more than **80 types** based on antigenic differences in the M protein (e.g., *S pyogenes* type 12 is a nephritogenic strain).

—is also classified into the β-hemolytic group of the following three types of enzymatic hemolysis of red blood cells produced by different streptococci on blood agar plates:

1. **Alpha (α)**-hemolytic group is characterized by incomplete lysis, with green pigment surrounding the colony.

2. **Beta (β)**-hemolytic group is characterized by total lysis and release of hemoglobin and a clear area around the colony.

3. **Gamma (γ)**-hemolytic group is characterized by absence of lysis.

—is **sensitive to bacitracin,** an antibacterial polypeptide, in contrast to other streptococci.

—is catalase negative.

—rarely becomes resistant to penicillin.

—can be detected by throat smears on blood agar, latex agglutination tests, or rapid (10-minute) test using a fluorescein-labeled monoclonal antibody.

—is compared with other serogroups in Table 3-1.

C. **Attributes of pathogenicity—**ary*Streptococcus pyogenes*

—possesses M proteins, **a potent virulence factor** found on fimbriae that **interferes with phagocytosis.**

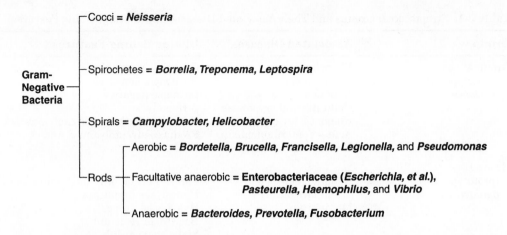

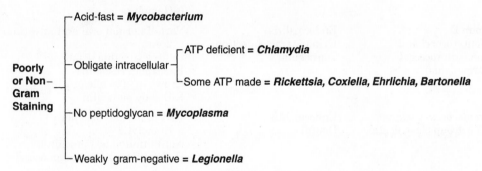

Figure 3-2. Flow chart for differentiating gram-negative and poorly or non–Gram-staining bacterial genera. (Reproduced with permission from Hawley LB: *High-Yield Microbiology and Infectious Diseases.* Philadelphia, Lippincott Williams & Wilkins, 2000, p 44.)

—has **a nonantigenic, antiphagocytic hyaluronic acid capsule** that promotes invasiveness.

—may secrete three serologic types of **erythrogenic exotoxins** that require lysogenic phage for production and cause the rash in scarlet fever. They are superantigens.

—produces two hemolysins: **streptolysin S** (a leukocidal protein responsible for β-hemolysis on blood agar plates) and **streptolysin O** (an antigenic, oxygen-sensitive, leukocidal protein).

—possesses multiple other enzyme systems (e.g., hyaluronidase, streptokinase, streptodornase, nicotinamide adenine dinucleotidase).

D. Clinical diseases

1. Streptococcal pharyngitis

—is characterized by sore throat, fever, headache, nausea, cervical lymphadenopathy, and leukocytosis.

—can result in complications (e.g., tonsillar abscesses, mastoiditis, septicemia, osteomyelitis, rheumatic fever).

—can result in **intense pharyngeal redness,** edema of the mucous membranes, and a purulent exudate.

Table 3-1. Streptococcal Groups and Their Associated Diseases and Distinguishing Features

Group	Associated Diseases	Distinguishing Features
Group A (prototype: *Streptococcus pyogenes*)	Pharyngitis Scarlet fever Impetigo Cellulitis and erysipelas Rhematic fever Acute glomerulonephritis Endocarditis	Contains M protein Bacitracin sensitive Catalase negative β-Hemolytic Produces erythrogenic exotoxins Produces streptolysins S and O
Group B (prototype: *Streptococcus agalactiae*)	Neonatal sepsis (early and late onset) Meningitis	Part of normal oral and vaginal flora Hydrolyzes hippurate Has five serotypes Bacitracin resistant Sialic acid capsule β-Hemolytic
Group D (enterococci and nonenterococcal organisms)	Endocarditis Urinary tract infections Septicemia	Part of normal oral and intestinal flora Causes variable hemolysis Bacitracin resistant Grows in 40% bile or pH 9.6 Killed by penicillin
Streptococcus viridans (no group classification)	Endocarditis Dental caries	Part of normal oral flora α-Hemolytic Not inhibited by optochin Differentiate from pneumococci
Streptococcus pneumoniae	Pneumonia	Large polysaccharide capsule Antiphagocytic Sensitive to optochin Lysed by bile

—can be treated with penicillin, preferably one that is effective for 3 weeks.

2. Scarlet fever

—exhibits symptoms resembling those of streptococcal pharyngitis.

—is accompanied by a rash caused by phage-coded erythrogenic toxins.

3. Rheumatic fever

—follows group A streptococcal throat infection in genetically predisposed individuals; however, 20% of patients may show no early signs or symptoms.

—results in a systemic inflammatory process involving the connective tissue, heart, joints, and central nervous system (CNS).

—may lead to progressive chronic debilitation.

—may **damage heart muscle and valves,** with **mitral stenosis** as a lesion hallmark.

—may result from antistreptococcal antibodies cross-reacting with sarcolemmal muscle and kidney. The resulting antigen–antibody complexes initiate a damaging inflammatory process.

—should be treated promptly with penicillin, which should be continued prophylactically to prevent recurring infections and increased damage.

II. *Haemophilus influenzae*

A. General characteristics—*Haemophilus influenzae*

—is a gram-negative, pleomorphic rod showing some very elongated forms in culture but short rods (coccobacilli) in cerebrospinal fluid (CSF).

—requires the **X (hemin)** and **V (NAD)** growth factors, which are both found in red blood cells but must be released by lysis; thus, *H influenzae* is isolated on chocolate agar.

—colonizes the upper respiratory tract.

—**Nonencapsulated** (nontypeable) strains are part of the normal upper respiratory tract flora and cause noninvasive mucosal infections (e.g., **otitis media, sinusitis, bronchitis, conjunctivitis, pneumonia**).

—**Encapsulated (typeable) strains (most commonly type b)** colonize mucosa of both immune and nonimmune individuals. In young, **unvaccinated** children, encapsulated strains may cause serious, invasive disease, primarily **septicemia, meningitis,** and **epiglottitis.**

B. Attributes of pathogenicity

1. Polysaccharide capsule (polyribitol phosphate)

—in a nonimmune child inhibits phagocytic uptake of *H influenzae,* allowing the organism to circulate in the blood stream.

—in an immune child will get coated with anticapsular antibody, which will promote phagocytosis, resulting in killing of the encapsulated *H influenzae.*

—Anticapsular antibodies promote phagocytosis and resultant killing of encapsulated strains, providing protection from invasive disease. Little or no antibody exists in unvaccinated children 3 months to 2 years of age, the period of the highest incidence of meningitis. In unvaccinated individuals older than 5 years of age, increasing antibody titers appear and infection incidence decreases.

2. Immunoglobulin A (IgA) protease

—facilitates upper respiratory tract colonization.

3. Endotoxin

—activates macrophages.

C. Clinical disease

1. Common infections (nonencapsulated strains)

a. **Otitis media** and **sinusitis** can occur in individuals of any age, even if vaccinated.

b. *H influenzae* causes **bronchitis** and **pneumonia,** particularly in people with chronic obstructive pulmonary disease.

2. Rare infections (type B encapsulated strains)

a. Acute bacterial **meningitis** (see Central Nervous System Infections) still occurs **in unvaccinated children** but is rare in vaccinated children.

b. **Epiglottitis** in unvaccinated children is rapidly progressive with severe problems within 2 hours; death may occur within 24 hours. Microabscesses and edema restrict breathing, causing respiratory blockage.

D. Laboratory diagnosis (respiratory infections)

1. **Specimens.** Otitis media is generally not cultured. Posterior pharynx cultures in epiglottitis are done only if a tracheostomy tray is immediately available. Blood and direct aspirates are cultured for other respiratory infections.

2. **Cultures.** Culture on **chocolate agar;** speciate using requirement for X (hemin) and V (NAD) factors on blood or nutrient agar. **Satellite phenomenon** is the growth of *H influenzae on blood agar next to Staphylococcus aureus,* which produces excess NAD and lyses blood, releasing hemin.

E. Control

1. **Treatment.** β-Lactamase production is seen in 20%–30% of strains of *H influenzae.*

2. **Prevention**

a. **Vaccination with conjugate vaccine** (the type B polysaccharide capsule complexed to protein) reduces the incidence of type b invasive disease; it has no effect on infections with nontypeable strains.

b. This vaccine and other important bacterial vaccines are listed in Table 3-2.

III. *Corynebacterium diphtheriae*

A. General characteristics—*Corynebacterium diphtheriae*

—is a **gram-positive, club-shaped rod** often occurring in V- and L-shaped

Table 3-2. Bacterial Vaccines

Organism	Component	Mechanism of Protection	Use
Streptococcus pneumoniae	23 Capsular polysaccharides	Antibodies to capsule	Elderly; compromised patients
Neisseria meningitidis	Capsular polysaccharides (A, C, W135, Y)	Antibodies to capsule	Infants; military settings
Haemophilus influenzae	Capsular polysaccharide conjugated to diphtheria toxoid or to *N meningitidis* outer membrane protein	Antibodies to capsule	Infants
Bordetella pertussis	Inactivated whole organism Acellular	Antibodies and cell-mediated immunity	Infants
Corynebacterium diphtheriae	Diphtheria toxoid	Antibodies to toxin	Infants
Clostridium tetani	Tetanospasmin toxoid	Antibodies to toxin	Infants

arrangements ("Chinese characters") that produces large **volutin (polyphosphate) granules.**

—causes diphtheria through upper respiratory colonization and elaboration of a potent exotoxin. (In immunized persons, this occurs without significant disease.)

B. Classification—*Corynebacterium diphtheriae*

—is related to the nocardia and mycobacteria.

C. Attributes of pathogenicity—diphtheria exotoxin

—is a potent **A-B ("two component") exotoxin,** with the B component binding to specific cell membrane receptors required to trigger uptake of the A component by the cell. Primary **target cells** include **upper respiratory tract, heart, and nerve cells.**

—Component A is an enzyme [adenosine diphosphate (ADP) ribosyl transferase] that **ADP ribosylates elongation factor 2 (EF-2)** inhibiting nascent peptide chain movement, thus **shutting down eukaryotic protein synthesis.**

—is **produced only in strains of *C diphtheriae*, which are stably infected (lysogenized) by β-corynephage.** The DNA of the bacteriophage resides in the bacterial cell (*tox*+ cells) and directs the synthesis of the toxin. Toxin production occurs at low iron concentrations.

—in its **inactivated form (toxoid)** is a component of the diphtheria, tetanus, and acellular pertussis (**DTaP**) vaccine as well as the tetanus and diphtheria toxoids (**Td**) vaccine.

D. Clinical disease—respiratory tract diphtheria (pseudomembranous pharyngitis)

—is rare (< 5 cases/year in the United States since 1983).

—begins as a **mild pharyngitis** with slight fever and chills.

—spreads up to the nasopharynx or down to the larynx and trachea. The **bacteria themselves do not disseminate** but elaborate the diphtheria **exotoxin, which circulates** and causes additional symptoms such as hoarseness and stridor.

—results in a **firmly adherent, dirty gray, spreading pseudomembrane** composed of inflammatory necrosis, fibrin, epithelial cells, neutrophils, monocytes, and bacteria. This pseudomembrane may cause **asphyxiation.**

—causes **cervical adenitis and edema** which, in severe cases, may produce the characteristic **"bull neck"** appearance.

—has the following **complications from systemic circulation of diphtheria toxin:**

    —**myocarditis** and, occasionally, more severe cardiotoxicity

    —paralysis of the soft palate and more severe **neuropathies**

E. Laboratory diagnosis

—requires notification of laboratory and culture on two special media:

—**Löffler's coagulated serum medium.** On this medium, *C diphtheriae* produces polyphosphate storage granules (called **volutin granules**) that stain variegated **blue/red (metachromatic).**

—**Tellurite-containing differential medium.** *C diphtheriae* imports and reduces tellurite, turning the colonies gray to black.

—**requires demonstration of toxin production,** generally done with the **agar diffusion Elek test.** Commercially prepared strips of filter paper containing diphtheria antitoxin are in the agar medium perpendicular to streaks of the patient's strain, a known toxin-producing strain and a non–toxin-producing strain. Where diffused toxin (if produced by the growth) and antitoxin meet at optimal concentrations, a precipitin line is seen in the agar.

F. **Control**

1. **Treatment** is with **antitoxin and erythromycin.**

2. **Prevention** is by proper vaccination with toxoid in DTaP followed by Td boosters. Vaccination does not prevent colonization but has resulted in greatly reduced incidence of colonization and disease.

IV. *Fusobacterium nucleatum*

A. **General characteristics—*Fusobacterium nucleatum***

—are gram-negative, polymorphic, long, slender filaments and fusiform rods.

—are non–spore-forming anaerobes sensitive to oxygen.

—occur normally in the mouth and occasionally in the stool.

—anaerobic growth is facilitated when oxygen is used by oral aerobic or facultative microorganisms, thereby lowering the redox potential.

—Anaerobes outnumber aerobes 100:1 in the mouth.

—Attributes of pathogenicity have not been clearly identified.

B. **Infections—*Fusobacterium nucleatum***

—acts synergistically with oral spirochetes, resulting in an ulcerating, necrotizing gingivitis (**Vincent's angina,** or trench mouth).

—is responsible for head, neck, and chest infections, and is a common microorganism isolated from brain abscesses.

C. **Treatment** is with penicillin G.

LOWER RESPIRATORY TRACT INFECTIONS

I. *Streptococcus pneumoniae*

A. **General characteristics—*Streptococcus pneumoniae***

—is part of the **normal oropharyngeal flora** in 40%–70% of human beings.

—is a gram-positive, α-hemolytic, lancet-shaped diplococcus.

—possesses a group-specific carbohydrate common to all pneumococci, which can be precipitated by a C-reactive protein found in the plasma during an inflammatory response. Quantitation of precipitate is a clinical laboratory index of the extent of inflammation, not an antigen–antibody reaction.

—possesses a type-specific polysaccharide capsule with more than 80 different T cell–independent antigenic types. Experimental injection of relatively large amounts of capsular polysaccharide leads to tolerance rather than immunity.

—types can be distinguished by swelling of the capsule in the presence of type-specific antiserum (**quellung reaction**).

—should be differentiated from nonpathogenic *Streptococcus viridans* because the latter also is gram-positive, is usually diplococcal, is found as part of the normal flora in the pharynx and sputum, and produces **α-hemolysis** on blood agar.

—is differentiated from other streptococci by:

1. Sensitivity to the quinine derivative ethyl hydrocuprine (**optochin**)

2. Sensitivity to bile, which solubilizes pneumococci by increasing an autolytic amidase

3. Fermentation of inulin

B. Attributes of pathogenicity

1. Little evidence exists for production of toxins; disease probably occurs through multiplication of the pneumococci and the resulting inflammatory response.

2. Virulence is attributed to the antiphagocytic capacity of the capsule.

C. Clinical disease

1. **Pneumococcal pneumonia** seldom occurs as a primary infection.

2. Pathogenicity is associated with disturbances of normal defense barriers of the respiratory tract.

3. Infants, elderly, immunosuppressed persons, and chronic alcoholics are most vulnerable.

4. Self-infection can occur by aspiration after epiglottal reflexes have been slowed due to chilling, anesthesia, morphine use, alcohol use, virus infection, or increased pulmonary edema.

5. Classic manifestations include an abrupt onset, fever, chills, chest pain, and productive cough, followed by a crisis on days 7–10 after infection.

6. In 50%–70% of untreated cases, **recovery** is associated with the appearance of an anticapsular antibody.

7. Two thirds of deaths occur in the first 5 days of clinical disease.

8. The disease is identified by **culture of lung sputum** (not saliva), followed by typing via the quellung reaction.

9. **Otitis media** and **septicemia** occur in infants older than 2 months of age.

   10. *S pneumoniae* is a leading cause of **bacterial meningitis,** mainly in infants and the aged (see Central Nervous System Infections).

D. Treatment

   1. Penicillin or other appropriate antibiotics are used; however, penicillin-resistant strains with modified penicillin-binding proteins are emerging.

   2. An effective vaccine for adults, which contains at least 23 different type-specific polysaccharides, is available. This vaccine is poorly immunogenic in infants; however, a polysaccharide–protein **conjugate** vaccine is available for infants.

II. *Mycoplasma pneumoniae*

A. General characteristics—*Mycoplasma pneumoniae* and all mycoplasmata

   —are the smallest of the bacteria.

   —**lack a cell wall** (unique for bacteria) and should not be confused with bacterial L forms, which lack a cell wall in the presence of antibiotics. (L forms revert back to cell wall forms after the antibiotic is removed.)

   —**require cholesterol** (unique for bacteria) for growth because, like all bacteria, they cannot make cholesterol.

   —are extracelluar, mucous membrane pathogens that do not invade other tissues.

B. Classification

   1. *M pneumoniae* [also termed pleuropneumonia-like organism (PPLO)], or Eaton agent causes respiratory tract infections.

   2. *Mycoplasma hominis* and *Ureaplasma urealyticum* appear to be involved in genital tract infections.

C. Attributes of pathogenicity—*Mycoplasma pneumoniae*

   —attaches to human mucosal cells by the P1 protein.

   —releases hydrogen peroxide, damaging epithelial cells and producing a long-lasting, hacking cough.

   —Fusion of the mycoplasma membrane with the host may deposit mycoplasma antigens, which then play a role in autoimmune-like reactions.

D. Clinical manifestations—*Mycoplasma pneumoniae*

   —causes pharyngitis and **tracheobronchitis.**

   —causes primary **atypical pneumonia** (i.e., **walking pneumonia**) characterized by a gradual onset of fever, throbbing headache, malaise, and severe cough (initially nonproductive); over several weeks, interstitial or bronchopneumonic pneumonia develops; radiographic appearances vary but most commonly reveal an infiltrative pattern.

   —is the most common cause of pneumonia from 5–15 years of age.

E. Laboratory diagnosis

1. Diagnosis is based on clinical presentation and **serology or polymerase chain reaction (PCR)** [very sensitive]. Serology is done on acute and convalescent sera.

   —**Cold agglutinins** (autoantibodies agglutinating red blood cells at 4°C) may be present after 1–2 weeks of clinical disease. Titers greater than 1:32 are generally considered positive.

   —Complement fixation is more sensitive.

2. When done, *Mycoplasma* **culture**

   —requires **special *Mycoplasma* or PPLO culture medium.**

   —is slow; tiny colonies with a "**fried egg**" appearance grow in 2–3 weeks.

   —Giemsa stain on cultured organisms reveals **small, pleomorphic** bacteria.

F. Control

1. **Treatment** is with erythromycin or doxycycline over a prolonged period to help resolve manifestations.

2. **Reinfections** with *M pneumoniae* are common.

III. *Legionella pneumophila*

A. General characteristics—*Legionella pneumophila*

—is a poorly staining, gram-negative, rod-shaped bacterium that may form longer filaments.

—stains well only with Dieterle's silver stain.

—is a facultative, intracellular parasite that causes a fibrinopurulent pneumonia.

—has a high density of cellular branched fatty acids.

—is catalase positive; most strains are weakly oxidase positive.

—hydrolyzes hippurate (unlike other species of *Legionella*).

—is a stream bacterium that contaminates air-conditioning cooling towers.

—is frequently harbored by amoeba.

B. Classification—*Legionella pneumophila*

—is classified in a new family and genus of **aquatic organisms.**

—is the major causative agent of **legionnaires' disease.**

C. Attributes of pathogenicity—*Legionella pneumophila*

—grows **intracellularly** and fails to activate the alternate complement pathway.

—produces **cytotoxin,** a small peptide, interfering with oxygen-dependent processes of phagocytosis.

—produces **β-lactamases** to inactivate cephalosporins and penicillins.

—produces an endotoxin.

D. Clinical disease

1. Pneumonia (legionnaires' disease)

—is acquired by **inhalation** of the organism from environmental sources.

—is most common in smokers and in the presence of an organ transplant, T-cell defect, or chronic lung disease.

—starts with abrupt onset of fever and chills, an initially nonproductive cough, headache (frequently accompanied by mental confusion), diarrhea, microscopic hematuria, and proteinuria.

—peaks in frequency from July to October (air-conditioning cooling towers are more susceptible to bacterial growth in hot months).

—often occurs in clusters.

—is not transmitted by person-to-person contact.

2. Pontiac fever

—is a mild disease consisting of headache, fever, and myalgia without pneumonia.

E. Laboratory diagnosis—*Legionella pneumophila*

—is often diagnosed by direct fluorescent antibody staining of specimens or by demonstration of Dieterle's silver-stained rods in a specimen demonstrated to be negative by Gram stain.

—may be grown and identified on buffered charcoal yeast extract agar (which provides the **required cysteine and iron**).

—may also be identified by an increase in antibody titer.

F. Control

1. Treatment

—is with erythromycin.

—is given concomitantly with rifampin therapy to immunocompromised patients.

2. Prevention

—Contaminated sources (e.g., cooling towers, shower heads, nebulizers) should be decontaminated with hyperchlorination, other disinfectants, or heat.

IV. *Bordetella pertussis*

A. General characteristics—*Bordetella pertussis*

—is a strict aerobic, gram-negative coccobacillus.

—causes whooping cough, predominantly in children younger than 1 year of age.

—is part of the highly effective DTaP vaccine.

—is a classic example of the need for continued vaccination; 2000–5000 cases occur yearly in the United States, despite a high rate of vaccination; in countries where vaccine compliance waned, major outbreaks followed within 5 years.

B. Classification

1. *B pertussis* causes classic **whooping cough.**
2. *Bordetella parapertussis* causes a mild form of whooping cough.
3. *Bordetella bronchiseptica* is primarily an animal pathogen that occasionally causes a mild whooping cough in humans.

C. Attributes of pathogenicity

1. **Pertussis toxin** (A-B type) is a single antigen causing local tissue damage associated with inflammation.
2. **Hemagglutinins** (adhesins) are responsible for specific attachment to the cilia of the upper respiratory tract epithelium.
3. An **undefined cough toxin** is probably active neurologically; the cough persists for weeks after organisms are killed by erythromycin.

D. Clinical disease—*Bordetella pertussis*

—is localized only in the respiratory tract and is highly contagious.

—is associated with a variety of symptoms; generally, the younger the patient, the more severe the disease.

—is associated with the following prognosis: one third of unvaccinated patients recover without problems, neurologic problems develop in one third, and one third exhibit severe neurologic deficits (coma, convulsions, blindness, and paralysis, probably associated with anoxia).

—occurs in three distinct stages:

1. **Catarrhal stage:** mild upper respiratory tract infection with sneezing, slight cough, low fever, and runny nose (lasts 1–2 weeks)
2. **Paroxysmal stage:** extends to the lower respiratory tract, with **severe cough** (5–20 forced hacking coughs per 20 seconds); little time to breathe **causes anoxia** and **vomiting;** tissue damage predisposes the patient to secondary bacterial infections and pneumonia (lasts 1–6 weeks)
3. **Convalescent stage:** less severe cough that may persist for several months

E. Laboratory diagnosis

1. Clinical suspicion is critical.
2. **Complete blood count** may reveal **lymphocytosis.**
3. **PCR** is now available to identify *B pertussis* from clinical specimens.
4. **Cultures.** Posterior nasopharyngeal specimens are plated on **Regan-Lowe** or Bordet-Gengou medium. Direct cough inoculation of plates can be done at bedside. The organism is both delicate and fastidious. Cultures in vaccinated individuals will not be positive. In unvaccinated individuals, the ability to culture decreases in the paroxysmal stage.

5. **Direct immunofluorescent antibody staining** for clinical specimens is more sensitive than culture.

F. Treatment

—is with erythromycin to eradicate *B pertussis.*

—is with other antibiotics to prevent secondary bacterial infection; 30% of patients develop pneumonias attributable to other organisms.

—is with supportive measures (e.g., secretions are removed, oxygen and humidity are provided, electrolytes and nutritional status are monitored).

—is not necessarily a failure when cough persists after erythromycin therapy (due to residual toxins).

G. Prevention

1. The disease is most contagious in the catarrhal stage when the highest concentration of organisms is present; the patient should be isolated (especially from infants 1 year of age or younger) for 4–6 weeks.

2. The attack rate is 90% in persons who are nonimmune to *B pertussis.*

3. Immune contacts who are younger than 4 years of age should be boosted with vaccine, and prophylactic erythromycin should be given.

4. Nonimmune contacts should be given erythromycin only (it is too late to give vaccine).

5. Vaccination should be started with the acellular vaccine (DTaP) at 2 months of age, and three boosters should be given (maternal antibodies are Igm and do not cross the placenta).

6. Continued routine use of the vaccine is necessary; severe adverse reactions are rare.

V. *Chlamydia psittaci*

A. General characteristics—*Chlamydia psittaci*

—is an **obligate intracellular pathogen** (cannot synthesize adenosine triphosphate).

—has a cell wall, but the cell wall lacks peptidoglycan.

—resembles gram-negative bacteria.

—exists in two forms:

1. An **elementary body,** which is infectious

2. A **reticular body,** which is the intracellular reproductive form

B. Attributes of pathogenicity

1. Some toxic effects of antigens kill the host cell.

2. The reticular body divides by binary fission in an intracellular vacuole.

3. The pathogen usually causes subclinical infections in the natural host.

C. Clinical disease—psittacosis

—is a natural disease of birds (ornithosis), particularly psittacine birds such as parrots.

—is also a zoonotic human disease of the lower respiratory tract that ranges from subclinical to fatal pneumonia.

—is an occupational disease associated with the raising and processing of poultry.

D. Laboratory diagnosis

—is usually made on the basis of patient history and clinical symptoms.

—may be aided by fluorescent monoclonal antibody staining of elementary bodies in exudates or complement fixation–based serology, which is group specific, but not species specific.

E. Control

1. **Treatment** is with doxycycline or tetracycline.

2. **Prevention** is by improved hygienic standards.

VI. *Chlamydia pneumoniae*

A. General characteristics—*Chlamydia pneumoniae*

—was formerly known as the TWAR agent.

—has the same general characteristics as those listed for *C psittaci*.

B. Attributes of pathogenicity

—Some toxic effects of antigens kill the host cell.

C. Clinical disease—*Chlamydia pneumoniae*

—causes various lower respiratory tract infections, including bronchitis and pneumonia.

—causes "walking pneumonia" in young adults.

D. Laboratory diagnosis

—requires organism isolation accompanied by fluorescent antibody staining or complement fixation–based serology, which is group specific, but not species specific.

E. Control

—is with doxycycline or tetracycline.

VII. *Mycobacterium tuberculosis*

A. General characteristics—*Mycobacterium tuberculosis*

—is a slender, slightly curved **rod.**

—has a complex **peptidoglycan–arabinogalactan mycolate cell wall** that is approximately 60% lipid, resulting in acid-fastness, poor Gram staining, and resistance to drying and many chemicals.

—**stains poorly with Gram stain** but has a highly cross-linked peptidoglycan (like gram-positives) and no endotoxin.

—**is an acid-fast bacillus** that retains the carbol fuchsin even when decolorized by acid alcohol (because of long-chain fatty acids called **mycolic acids** in the cell wall).

—is resistant to acid and alkali, which allows treatment of sputum to reduce normal contaminating bacteria before culture.

—is a slow grower because it has single copies of ribosomal genes.

—stimulates a strong cell-mediated immune response in a healthy host.

B. Classification

1. Mycobacteria are related to the corynebacteria, actinomycetes, and nocardiae. See Table 3-4 for a comparison.

2. *M tuberculosis* is distinguished from other mycobacteria by substantial **niacin production** and the presence of a **heat-sensitive catalase,** which is functional at body temperature but not at 68°C.

C. Attributes of pathogenicity

1. **Cord factor (trehalose mycolate)** on the cell surface is a **virulence factor** that

—disrupts mitochondrial membranes, interfering with respiration and oxidative phosphorylation.

—inhibits neutrophil migration and causes the organism to grow in a cord or serpentine fashion in culture.

—is associated with **granuloma formation.**

2. **Sulfatides** (sulfur-containing glycolipids) potentiate the toxicity of cord factor and promote **intracellular survival** by inhibiting the phagosome–lysosome fusion and suppressing superoxide formation.

D. Clinical disease—tuberculosis

—is caused by *M tuberculosis* (or *Mycobacterium bovis* in countries that do not pasteurize milk.)

—exposure occurs most commonly through inhalation of organisms in respiratory droplets or the dried **droplet nuclei** from an infected individual.

—is more common in persons of lower socioeconomic class, recent immigrants, and persons infected with the human immunodeficiency virus.

1. **Primary tuberculosis** occurs in the **lungs of immunologically** naive individuals.

   a. The mycobacteria are picked up by phagocytic cells but are not killed; they replicate, killing the phagocytes.

   b. Ultimately, the activation of macrophages and sensitization of T cells leads to granuloma formation.

   c. Caseous necrosis occurs in the center of the granuloma. Viable organisms often remain on the outer edges of the necrosis, inside the granuloma.

   d. Leakage of antigens from these granulomas maintains activated immune state.

   e. Clinical findings are insignificant at this stage.

2. Secondary tuberculosis occurs in previously sensitized individuals with a weakened immune response.

   a. Secondary tuberculosis may be from reinfection or reactivation of primary tuberculosis.

   b. An old granuloma may "weaken" and erode into a bronchus or blood vessel and spread in an individual no longer able to contain the infection.

   c. Symptoms are cough (often with bloody sputum), night sweats, fever, anorexia, and weight loss.

E. Laboratory diagnosis—the diagnosis of **tuberculosis** is aided by

—**microscopic demonstration of acid-fast bacteria** in sputum, induced sputum, or gastric washings.

1. Sputum may be screened with auramine-rhodamine fluorescent stain; this stain is a nonspecific interaction with the waxy wall. (No antibody is involved.)

2. Positive specimens are confirmed with Ziehl-Neelsen acid-fast stain (Table 3-3).

—**culture** in a radiolabeled broth demonstrating the metabolism of ^{14}C-**labeled palmitic acid** with release of $^{14}CO_2$. (These specimens were formerly plated on **Lowenstein–Jensen medium**.) Drug susceptibilities may also be determined in the broth system.

—**skin testing** with a purified protein derivative (PPD) of *M tuberculosis*.

1. A positive test indicates **infection at some time** but not necessarily current disease. (Disease is indicated by clinical symptoms and positive sputum and culture.) The skin test is considered positive if the zone of **induration** measures:

   a. ≥ 15 mm in a person not known to have exposure

   b. ≥ 10 mm in individuals from countries of high risk

   c. ≥ 5 mm in a person infected with the human immunodeficiency virus or with recent known exposure

Table 3-3. Ziehl-Neelsen Acid-Fast Stain

Steps	Color at End of Each Step	
Reagent	**Acid-Fast Bacteria**	**Non–Acid-Fast Bacteria***
Carbol fuchsin with heat[†]	Red (hot pink)	Red (hot pink)
Acid alcohol	Red	Colorless
Methylene blue (pale blue)[‡]	Red	Blue

Mycobacterium is acid-fast; *Nocardia* is partially acid-fast. Most bacteria are non–acid-fast.
[†]Without heat, the dye would not enter mycobacterial cells.
[‡]Sputa and human cells appear blue.

2. Individuals with known tuberculous disease and a negative PPD test are **anergic** to the antigen (a poor prognostic sign).

F. **Control**

1. **Prophylaxis. Isoniazid** is given to individuals with known exposure to tuberculosis and conversion of the skin test to positive but no clinical signs, or to anyone with a positive skin test who is younger than 35 years of age and has never been treated.

2. **Treatment for uncomplicated pulmonary tuberculosis in a previously untreated, cooperative patient.** Isoniazid, rifampin, pyrazinamide, and ethambutol are administered for 2 months followed by 4 months of isoniazid and rifampin (unless susceptibilities indicate drug resistance).

3. Multiple drug-resistant strains are emerging and complicating treatment.

VIII. *Mycobacterium avium-intracellulare* (MAI or MAC for *M avium* complex)

A. **General characteristics**—*Mycobacterium avium-intracellulare*

—is a *Mycobacterium;* thus, it is acid-fast.

—does not produce niacin nor reduce nitrate.

—is generally nonchromogenic.

—is an environmental organism found in water, soil, birds, and other animals.

B. **Attributes of pathogenicity**—*Mycobacterium avium-intracellulare*

—is an **opportunist** rather than a pathogen, causing diseases resembling tuberculosis in compromised patients.

—is **not contagious** from person to person.

—is **intracellular.**

C. **Clinical disease**

—is a **chronic bronchopulmonary disease** in adults with preexisting chronic pulmonary problems.

—disseminates in patients with acquired immunodeficiency syndrome (AIDS) with low $CD4^+$ counts (i.e., generally <50 cells/mm^3). (This condition is common in AIDS patients and is an AIDS-defining condition with a poor prognosis.) It is characterized by fever, night sweats, anorexia, weight loss, and diarrhea. Although the lungs are involved, the gastrointestinal tract may be the initial site of infection.

D. **Laboratory diagnosis** is with blood cultures using a variety of procedures, including radiometric techniques with probes for rapid identification of growth.

E. **Control**

1. **Antibiotic prophylaxis in AIDS patients** is started when CD4$^+$ cell counts are < 100 cells/mm^3.

2. Treatment response in AIDS patients is poor because of their compromised immune status.

IX. *Nocardia*

A. General characteristics—*Nocardia*

—is a filamentous **soil bacterium** that fragments into rods.

—is **gram-positive** and **partially acid-fast.**

—is **aerobic.**

—is related to *Corynebacterium, Mycobacterium,* and *Actinomyces* (Table 3-4).

B. Clinical manifestations—pulmonary infection

—from inhalation of *Nocardia* is **acute in children and compromised adults** and is chronic in other adults.

—may **metastasize** to the brain.

C. Laboratory diagnosis

—is often made at autopsy.

—tests include gastric washings, lung biopsy, and brain biopsy with culture and cytologic testing.

D. Treatment. Sulfonamides are used as treatment.

X. *Prevotella melaninogenica* (formerly *Bacteroides melaninogenicus*)

A. General characteristics—*Prevotella melaninogenica*

—is a **small, gram-negative, anaerobic coccobacillus** with occasional long forms.

—has distinctive **black colonies** on agar.

—is mainly a part of the normal flora of the mouth; saliva has 10^9 anaerobes/mL.

—is found in low numbers in the gastrointestinal and genitourinary tracts.

Table 3-4. Characteristics of Mycobacteria and Related Organisms

Genus	Anaerobic	Acid-Fast	Morphologic Features
Actinomyces	Yes	No	Rods, filaments, some branching
Corynebacterium	No	No	Rods
Mycobacterium	No (obligate aerobe)	Yes	Rods (slightly curved or straight)
Nocardia	No	Partially	Filaments fragmenting into rods

B. Attributes of pathogenicity—*Prevotella melaninogenica*

—produces a potent endotoxin and a collagenase.

C. Infections—*Prevotella melaninogenica*

—causes lung abscesses; **putrid sputum** is a clue to anaerobic lung infection.

—causes infections of the female genital tract.

D. Treatment is with metronidazole and clindamycin. Carbapenems are the most potent β-lactam.

XI. OTHER

A. *Staphylococcus aureus* pneumonia

—has a mortality rate up to 65% depending on underlying health.

—is associated with the following underlying conditions:

1. Postinfluenza

2. Ventilator use

3. *S aureus* endocarditis in intravenous drug abusers

4. Cystic fibrosis

—has a patchy pattern on radiograph with necrotic focal lesions consisting of multiple abscesses; empyema may occur.

B. *Haemophilus influenzae* pneumonia

—is the **second most common cause of community-acquired bacterial pneumonia.** It is particularly seen in those with chronic obstructive pulmonary disease, alcoholics, and infants younger than 2 years of age.

—Increased incidence is seen following influenza outbreaks.

C. *Pseudomonas aeruginosa* pneumonia

—**Mucoid strains colonize the lungs of patients with cystic fibrosis** and cause repeated infections. (*Pseudomonas* is detailed in Skin and Soft Tissue Infections, III.)

—is common in intubated patients.

—often results in mental confusion, cyanosis of increasing severity, and gram-negative septic shock.

GASTROINTESTINAL TRACT INFECTIONS

I. Enterobacteriaceae Family (Enterics)

A. General characteristics—Enterobacteriaceae family

—is composed of hundreds of closely related species and strains inhabiting the large bowel of humans and animals.

—plasmids and DNA are exchanged frequently, resulting in new antigens and, thereby, new serologic strains.

—includes the medically important tribes of Escherichieae, Serratieae, Salmonelleae, Klebsielleae, Proteeae, and Yersinieae.

—is characterized by gram-negative, non–spore-forming rods (generally facultative anaerobes) that ferment glucose to acid and reduce nitrates to nitrites.

    —may be differentiated according to genera and species by antigens (serology), biochemical fermentations, carbohydrate fermentation, or growth on differential and selective media.

    —causes two major disease syndromes: **nosocomial infections** and **gastrointestinal disturbances.**

B. Identification of pathogens among normal flora

—is difficult because the normal flora in the intestine vastly outnumber any pathogen.

—is aided by the knowledge that most pathogens, except *Escherichia coli,* **do not ferment lactose.**

—is facilitated by plating the specimen onto differential or selective media tailored to the pathogen.

1. **Examples of differential media** include:
    a. **Eosin methylene blue**
        —differentiates *E coli* as metallic green colonies, whereas pathogenic, non–lactose-fermenting *Salmonella* and *Shigella* organisms are translucent.
        —inhibits gram-positive organisms via aniline dyes.
    b. **MacConkey agar**
        —differentiates lactose fermenters such as *E coli* colonies (which appear pink) from non–lactose-fermenting pathogenic colonies (which appear translucent).
        —inhibits other organisms by its content of bile salts and crystal violet.

2. **Examples of selective media** include:
    a. **Hektoen enteric media**
        —inhibits gram-positive and many commensal nonpathogenic organisms.
        —permits direct plating of feces and selective growth of the pathogen.
        —differentiates lactose fermenting from non–lactose-fermenting organisms.
    b. **Salmonella–Shigella agar** contains a high concentration of bile salts and sodium citrate, which inhibit gram-positive and many gram-negative bacteria, including coliforms.

3. **Other differential tests** include:
    a. **Fluorescent antibody** added directly onto the specimen
    b. **Agglutination**

    c. **Packaged systems** containing multiple carbohydrates and other biochemicals to detect differential fermentations

C. **Antigenic structure** (see Figure 1-2)

  1. **Capsular (K) antigens**

    —are generally polysaccharide in nature.

    —are exemplified by *Klebsiella pneumoniae* and *Salmonella typhi.*

  2. **Flagellar (H) antigens** are proteins with antigenically specific and nonspecific phase variations.

  3. **Fimbriae (pili)** are responsible for attachment and, thereby, colonization of the organism.

  4. **Somatic (O) antigens**

    —are lipopolysaccharides (LPS), with the terminal sugars as the dominant, determinant group in serologic classification.

    —can be classified within the Salmonelleae tribe into a wide variety of serotypes by the Kauffmann-White schema.

D. **Attributes of pathogenicity**

  1. **The capsule** suppresses phagocytosis.

  2. **Enterotoxins (exotoxins)**

    —cause transduction of fluid into the ileum.

    —Both a heat-labile and heat-stable exotoxin can occur under the genetic control of transmissible plasmids produced by *E coli* (and *Vibrio cholerae*). The **heat-labile toxin** has two subunits, A and B.

    a. **Subunit B** binds to the G_{M1} ganglioside at the brush border of small intestinal epithelial cells, facilitating entrance of subunit A.

    b. **Subunit A** activates adenylate cyclase, which increases cyclic adenosine monophosphate (cAMP).

      (1) Hypersecretion of water and chloride and inhibition of sodium resorption result, leading to **electrolyte imbalance.**

      (2) The gut lumen becomes distended with fluid, causing hypermotility and diarrhea.

    —The **heat-stable toxin** activates guanylate cyclase in epithelial cells, stimulating fluid secretion via cyclic guanosine monophosphate (cGMP).

  3. **Endotoxins** are an LPS complex in the outer membrane, which differs serologically in terminal end sugars (O antigen) but has a common toxic lipid A core, causing:

    a. **Hypotension** from release of endogenous hypotensive agents from platelets and other cells, mainly tumor necrosis factor, interleukin 1 (IL-1), and interleukin 6 (IL-6)

    b. **Fever** because minute amounts (micrograms) induce the endogenous pyrogens IL-1 and IL-6 in humans

    c. **Hemorrhage** in the adrenal glands, intestine, heart, and kidneys, which can be reproduced experimentally in animals in two ways:

      (1) **Local Shwartzman reaction,** in which two injections of endo-

toxin are given (the first given intradermally, followed in 1–2 days by the second given intravenously)

—results in hemorrhage at the intradermal site of first injection. Capillaries become plugged with a thrombus of platelets, white blood cells, and fibrinoid material.

—resembles hemorrhage seen in humans during gram-negative bacteremia.

(2) Generalized Shwartzman reaction, in which two injections of endotoxin are given intravenously, 1–3 days apart

—results in **bilateral renal cortical necrosis** resembling disseminated intravascular coagulation (DIC).

—may act by the following mechanism: the first injection causes conversion of fibrinogen to fibrin; the second injection inhibits phagocytosis of fibrin, and fibrin deposits interrupt circulation in the kidney.

—may be produced by only one exposure to endotoxic bacteria during pregnancy or cortisone treatment.

d. Adjuvant action on the immune response by substantially increasing antibody response to unrelated antigens and stimulating B cells as a mitogen

e. Increased resistance to other infectious agents and tumors by causing secretion of protective cytokines

f. Cytokine secretion, in which many diverse, physiologically active molecules are released from macrophages, T cells, and other cells under varying conditions

E. Disease syndromes

1. Nosocomial (hospital-acquired) infections

—occur frequently, affecting approximately 2 million people yearly, or 5%–10% of the hospital population.

—can cause bacteremia, which frequently results in shock.

—have a high fatality rate (40%–60%) because many of these organisms are relatively resistant to antibiotics.

—are normally noninvasive in healthy individuals; however, patients who are immunocompromised (such as those with cancer or heart or lung disease) or immunosuppressed are at particular risk.

—have outcomes dependent on the extent of preexisting debilitating disease.

2. Gastrointestinal disturbances

—are usually due to enterotoxins secreted by Enterobacteriaceae organisms.

—must be differentiated from gastrointestinal upsets caused by staphylococci, which have a shorter incubation period (6 hours); Enterobacteriaceae organisms generally have an incubation period of 1–2 days.

—caused by pathogenic ***E coli*** may exhibit three distinct disease syndromes: **enterotoxigenic syndrome** (traveler's diarrhea), **entero-**

pathogenic syndrome (occurs in infants), and **enteroinvasive syndrome** (dysentery) [see Gastrointestinal Tract Infections, IV C].

II. *Salmonella*

A. General characteristics—*Salmonella*

—have a **wide host range,** including humans, animals, and birds.

—are gram-negative motile rods indistinguishable microscopically from other Enterobacteriaceae organisms.

—are categorized into more than 1800 serotypes; most human disease results from *Salmonella typhi, Salmonella enteritidis, Salmonella typhimurium, Salmonella paratyphi A, Salmonella schottmuelleri,* or *Salmonella choleraesuis.*

—**do not ferment lactose;** species are differentiated by production of acid, gas, and hydrogen sulfide from glucose.

B. Classification—*Salmonella*

—are grouped via the Kauffmann-White schema into more than 40 groups based on differences in the oligosaccharide ligands (determinant groups) of the somatic (O) antigens found in the outer membrane.

1. Assignment of an organism to a particular group is based on the common possession of a major O antigen, which is identified by an Arabic numeral.

2. For example, *S typhi* 9 and 12 and *S enteritidis* 1, 9, and 12 are assigned to Group D because they possess the major antigen, number 9.

   —may possess a **capsular (K) antigen,** exemplified by the virulence (Vi) antigen of *S typhi.*

   —are identified further by the presence of different **flagellar (H) antigens.**

C. Attributes of pathogenicity—*Salmonella*

—possess an endotoxin that causes diverse toxic manifestations, including fever, leukopenia, hemorrhage, hypotension, shock, and DIC.

—may possess an exotoxin (enterotoxin).

—are aided by antiphagocytic activity of the capsule.

—can survive within macrophages by an unknown means.

D. Clinical disease

1. Enterocolitis (gastroenteritis or food poisoning)

   —is the most common form of salmonella infection in the United States (approximately 2 million cases per year).

   —results from multiple **sources of contamination,** including food (most commonly poultry and poultry products), human carriers (particularly food handlers), and exotic pets (turtles and snakes).

—is commonly caused by *S typhimurium* and *S enteritidis,* which usually require a high infecting dose with an 8- to 48-hour incubation period.

—is a **self-limiting illness** manifested by fever, nausea, vomiting, and diarrhea.

—may result in an increased carrier rate after antibiotic therapy.

—is usually characterized by the following pattern:

a. Ingestion of organisms in contaminated food

b. Colonization of the ileum and cecum

c. Penetration of epithelial cells in the mucosa and invasion, resulting in acute inflammation and ulceration

d. Release of prostaglandin by enterotoxins, resulting in activation of adenyl cyclase and increased cAMP

e. Increased fluid secretion in the intestines

2. **Septicemic (extraintestinal) disease**

—is an acute illness, most often of nosocomial origin, with abrupt onset and early invasion of the blood stream.

—is characterized by a precipitating incident that introduces bacteria (e.g., catheterization, contaminated intravenous fluids, abdominal or pelvic surgery), followed by a triad of chills, fever, and hypotension.

—may cause local abscesses, osteomyelitis, and endocarditis if the organisms are disseminated widely.

—may be caused by many *Salmonella* species as well as other Enterobacteriaceae organisms.

—has a high mortality rate (30%–50%), depending on the degree of pre-existing debilitation.

3. **Enteric fevers**

—are produced mainly by *S typhi* (typhoid fever) and, to a lesser degree, by *S paratyphi* and *S schottmuelleri,* all of which are strictly human pathogens.

—occur through ingestion of food or water, usually contaminated by an unknowing carrier.

—are highly infective even with small numbers of bacteria (e.g., 200).

—progress as follows:

a. During an incubation period of 7–14 days, the organisms multiply in the small intestine, enter the intestinal lymphatics, and are disseminated via the blood stream to multiple organs.

b. Blood cultures then become positive and the patient experiences malaise, headache, and gradual onset of a fever that increases during the day, reaching a plateau of 102°F–105°F each day.

c. Multiplication takes place in the reticuloendothelial system and lymphoid tissue of the bowel, producing hyperplasia and necrosis of the lymphoid Peyer's patches.

d. A characteristic rash ("rose spots") may appear in the second to third week.

    e. Typically, the disease lasts 3–5 weeks; the major complications are gastrointestinal hemorrhage and bowel perforation with peritonitis.

    f. After recovery, 3% of patients become carriers; the organism is retained in the gallbladder and biliary passages, and cholecystectomy may be necessary.

E. Laboratory diagnosis

    1. Enterocolitis. Blood cultures are usually negative, and agglutination reactions are not helpful.

    2. Septicemic disease. Diagnosis is usually by blood culture because the organisms do not localize in the bowel and stool cultures are often negative.

    3. Enteric fevers

        a. Diagnosis is usually by isolation of the organism from the blood or stool after 1–2 weeks by plating onto differential media, selective media, or both.

        b. Diagnosis by serology, showing increasing titers of O antibody, is of lesser significance.

F. Control

    1. Enterocolitis

    —requires no specific therapy except replacement of fluid loss.

    —Antibiotic therapy may increase the carrier rate.

    2. Septicemic disease

    —has no specific therapy other than maintenance.

    —can be controlled with antibiotics.

    3. Enteric fevers

    —Chloramphenicol is usually the drug of choice, but ampicillin is also effective against most strains.

III. *Shigella*

A. General characteristics—*Shigella*

—is a gram-negative, facultative anaerobic, nonmotile rod.

—species are pathogenic in small numbers for humans.

—species have no known animal reservoir and are not found in soil or water unless contaminated with human fecal material.

—infection is spread rapidly, largely because of unrecognized clinical cases and because carriers are convalescent or healthy (< 1% of carriers are under the care of a physician).

—disease spreads through poor sanitation and is readily transmitted from person to person via food, fingers, feces, and flies.

—species ferment glucose with acid, but rarely with gas; only *Shigella sonnei* ferments lactose.

B. Classification. *Shigella* is classified into four groups based on differences in somatic (O) antigens:

1. **Group A,** *Shigella dysenteriae* (rarely found in the United States, unless imported)

2. **Group B,** *Shigella flexneri* (common in the United States)

3. **Group C,** *Shigella boydii* (rarely found in the United States)

4. **Group D,** *Shigella sonnei* (the most common cause of shigellosis in the United States)

C. Virulence attributes

1. All shigellae contain an endotoxic LPS.

2. *S dysenteriae* type 1 secretes a potent, heat-labile protein exotoxin (Shiga toxin) that causes diarrhea and acts as a neurotoxin.

3. Organisms possess the capacity to multiply intracellularly, resulting in focal destruction and ulceration.

D. Clinical disease

1. **Shigellosis** (bacillary dysentery) is characterized by acute inflammation of the wall of the large intestine and terminal ileum; blood stream invasion is rare.

2. **Complications** include necrosis of the mucous membrane, ulceration, and bleeding.

3. Disease is characterized by sudden onset of **abdominal pain, cramps, diarrhea, and fever** after a short incubation period (1–4 days).

4. Stools are liquid and scant; after the first few bowel movements, they contain mucus, pus, and occasionally blood.

E. Laboratory diagnosis

—is made from stool culture of the organism onto differential and selective media.

—cannot be made by using serology and blood culture.

F. Control

1. Only *S dysenteriae* infections require antibiotic therapy; however, resistance to antibiotics has been developing.

2. **Fluid replacement** is the most important therapy.

3. **Vaccines** are under development.

4. Epidemiologic control by isolation of carriers, disinfection of excrement, and proper sewage disposal can be effective.

IV. *Escherichia coli*

A. General characteristics—*Escherichia coli*

—is a gram-negative short rod.

—is a facultative anaerobic member of the Enterobacteriaceae family.

—is present without incident in high concentrations (10^8/g) in normal human feces.

B. Attributes of pathogenicity—*Escherichia coli*

—can result in serotypic changes and associated pathogenicity through plasmid exchange of virulence (toxin) genes.

—can cause damage to intestinal epithelium after adherence through pili.

C. Clinical disease—diarrhea

—is caused by four different strains:

1. Enteropathogenic *E coli* (EPEC)

—is nontoxigenic; adhesion to enterocytes damages villi.

—affects mainly infants and children.

2. Enterohemorrhagic *E coli* (EHEC)

—occurs as a contaminant in undercooked meats.

—has a dominant serotype of 0157:H7, with cattle being the main reservoir.

—secretes a Shiga-like toxin (a cytotoxin also called verotoxin) responsible for inflammation of the colonic mucosa, resulting in bloody diarrhea.

3. Enteroinvasive *E coli* (EIEC)

—causes bloody diarrhea in children similar to shigellosis.

—rarely occurs in the United States.

4. Enterotoxigenic *E coli* (ETEC)

—causes "traveler's diarrhea" in all age-groups.

—spreads through contaminated food and water.

—adheres to the small intestine via pili.

—secretes a heat-labile (LT) and a heat-stable (ST) exotoxin.

  a. LT toxin is an A-B toxin acting similarly to cholera toxin (see Table 1-3); it catalyzes ADP ribosylation, increasing adenylate cyclase activity and resulting in increased cAMP and loss of water and ions into the intestinal lumen.

  b. ST toxin activates guanylate cyclase, increasing cGMP and resulting in hypersecretion of fluids and electrolytes.

D. Treatment is with antibiotics; selection depends on site of infection and age of patient.

V. *Vibrio cholerae*

A. General characteristics—cholera

—is one of the most devastating pandemic diseases.

—outbreaks of small, sporadic nature have been linked to ingestion of contaminated seafood along the coast of the Gulf of Mexico in the United States.

—occurs in individuals who are predisposed to the infection by poor nutrition and debilitation.

—is a prototype of an enterotoxin-induced diarrhea.

—is endemic in several countries.

B. Classification

1. *V cholerae* causes classic cholera; most epidemics are due to biotypes cholerae, El Tor, and 0139.

2. *Vibrio parahaemolyticus* causes relatively mild gastroenteritis.

C. Attributes of pathogenicity

1. Almost all pathology is attributed to **choleragen,** a protein enterotoxin.

2. Choleragen has an A fragment (toxic action) and a B fragment (binding to cells); it specifically attaches to epithelial cells of microvilli at the brush borders of the small intestine.

3. Choleragen stimulates adenyl cyclase to overproduce cAMP, which upsets the fluid and electrolyte balance; this causes hypersecretion of chloride and bicarbonate.

4. Choleragen is similar to *E coli* LT toxin.

D. Clinical manifestations

—result from ingestion of contaminated water or food.

—have an abrupt onset of **intense vomiting and diarrhea** as the key finding. **Copious fluid** loss (15–20 L/day) leads to rapid metabolic acidosis and hypovolemic shock.

—include sunken eyes and cheeks with diminished skin turgor.

—result in remission or death after 2 or 3 days.

E. Laboratory diagnosis

1. Identification

a. Diagnosis relies on clinical manifestations, combined with a history of residence in or recent visit to an endemic area.

b. Gram-negative, short-curved ("comma-shaped") rods appear in the stool specimen.
   A fluorescent antibody test should be performed on the stool specimen.

c. Culture the stool specimen on a selective medium and then perform a fluorescent antibody test or slide agglutination test on organisms from isolated colonies.

2. Clinical specimens

a. Stool specimens are clear and watery (**"rice-water" stools**).

b. Organisms are sensitive to acid pH; therefore, stools should be cultured immediately.

F. Treatment

1. The key is **prompt replacement of fluids and electrolytes;** the patient should appear healthier within 1–3 hours.

2. Fluids should initially be administered intravenously; as the patient responds, they should be administered orally.

3. Fluid and electrolyte therapy reduces the fatality rate from 60% to 1%.

4. Tetracycline should be given to prevent the patient from infecting others; if antibiotics are not given, the patient will recover but will shed organisms for as long as 1 year.

G. **Prevention** can be achieved by:

—**adequate sewage disposal** and **water purification**

—hospitalizing the patient (rice-water stools are highly contagious)

—identifying and treating carriers with **tetracycline**

VI. *Staphylococcus aureus* (see Skin and Soft Tissue Infections, I)

A. **General characteristics—*Staphylococcus aureus***

—is a β-hemolytic, catalase-positive, gram-positive coccus that grows in clusters.

—is found in the oropharynx and on skin and is **spread to food from the nares or from cutaneous lesions of food preparers.**

—**produces heat-stable (60°C) enterotoxins in poorly refrigerated, high-protein foods** (e.g., ham, custard-filled pastries, potato salad).

B. **Clinical disease**

—is characterized by **rapid onset (2–6 hours** after ingestion of the toxin-containing food) of **nausea, gastrointestinal pain, vomiting, and diarrhea.**

—Symptoms resolve quickly (generally in less than 24 hours).

C. **Control**

1. No treatment is generally necessary.

2. Prevention is by properly refrigerating foods and by preventing contamination of foods through glove use.

VII. *Campylobacter jejuni*

A. **General characteristics—*Campylobacter jejuni***

—is a **gram-negative, curved rod** with polar flagella.

—is positive for oxidase and catalase and is ***microaerophilic.***

—is sometimes seen in "nose-to-nose" pairs with extending polar flagella described as having the appearance of "**seagull's wings.**"

—has an incidence in the United States as high as *Salmonella* and *Shigella* infections combined.

—is found in a wide variety of wild and domestic animals and is transmitted to humans most commonly through **dogs** or by **poultry products.** Outbreaks have been caused by **unpasteurized milk and contaminated rural wells.**

B. **Attributes of pathogenicity—***Campylobacter jejuni*

—has flagellated forms, which are more virulent than nonflagellated forms.

—**invades tissue,** causing **fever, abdominal pain,** and **bloody diarrhea.**

C. **Clinical disease—acute enteritis**

—results from oral **ingestion of the organism,** leading to colonization and **invasion** of the intestinal lining and "inflammatory diarrhea."

—may lead to extraintestinal and postinfective complications, including **reactive arthritis** and **Guillain-Barré syndrome.** (About 30% of cases of Guillain-Barré syndrome are due to *C jejuni*).

D. **Laboratory diagnosis—***Campylobacter jejuni*

—is found in the stool as numerous darting organisms along with blood and excess neutrophils (indicating inflammation).

—is isolated on special agar (**Campy or Skirrow's agar**) grown at **42°C** (which suppresses most of the growth of other gastrointestinal tract flora) under **microaerophilic conditions.**

E. **Control**

1. **Treatment** is with fluid and electrolytes; however, the disease is generally self-limiting (lasts < 1 week). In severe cases, treatment is with ciprofloxacin or erythromycin.

2. **Prevention** is by sanitation and pasteurization.

VIII. *Helicobacter pylori*

A. **General characteristics—***Helicobacter pylori*

—is associated with **gastritis, gastric and duodenal ulcers, and gastric carcinomas.**

—is **gram-negative, urease-positive,** and motile.

B. **Classification.** *H pylori* is now classed by the World Health Organization as a **type I carcinogen.**

C. **Attributes of pathogenicity—***Helicobacter pylori*

—produces **urease** to neutralize stomach acid on its migration to the stomach lining.

—produces a **mucinase** and is **flagellated,** which improves penetration of the mucous layer.

—**adheres to fucose-containing receptors;** these may be the ABO(H) and Lewis blood group antigens that are expressed on the gut epithelia, possibly explaining the **increased incidence of ulcers in Lewis and type O individuals.** Pili appear involved in adherence.

—type I strains (and not type II) also produce a vacuolating cytotoxin.

D. Clinical disease occurs as epigastric pain, sometimes with nausea, vomiting, anorexia, and gas production.

E. Laboratory diagnosis may be made by:

—endoscopic biopsy with urease test, microscopic examination, or culture on *Campylobacter* medium, **or**

—demonstration of serum antibodies, **or**

—radioactive breath test to reveal urease activity on swallowed-labelled urea

F. Control. Treatment is generally with:

—omeprazole and amoxacillin and clarithromycin, **or**

—bismuth subsalicylate, metronidazole, tetracycline, and omeprazole

IX. *Clostridium botulinum*

A. General characteristics—*Clostridium botulinum*

—is a gram-positive, spore-forming, anaerobic rod.

—requires a low redox potential in tissues; clostridia cannot infect healthy tissues.

—spores are ubiquitous in soil and are highly resistant to environmental conditions.

B. Attributes of pathogenicity—*Clostridium botulinum*

—produces a potent exotoxin that acts at the myoneural junction to produce flaccid muscle paralysis due to suppression of acetylcholine release from the axon terminals of peripheral nerves.

—is compared with other clostridial toxins in Table 3-5.

C. Clinical manifestations. *C botulinum* causes two types of infection:

1. Food poisoning follows ingestion of the preformed toxin in contami-

Table 3-5. Clostridia

Organism	Toxin	Mechanism of Action
Clostridium tetani	Tetanospasm exotoxin	Obliterates inhibition reflex response at synaptosomes of brainstem and spinal cord
Clostridium botulinum	Botulinum exotoxin	Paralysis of cholinergic nerve fibers at myoneural junction suppresses acetylcholine release
Clostridium difficile	Enterotoxin, cytotoxin	Gastrointestinal distress, kills mucosal cells
Clostridium perfringens	α-Toxin (11 other toxins)	Lecithinase, destroys cell membranes

nated food. **Clinical findings** include nausea, vomiting, dizziness, cranial palsy, double vision, swallowing and speech problems, muscle weakness, respiratory paralysis, and death (in 20% of cases).

2. **Intestinal (infant) botulism** occurs in infants after spore ingestion and subsequent germination in the gastrointestinal tract.

   a. The exotoxin disseminates, causing constipation, generalized weakness, and loss of head and limb control (resulting in a floppy appearance).

   b. This type of infection rarely is fatal.

3. In rare cases, **wound infection** occurs, with manifestations similar to those of soft-tissue wounds.

D. **Laboratory diagnosis.** The presence of the toxin in food, stool, blood, and vomitus is demonstrable by injection of sample into mice; botulinum **antitoxin** protects against lethality.

E. **Treatment**

—For food poisoning, give antitoxin and use supportive measures for respiratory control, stomach lavage, and enemas. Antibiotics should not be given and the caregiver should act rapidly.

—For **intestinal botulism** in infants, only supportive care is needed; there should be complete recovery without deficits.

F. **Prevention**

—Give antitoxin to all persons who ate contaminated food, even if symptoms have not developed.

—Heat food to 80°C–100°C for 10 minutes to inactivate the toxin (but not the spores).

—Use proper sterilization techniques for home canning.

—Refrain from giving honey, which may contain organisms, to infants younger than 1 year of age.

X. *Clostridium difficile*

A. **General characteristics—*Clostridium difficile***

—is a gram-positive, spore-forming, anaerobic rod.

—is a component of the normal intestinal flora of infants and some adults.

—contamination of hospitals and hospital personnel persists via asymptomatic carriers.

B. **Attributes of pathogenicity—*Clostridium difficile***

—has many strains that are resistant to antibiotics relative to other members of the gut flora.

—Antibiotic treatment kills organisms that normally restrict growth of *C difficile,* resulting in overgrowth of the latter.

—produces two toxins: an enterotoxin that causes gastrointestinal upset and a cytotoxin that kills mucosal cells.

C. **Clinical manifestations** occur as severe gastroenteritis, termed **pseudo-membranous colitis** or **antibiotic-associated** colitis, and follows antibiotic therapy to treat other bacterial infections.

D. **Treatment** is with vancomycin or metronidazole and fluid and electrolyte status should be monitored.

XI. *Bacteroides fragilis*

A. **General characteristics—*Bacteroides fragilis***

—is a gram-negative, anaerobic rod, usually pleomorphic, with vacuoles and swelling.

—grows rapidly under anaerobic conditions and is stimulated by bile.

—contains levels of superoxide dismutase and catalase, which make it somewhat resistant to short exposure to oxygen.

—accounts for 1% of gut anaerobes, most of which are bacteroides.

—is found in the female genital tract but rarely in the oral cavity.

—is usually involved in **polymicrobic infections** that involve more than one genus or species; consequently, therapy with several antibiotics may be necessary.

—is compared with other non–spore-forming anaerobes in Table 3-6.

B. **Attributes of pathogenicity—*Bacteroides fragilis***

—possesses a **capsule** that inhibits phagocytosis.

Table 3-6. Properties of Non–Spore-Forming Anaerobic Bacteria

Organism	Distinguishing Bacteriologic Feature	Habitat	Clinical Correlation	Treatment
Bacteroides fragilis	Pleomorphism	Gut; female genital tract	Brain abscess; gastrointestinal abscess; pelvic inflammatory disease; cellulitis	Débridement and drainage; metronidazole (clindamycin as second-line agent)
Prevotella melaninogenica	Black colonies on agar; putrid sputum	Mouth; gastrointestinal and genitourinary tracts (occasionally)	Lung abscess; female genital tract infections	Débridement and drainage; metronidazole (clindamycin as second-line agent)
Fusobacterium nucleatum	Cigar shape	Mouth	Necrotizing gingivitis; head, neck, and chest infections	Penicillin; cephalosporin

—has a weak endotoxin (in contrast to *Prevotella*) and no exotoxin.

—also possesses a collagenase and hyaluronidase, which aids its spread.

C. Clinical manifestations

—are a frequent cause of gastrointestinal **abscesses** after damage to mucosal barriers.

—are **foul smelling.**

—are the leading cause of **pelvic inflammatory disease.**

—are a frequent cause of brain abscesses and cellulitis.

—are not communicable or transmissible.

D. Treatment

—with tetracyclines is generally ineffective because most organisms are resistant; they possess a **β-lactamase** that destroys penicillins and cephalosporins.

—is with metronidazole; clindamycin, kanamycin, and chloramphenicol also are suggested as therapeutic agents for this relatively resistant organism.

GENITOURINARY TRACT INFECTIONS

I. *Escherichia coli*

A. General characteristics—*Escherichia coli* (see Gastrointestinal Tract Infections, IV)

—is the most common infection of the urinary tract.

—occurs after contamination of the genital area with feces.

—is more common in women due to shortness of the urethra and its proximity to the anal area.

B. Attributes of pathogenicity

1. Organisms adhere readily to the mucosa via pili, causing damage.

2. Endotoxin (LPS) induces inflammation.

3. Host factors include obstructions, sexual intercourse, catheters, diaphragms, and voiding impairment.

C. Clinical disease

1. **Cystitis** is characterized by painful, frequent urination; hematuria; and urgency.

2. **Pyelonephritis** infection of the kidneys follows ascending urinary tract infection; it is characterized by fever, flank pain, and tenderness and may lead to endotoxic shock.

3. **Prostatitis** can occur in older men.

D. Treatment is with an appropriate antibiotic. Most *E coli* strains are susceptible to penicillin and ciprofloxacin.

II. *Staphylococcus saprophyticus*

A. General characteristics—*Staphylococcus saprophyticus*

—belongs to the genus *Staphylococcus*. Staphylococci are all **catalase-positive, gram-positive cocci** usually arranged in clusters (singles, diplococci, and short chains in tissues).

—is **nonhemolytic, coagulase negative,** and **resistant to novobiocin** when cultured on blood agar.

—is **nitrite negative.**

B. Attributes of pathogenicity. *S saprophyticus* adheres to uroepithelial cells.

C. Clinical disease. Urinary tract infections occur in sexually active young women ("honeymoon cystitis"). *E coli* is still more common in this population.

III. *Proteus mirabilis*

A. General characteristics—*Proteus mirabilis*

—is a gram-negative, motile short rod.

—produces a typical "swarming" growth on blood agar.

—is primarily an opportunist, transmitted via catheters.

B. Attributes of pathogenicity—*Proteus mirabilis*

—produces a powerful urease that hydrolyzes urea to ammonia and CO_2.

—results in stones and calculi, leading to urinary tract obstruction.

C. Clinical disease. Infection is a major cause of urinary tract infections, both community acquired and nosocomial.

D. Treatment is with ampicillin and cephalosporin; the organism is resistant to tetracyclines.

IV. *Enterococcus faecalis*

A. General characteristics—*Enterococcus faecalis*

—was formerly classified as group D streptococci.

—occurs as part of the normal intestinal and oral flora in humans and animals.

—is a facultative anaerobic, gram-positive coccus.

—produces β-hemolysis on blood agar; other strains exhibit variable hemolysis, but most are α- or γ-hemolytic.

—can be differentiated by reactivity with antiserum, bacitracin resistance, and growth in 40% bile, pH 9.6 or 6.5% salt solution.

B. Attributes of pathogenicity

   1. Attributes of pathogenicity have not been identified.

   2. Organisms are generally noninvasive opportunists; however, they are a leading cause of nosocomial infections.

   3. Clinical significance needs to be established over mere contamination.

C. Clinical disease includes urinary tract infections, septicemia, and associated endocarditis.

D. Treatment

   1. Antibiotic sensitivity should be tested to determine appropriate treatment.

   2. The organism is relatively **resistant to many antibiotics;** it is inhibited but not killed by penicillin.

V. *Neisseria gonorrhoeae*

A. General characteristics—*Neisseria gonorrhoeae*

   —is an oxidase-positive, gram-negative diplococcus with a "kidney bean" morphologic appearance.

   —is **epidemic,** with the highest incidence in the most sexually active group (15–25 years of age).

B. Classification

   1. *N gonorrhoeae* does not ferment maltose, which distinguishes it from *Neisseria meningitidis.*

   2. Differentiation is by **auxotyping** (nutritional requirements) or **colonial morphology** (types 1 and 2 are virulent; types 3, 4, and 5 are much less virulent).

C. Attributes of pathogenicity—*Neisseria gonorrhoeae*

   —produces an IgA protease that degrades IgA_1; this antibody probably plays a key early role in mucosal infections. (IgA proteases are also found in *Haemophilus* and streptococcal organisms.)

   —possesses a plasmid that codes for penicillinase production.

   —possesses pili, which are protein surface fibrils that mediate attachment to the mucosal epithelium.

   1. Pili undergo phase variation (on/off switch of pili production). Nonpiliation greatly reduces virulence.

   2. Pili also exhibit antigenic variation and have the capacity to produce millions of variants, which is partly responsible for the lack of protection against subsequent infections.

      —possesses outer membrane proteins that form porins (PI and PIII) and that determine clumping (PII) or opacity. PII⁻ strains are isolated from disseminated forms. Pili and PII play major roles in adherence.

      —possesses endotoxin activity that damages mucosal cells. Unlike most LPS, *N gonorrhoeae* lacks lengthy O-antigenic side chains and is termed lipo-oligosaccharide (LOS).

D. Clinical disease

—results in **mucous membrane infections,** primarily in the anterior urogenital tract.

—is **absent** in 20%–80% of infected women and 10% of infected men; these asymptomatic carriers may transmit the bacteria to consorts, causing **symptomatic gonorrhea.**

—is compared with other sexually transmitted diseases in Table 3-7.

—Repeated infection may cause scarring with subsequent **sterility** in either gender and may predispose women to ectopic pregnancy.

—reflects various types of infections, including:

1. **Urethritis** in men is characterized by thick, yellow, purulent exudate containing bacteria and numerous neutrophils; frequent, painful urination; and possibly an erythematous meatus. Complications include epididymitis and prostatitis in males.

2. **Endocervicitis or urethritis** in women is characterized by a purulent vaginal discharge; frequent, painful urination; and abdominal pain. Approximately 50% of cases go undiagnosed. Complications include arthritis, pelvic inflammatory disease, and sterility.

3. **Rectal infections** (prevalent in homosexual males) are characterized by painful defecation, discharge, constipation, and proctitis.

4. **Pharyngitis** is characterized by purulent exudate; the mild form mimics viral sore throat, whereas the severe form mimics streptococcal sore throat.

5. **Disseminated infection** (blood stream invasion) is infection in which organisms initially localize in the skin, causing **dermatitis** (a single maculopapular, erythematous lesion), then spread to the joints, causing overt, painful arthritis of the hands, wrists, elbows, and ankles.

Table 3-7. Bacterial Sexually Transmitted Diseases

Organism	Prominent Clinical Feature	Complication	Complications in Pregnancy
Neisseria gonorrhoeae	Urethritis	Pelvic inflammatory disease; arthritis	Newborn conjunctivitis (severe)
Chlamydia trachomatis serotypes D–K	Urethritis	Pelvic inflammatory disease	Newborn pneumonia or conjunctivitis
Chlamydia trachomatis (lymphogranuloma venereum)	Regional adenopathy	Genital fistulas, ulcers, and elephantiasis	. . .
Treponema pallidum	Hard chancre, primary stage	Nerve; aorta; brain damage of tertiary stage	Congenital infection causing stillbirth or birth defects
Haemophilus ducreyi	Soft chancre with multiple ulcers	. . .	. . .
Group B streptococci	Mild genital tract infection	. . .	Fulminant meningitis in baby

6. **Infant eye infection (ophthalmia neonatorum),** which is contracted during passage through the birth canal, is characterized by severe, bilateral purulent **conjunctivitis** that may rapidly lead to blindness.

E. Laboratory diagnosis

1. **Identification**
   a. Organisms are gram-negative, intracellular and extracellular diplococci. Numerous neutrophils appear in purulent exudate in men. Because of endocervical localization, a characteristic Gram stain of organisms is less likely in females.
   b. Culture should be immediately placed on warm Thayer-Martin chocolate agar in a candle jar.
   c. Oxidase test is positive.
   d. Organisms use glucose but not maltose.
   e. Newer techniques involve immunofluorescence, enzyme-linked immunosorbent assay (ELISA), or gene probes on a clinical swab.

2. **Clinical specimens**
   a. In women, both genital and rectal cultures should be obtained.
   b. If a speculum or anoscope is used, lubricant should not be used because it kills many organisms and reduces the chance for a successful culture.
   c. The organisms are labile, and specimens should be plated immediately.
   d. If disseminated gonorrhea is present, blood and synovial fluid should be cultured; culture of skin lesions is rarely successful.

F. Control

1. **Treatment**
   a. Ceftriaxone should be given, followed by a tetracycline to treat possible chlamydial infection.
   b. In approximately 50% of cases, pelvic inflammatory disease is severe enough to warrant hospitalization.
   c. Pelvic inflammatory disease predisposes the patient to repeated episodes caused by other bacteria and to ectopic pregnancy.

2. **Prevention**
   a. The patient's sexual partners should be treated and **condom** use should be encouraged.
   b. Asymptomatic patients should be identified by culture and treated.
   c. To prevent neonatal gonococcal conjunctivitis, topical silver nitrate or tetracycline should be used.

VI. *Treponema pallidum*

A. General characteristics—*Treponema pallidum*

—is a corkscrew-shaped, motile organism with unusual morphologic appearance of the outer envelope, three axial filaments, a cytoplasmic membrane–cell wall complex with endotoxin, and a protoplasmic cylinder.

—causes chronic, painless infections that may last 30–40 years if untreated.

—decreases in number as host defenses are stimulated, causing disappearance of symptoms; subsequently, organisms multiply and symptoms reappear.

B. Classification

    1. Subspecies *pallidum* causes **syphilis,** which is sexually transmitted, epidemic worldwide, and may affect any tissue.

    2. Subspecies *pertenue* causes **yaws** (seen in hot tropical climates, not in the United States). Yaws involves bone and soft tissues.

    3. Subspecies *carateum* causes **pinta** (seen in Central and South America). Pinta involves the skin only.

    4. All three subspecies are morphologically and antigenically identical; differentiation is based solely on clinical manifestations.

C. Attributes of pathogenicity. Immunosuppressive treponemal components are responsible for the chronic nature of syphilis and for subsequent emergence of different stages.

D. Clinical disease—syphilis

    1. Vascular involvement leads to endarteritis and periarteritis, resulting in inhibited blood supply and necrosis.

    2. Lymphocyte and plasma cell infiltration occurs at sites of infection.

    3. The pathogenesis of syphilis varies considerably. It may involve many tissues of the body and is generally divided into three stages:

        a. Primary—localized infection with erythema, induration with a firm base (a **hard chancre**), and ulceration

        b. Secondary—disseminated infection with lesions in almost all tissues; mucocutaneous rash; may recur if untreated

        c. Tertiary—aortitis and CNS problems may be fatal

    4. In utero infection has severe manifestations, including abortion, stillbirth, birth defects, or latent infection (most common) with the snuffles (rhinitis) followed by a rash and desquamation.

E. Laboratory diagnosis

    1. Identification

        a. Syphilis is identified partly on the basis of **clinical manifestations.**

        b. Darkfield microscopy of lesion exudate may demonstrate **corkscrew-shaped spirochetes** (the organisms are too thin to identify by Gram stain).

        c. Serology. Two antibodies are produced in response to *T pallidum* infection:

            (1) Nontreponemal (reaginic) antibodies (these are not IgE)

                —are nonspecific (positive in many related or chronic diseases) but economical as a screening test.

                —are identified by other screens: Venereal Disease Research Laboratory (VDRL) test, rapid plasma reagin (RPR) card test, or automated reagin test (ART).

—titers are decreased in tertiary syphilis (even if untreated). If treated, a positive reagin test after 1 year suggests persistent infection, reinfection, or a false-positive result.

(2) Specific treponemal antibodies

—are more specific, but tests are costly and are used only to confirm a positive reagin test.

—are screened for by fluorescent treponemal antibody absorption (FTA-abs) test, *T pallidum* hemagglutination (TPHA) test, and the rarely used *T pallidum* immobilization (TPI) test.

—titers remain positive in most people, even with proper treatment.

—biologic false-positive results may confuse the diagnosis (positive serology in the absence of treponemal disease).

2. Clinical specimens

a. Lesion exudate should be obtained from a pustule or an ulcer for dark-field microscopy.

b. The organism cannot be grown in vitro.

F. Control

1. Treatment

a. Long-acting **penicillin** should be given.

b. **Jarisch-Herxheimer** reaction immediately after antibiotic therapy for secondary syphilis involves intensification of manifestations for 12 hours; this indicates that penicillin is effective.

c. With treatment, reagin-based serologic tests become negative 6 months after primary syphilis and 12 months after secondary syphilis; beyond the secondary stage, the patient may remain seropositive for years.

2. Prevention

a. Use of a **condom** minimizes transmission.

b. **All sexual contacts** should be treated prophylactically with **penicillin.**

c. In **pregnant patients,** serologic syphilis tests should be performed during the first and third trimesters.

VII. *Chlamydia trachomatis*

A. General characteristics—*Chlamydia trachomatis*

—is differentiated into 15 serotypes.

—has characteristics similar to those of *C psittaci* (see Lower Respiratory Tract Infections, V).

B. Attributes of pathogenicity. Toxic effects of antigens kill host cells.

C. Clinical disease

1. Subtypes D–K

—cause a **sexually transmitted disease** that may involve an associated inclusion conjunctivitis.

—are a prominent cause of **nongonococcal urethritis** in men and ure-thritis, cervicitis, salpingitis, and **pelvic inflammatory disease** in women.

—produce a relatively high incidence of asymptomatic or relatively in-apparent infections.

—can produce a self-limiting **inclusion conjunctivitis in neonates** de-livered through an infected birth canal.

—may cause neonatal pneumonia.

2. **Subtype L1, L2, L3**

—causes a sexually transmitted disease called **lymphogranuloma venereum,** which is characterized by a suppurative inguinal adenitis.

—may cause **lymphadenitis** to progress to lymphatic obstruction and rectal strictures if the disease is untreated.

D. **Laboratory diagnosis**

—is frequently made by direct staining of genital tract specimen with fluo-rescence-conjugated monoclonal antibodies.

—is made by enzyme immunoassays for chlamydial antigens and non-radioisotope probes for 16s RNA sequences.

E. **Control**

1. **Treatment** is with doxycycline or erythromycin.

2. **Prevention** is by diagnosing mothers of infected neonates and urging standard control measures (e.g., use of condoms) to help prevent sexual transmission.

VIII. *Bacteroides fragilis*

—is a leading bacterial cause of **pelvic inflammatory disease.**

—is characterized as described in Gastrointestinal Tract Infections, XI.

CENTRAL NERVOUS SYSTEM INFECTIONS

I. *Streptococcus agalactiae*

A. **General characteristics—Streptococcus agalactiae**

—occurs frequently as part of the normal vaginal and oral flora in adult women.

—colonization of the female genital tract predisposes newborns to infection, sepsis, and meningitis.

—occurs as five serotypes (Ia, Ib, Ia/c, II, and III) based on antigenic differ-ences in capsular polysaccharides.

—is a β-hemolytic, gram-positive coccus.

—can be differentiated from other streptococci with group B antiserum, sodium hippurate hydrolysis, and resistance to bacitracin.

—acts synergistically with a staphylococcal hemolysin.

B. Attributes of pathogenicity

1. A **capsule** is the major virulence component.

2. An anticapsular antibody is protective in the presence of competent phagocytic cells and complement.

3. Peptidase inactivation of C′5a can occur, negating a beneficial polymorphonuclear (PMN) influx.

C. Clinical disease

1. **Early-onset neonatal sepsis** (birth to 7 days)

    —occurs readily in newborns, but only 1 in 100 infected newborns becomes clinically ill.

    —is associated with obstetric complications, premature birth, and respiratory distress.

    —has a fatality rate of more than 50%.

2. **Late-onset neonatal sepsis** (7 days to 4 months)

    —is characterized by meningitis.

    —commonly leads to permanent neurologic damage.

    —is caused mainly by serotype III.

    —has a fatality rate of 15%–20%.

D. Treatment

1. Penicillin G generally is given.

2. Vaccine use is limited because of poor response of children to polysaccharide antigens.

II. *Neisseria meningitidis*

A. General characteristics—*Neisseria meningitidis*

—is a gram-negative, oxidase-positive bacterium with the ability to use both glucose and maltose.

—causes a highly fulminant but generally sporadic disease prevalent at 6 months to 2 years of age, with occasional outbreaks in young adults.

—colonizes upper respiratory membranes before causing **meningococcemia.**

B. Classification. There are nine different capsular serogroups of *N meningitidis;* most infections in the United States are caused by the B, C, and Y serogroups.

C. Attributes of pathogenicity—*Neisseria meningitidis*

—possesses a capsular polysaccharide that inhibits phagocytosis.

—possesses an LPS, causing extensive tissue necrosis, hemorrhage, circulatory collapse, intravascular coagulation, and shock.

—possesses an IgA protease that degrades IgA_1; this is probably important because infections begin on mucosal membranes (streptococci and *Haemophilus* organisms also have this enzyme).

D. Clinical manifestations

1. The disease begins as **mild pharyngitis** with occasional slight fever.

2. In the susceptible age-group, organisms disseminate to most tissues (especially the skin, meninges, joints, eyes, and lungs), resulting in a **fulminant meningococcemia** that can be fatal in 1–5 days.

3. Initial signs and symptoms are fever, vomiting, headache, and stiff neck.

4. A **petechial eruption** then develops that progresses from erythematous macules to frank purpura; **vasculitic purpura** is the hallmark.

5. The LPS of the organism causes intravascular coagulation, circulatory collapse, and shock.

6. Death may occur with or without spread to the meninges.

7. **Waterhouse-Friderichsen syndrome** is fulminating meningococcemia with hemorrhage, circulatory failure, and adrenal insufficiency.

8. Sequelae after recovery involve eighth-nerve deafness, CNS damage (learning disabilities and seizures), and severe skin necrosis that may warrant skin grafting or amputation.

E. Laboratory diagnosis

1. **Identification**

   a. Gram-negative diplococcus are identified by Gram stain of CSF and skin lesion aspirates.

   b. Identification should be rapid; countercurrent immunoelectrophoresis or agglutination reactions detect capsular polysaccharide in blood and CSF.

   c. Nutrient broth (blood and CSF) or Thayer-Martin chocolate agar (skin lesion or pharyngeal swab) should be inoculated and incubated in high CO_2.

   d. Meningococcus is oxidase positive.

   e. *N meningitidis* uses glucose and maltose; *N gonorrhoeae* uses only glucose.

2. **Clinical specimens**

   a. Organisms are delicate and must be transported to the laboratory and processed quickly.

   b. For Gram stain of CSF, centrifuging may be needed to concentrate organisms.

F. Control

1. **Treatment**

   —requires **early diagnosis** and **prompt hospitalization** to be successful; problems with differential diagnosis may occur because the rash resembles those caused by Rocky Mountain spotted fever, secondary syphilis, rubella, and rubeola.

   —is with **high-dose intravenous penicillin,** which passes through the inflamed blood–brain barrier.

—requires **supportive measures** against shock and intravascular co-agulation.

2. Prevention

—is by giving **rifampin** or ciprofloxin to the patient (following penicillin) and to all family members and close contacts to eradicate the carrier state.

—is with vaccine, which is a capsular polysaccharide from A, C, W-135, and Y serogroups (B serogroup polysaccharide is poorly immunogenic). The major problem is vaccine failure in the target group (6 months to 2 years of age) in whom most infections occur. Infants are not routinely vaccinated in the United States. The vaccine is used routinely in the military, in asplenic individuals, and in individuals deficient in late complement components (C5–C8).

III. *Clostridium tetani*

A. General characteristics—*Clostridium tetani*

—is a gram-positive, spore-forming anaerobe.

—possesses a terminal spore, resulting in a characteristic "tennis racquet" morphologic appearance.

—spores are ubiquitous in soil.

—is of major concern during wars.

B. Attributes of pathogenicity

1. Toxigenicity is mediated by a large plasmid.

2. The organism secretes an exotoxin (tetanospasmin) that acts as synaptosomes to obliterate the inhibitory reflex response of nerve fibers, thus producing uncontrolled spasms; its main action is against the brainstem and anterior horns of the spinal cord. Release of acetylcholine is also impaired.

3. Tetanus toxin and botulinum toxin are two of the most potent toxins known.

C. Clinical disease

1. Infection follows minor trauma (such as a laceration or puncture) or occurs as umbilical cord stump infection in a neonate.

2. Manifestations include muscle stiffness, **tetanospasms** of **lockjaw** and back arching, and short, frequent spasms of voluntary muscles.

3. Death occurs after several weeks from exhaustion and respiratory failure.

D. Control

1. Treatment

a. The patient should be hospitalized and treatment begun without waiting for definitive diagnosis.

b. Antitoxins are effective only if toxins have not yet bound to tissues; therefore, administration should not be delayed.

c. Antitoxin and penicillin should be given, tissue should be débrided, a tracheotomy should be performed to aid breathing, and a quiet, dark environment should be provided to minimize external stimuli that can induce spasms.

2. **Prevention**

a. The **toxoid** is a component of the DTP vaccine. A booster should be given every 10 years; for major trauma, a booster should be given if the patient has not had one within the last 5 years.

b. Boosters should be given to pregnant women to stimulate maternal antibodies that will protect the newborn.

IV. Other

A. *Escherichia coli*

—is a common cause of meningitis in newborns and is similar to meningitis caused by group B streptococcus.

—infection generally occurs from the vaginal tract during childbirth.

—causative strains are generally encapsulated.

—is counteracted by the following drugs of choice: penicillin, third-generation cephalosporin, imipenem, cilastatin, or ciprofloxacin.

B. *Haemophilus influenzae*

—is a **gram-negative,** fastidious rod requiring the **X (hemin) and V (NAD) factors;** it is routinely grown on chocolate agar, which provides both (see Upper Respiratory Tract Infections, II D 2).

—strains that cause meningitis have the **type b polyribitol capsule.**

1. **Clinical disease—meningitis**

—occurs primarily **in unvaccinated children 3 months to 2 years** of age, so it is uncommon in the United States.

—is **rapidly progressive;** CNS deficits result in one third of cases (hydrocephalus, mental retardation, paresis, and speech and hearing problems).

2. **Diagnosis. Gram stain** of CSF shows gram-negative, **short bacilli.** Rapid diagnosis can be made by identifying the polyribitol phosphate (PRP) capsular antigen in CSF using latex particle agglutination (latex beads coated with specific anti-*Haemophilus* capsular antibodies) or counter-immunoelectrophoresis.

3. **Control**

a. **Vaccination** with conjugated vaccine (**capsular PRP linked to protein,** either diphtheria toxoid or *N meningitidis* outer membrane protein) has been 95% effective in preventing meningitis.

b. **Prophylaxis** of unvaccinated, close contacts younger than 5 years of age is with **rifampin** or ciprofloxacin.

C. *Streptococcus pneumoniae* is a common cause of meningitis following pneumococcal pneumonia, particularly in aging individuals.

D. *Bacteroides fragilis*

—is a pleomorphic **anaerobe.**

—is a frequent cause of brain abscesses.

—virulence factors include a polysaccharide capsule and an endotoxin.

—is usually associated with mixed infections.

—is resistant to penicillin; contains a β-lactamase.

—is sensitive to metronidazole.

E. *Fusobacterium nucleatum*

—is a common **anaerobe** isolated from brain abscesses and anaerobic meningitis.

—is associated with mixed infections.

—is sensitive to penicillin, in contrast to *Bacteroides.*

F. *Listeria monocytogenes*

—causes **meningitis and septicemia in immunocompromised patients,** particularly in renal transplant patients.

—may cause diarrhea in immunocompetent patients.

—causes clinical infections in pregnant patients, which may result in **fetal meningitis or systemic disease.**

—is characterized under Multisystem Infections.

CARDIOVASCULAR INFECTIONS

I. Viridans streptococci

A. General characteristics—viridans streptococci

—predominate in the normal human oral cavity.

—unlike other streptococci, cannot be classified by group-specific antigens.

—include 19 species differentiated by biochemical tests; the most common species are *Streptococcus salivarius, Streptococcus mutans, Streptococcus mitis,* and *Streptococcus sanguis.*

—are α-hemolytic, are uninhibited by optochin, and are not bile soluble. The latter two properties differentiate them from *S pneumoniae.*

B. Attributes of pathogenicity

1. No attributes of pathogenicity have been identified.

2. Organisms are generally noninvasive opportunists, commonly disseminated intravascularly by dental or other oral manipulation.

3. Secreted biotins promote adherence.

C. Clinical disease

1. On access to the blood stream, these organisms are the most frequent cause of subacute bacterial endocarditis, which can result from inflammation induced by deposition of viridans streptococci or any of several other bacterial genera on heart valves damaged by previous group A streptococcal (or congenital) disease.

2. Viridans streptococci are a major cause of dental caries.

D. Treatment

—is with penicillin, which generally is effective; resistant strains require an aminoglycoside as well.

—requires prophylactic penicillin in dental patients or other patients with preexisting valvular damage.

II. Enterococci (see Genitourinary Tract Infections, IV)

—are a common nosocomial cause of subacute bacterial endocarditis in a manner similar to viridans streptococci.

III. *Staphylococcus aureus* (see Skin and Soft Tissue Infections, I)

A. General characteristics—*Staphylococcus aureus*

—is a **β-hemolytic, catalase-positive, gram-positive coccus.**

—causes **bacterial endocarditis, usually acute,** often in a "normal" heart.

—like many streptococci, has properties that allow it to adhere to heart valves as well as prosthetic replacement valves.

B. Clinical disease—*Staphylococcus aureus* bacterial endocarditis

—occurs sometimes with **native valves** not known to be damaged.

—infection rapidly damages the heart.

1. **Coagulase** allows formation of platelet and fibrin clots, which reduces access of phagocytic cells to *S aureus*.

2. **Cytolytic toxins damage heart cells.**

—is common in **intravenous drug abusers** because of increased *S aureus* colonization of skin.

IV. *Staphylococcus epidermidis*

A. General characteristics—*Staphylococcus epidermidis*

—is a **coagulase-negative** *Staphylococcus* that is **sensitive to novobiocin.**

—has a remarkable ability to adhere to artificial materials in the body (e.g., catheters and prosthetic heart valves).

B. Clinical disease—bacterial endocarditis

—occurs generally with **prosthetic valves** or in intravenous drug abusers.

—is generally a chronic infection.

V. *Pseudomonas aeruginosa*

—causes endocarditis in **intravenous drug abusers** as a result of *Pseudomonas* contaminating drug paraphernalia or drug diluents.

—affects the **tricuspid valve** in most cases.

SKIN AND SOFT TISSUE INFECTIONS

I. *Staphylococcus aureus*

A. General characteristics—*Staphylococcus aureus*

—is a **catalase-positive, gram-positive coccus** arranged in **clusters.**

—is the only **coagulase-positive** and **β-hemolytic** *Staphylococcus.*

—may be part of the normal flora of carriers, usually in the nares or perineum. Carriage rate is 25%–75%, with hospital staff having the higher carriage rates and being more likely to carry drug-resistant strains. Surgical staff is an important source of staphylococci in surgical infections. Food handlers who sneeze or who have staphylococcal hand lesions are the major source infecting food that may lead to staphylococcal food poisoning.

—is a major cause of infections in hospitalized patients, especially surgical patients or patients with intravenous lines.

—has a **high incidence of drug resistance,** with methicillin-resistant strains resistant to β-lactams and most other antibiotics.

—is controlled primarily by phagocytic destruction (a major problem in chronic granulomatous disease).

—infection is enhanced in the presence of artificial materials in the body (e.g., sutures, tampons, surgical packing, intravenous catheters).

B. Classification

1. Staphylococci are **catalase positive** whereas streptococci are catalase negative.

2. *S aureus* (β-hemolytic and coagulase positive) is distinguished from the coagulase-negative staphylococci, which are nonhemolytic.

C. Attributes of pathogenicity

1. Coagulase enhances fibrin deposition and abscess formation. There is also a surface clumping factor that coats the cell with fibrin.

2. Cytolytic toxins (α, β, δ, γ, and leukocidin) are all hemolytic (except leukocidin) and destroy cellular membranes.

3. Enterotoxins secreted by some strains are fast acting, producing gas-

trointestinal symptoms in 2–6 hours. They are heat and acid resistant and bind to neural receptors causing vomiting.

4. TSST-1, formerly termed enterotoxin F, is a superantigen and toxin produced under certain environmental conditions, most commonly associated with tampon use and surgical packing. TSST-1 reduces liver clearance of endogenous endotoxin.

5. Exfoliatins produced by phage group II *S aureus* cause surface cell layers of the skin to separate (probably through disruption of intracellular junctions) leading to desquamation.

6. Protein A (a surface protein) is antiphagocytic (binding to the Fc portion of antibody, making it unavailable to attach to phagocytes).

7. Teichoic acids aid in attachment and stimulate the inflammatory response when complexed with peptidoglycan.

D. Clinical disease

1. **Skin infections** include impetigo (often bullous), folliculitis of the bearded region, boils (furuncles), carbuncles (more extensive), styes, and surgical wound, burn, or traumatic-lesion infections.

2. Scalded skin syndrome, with its characteristic bullae and desquamation of body surfaces, occurs most commonly in children younger than 5 years of age, sometimes with fairly minor infections but circulating exfoliatins.

3. Other *S aureus* infections include toxic shock syndrome, food poisoning, pneumonia, osteomyelitis, and endocarditis.

E. Laboratory diagnosis—*Staphylococcus aureus*

—is a gram-positive coccus found in tissue infections in pairs and short chains (clusters typical of solid media growth) with numerous neutrophils.

—is the only *Staphylococcus* to grow on **mannitol salt agar** with fermentation of the mannitol and production of acid. (This is a surveillance medium.)

—grows with β-hemolysis on blood agar.

—is catalase positive (as are all staphylococci) and coagulase positive.

—was formerly phage typed for epidemiologic identification of strains; newer methods include plasmid typing and ribotyping.

F. Control

1. **Treatment**

   a. Drainage of lesions is important along with antibiotic treatment.
   b. Antibiotic susceptibilities must be determined.
   c. Nonpenicillinase producers are treated with penicillin G.
   d. Penicillinase (plasmid-mediated) producers are treated with a penicillinase-resistant penicillin.
   e. Methicillin-resistant staphylococci strains have a mutated (chromosomal) penicillin-binding protein, making them resistant to all β-lactam drugs and must be treated with vancomycin or vancomycin plus other antibiotics.

      f. Penicillin-tolerant strains fail to stimulate autolysis.

      g. Drug resistance is often transferred by transduction.

  2. Prevention

    —disrupt transmission (hand washing, effective disinfectants) and reduce *Staphylococcus* on sheets and clothing (drying at > 70°C or dry cleaning).

    —reduce carriage.

    —use brief, high-dose perioperative antibiotics.

II. *Clostridium perfringens*

A. General characteristics—*Clostridium perfringens*

—is an **anaerobic,** spore-forming, large gram-positive rod.

—spores can be central or subterminal and are relatively heat resistant.

—produces 12 exotoxins causing food poisoning.

—has soil as a natural habitat; contamination can occur in home-canned goods, smoked fish, and honey.

—requires germination of spores and emergence of vegetative cells for toxin production.

B. Attributes of pathogenicity—*Clostridium perfringens*

—produces **α-toxin,** a potent lecithinase that damages cellular membranes and is identified in vitro by the Nagler reaction.

—produces 11 other toxins or enzymes that damage eukaryotic cells.

—produces an enterotoxin associated with food poisoning.

C. Clinical manifestations. *C perfringens* causes two types of infection:

  1. Soft tissue (muscle) wound infection following severe trauma (gunshot, car and industrial accidents, compound fractures, septic abortion, hypothermia); organisms elaborate toxins and enzymes to produce gas, edema, and impaired circulation; vascular destruction and lactic acid accumulation lower the redox potential, with two consequences:

    a. Anaerobic cellulitis, causing destruction of traumatized tissue only

    b. Myonecrosis (gas gangrene) or destruction of traumatized tissue and surrounding healthy tissue; progresses rapidly to shock and renal failure; is fatal in 30% of cases

  2. Food poisoning following ingestion of contaminated food containing a **preformed enterotoxin;** abdominal pain with severe cramps and diarrhea occur for 1 day

D. Treatment

  1. For **anaerobic cellulitis,** penicillin and additional antibiotics are given to prevent secondary bacterial infections; necrotic tissue should be débrided.

  2. For **myonecrosis,** penicillin and antitoxin are given and necrotic tissue is débrided. Surgery is likely. Bandages should not be too tight. Hyperbaric oxygen may be helpful.

3. For **food poisoning,** treatment usually is not necessary because the infection is self-limiting.

III. *Pseudomonas aeruginosa*

A. **General characteristics—*Pseudomonas aeruginosa***

—is a small, polarlly **flagellated, gram-negative rod** with pili.

—is a nonfermentative, oxidase-positive bacterium.

—is a ubiquitous environmental organism widely distributed in water, soil, and on plants. It can grow to large numbers overnight in either distilled or tap water.

—may produce clinically useful pigments, such as **fluorescein,** a greenish fluorescent pigment, and **pyocyanin, a blue-green pigment. Blue-green pus is a classic sign of *P aeruginosa* cellulitis (mainly in burn patients).**

B. **Classification.** *P aeruginosa* is only one of a large number of pseudomonads (many of which also cause opportunistic infections).

C. **Attributes of pathogenicity**

1. **Invasive factors** include:

a. **Pili,** which aid adherence to epithelial surfaces

b. **A mucoid exopolysaccharide layer (slime),** which increases adherence to tracheal epithelium and mucin, thereby inhibiting opsonophagocytic clearance and reducing aminoglycoside effectiveness; *P aeruginosa* strains isolated from cystic fibrosis patients are prominent slime producers

2. **Virulence factors** of *P aeruginosa* include:

a. ***Pseudomonas* exotoxin A,** an **ADP-ribose transferase** similar to diphtheria toxin that **inactivates EF-2** (elongation factor), halting protein synthesis and resulting in liver necrosis

b. **Exoenzyme S,** an ADP-ribose transferase capable of inhibiting eukaryotic protein synthesis

c. **Endotoxin (lipopolysaccharide),** which plays the usual role in triggering inflammation and systemic symptoms

d. **Phospholipase C,** which damages membranes, causing tissue necrosis

e. **Elastase and other proteolytic enzymes,** which damage elastin, human IgA, IgG, complement components, and collagen

D. **Clinical disease**

1. **Cellulitis**

—occurs in patients with **burns, wounds,** or **neutropenia.** *Pseudomonas* is the most common cause of osteochondritis (usually with overlying cellulitis) in foot puncture wounds.

—is indicated by **blue-green pus** and a **grape-like, sweet odor.**

—may be highly **necrotic.**

2. Septicemia

—results from hematogenous spread of the infection from local lesions or the gastrointestinal tract and causes gram-negative shock.

—may result in **ecthyma gangrenosum,** a distinctive **skin lesion** with central necrosis and an erythematous margin.

3. Recurring pneumonia

—occurs in individuals with cystic fibrosis.

E. Laboratory diagnosis—*Pseudomonas aeruginosa*

—is cultured on blood agar.

—is a **nonfermenter** on MacConkey (or any other) medium.

—is **oxidase positive** and produces a blue-green pigment and a grape-like odor.

F. Control

1. Treatment

—is difficult because of frequent resistance to antibiotics.

—requires **combination therapy:** an aminoglycoside and an antipseudomonal β-lactam agent until drug susceptibilities are determined.

2. Prevention is difficult, but the incidence of infection can be reduced by careful sanitization of drains, aerators, and whirlpools in burn units, by a hospital ban on plants and raw vegetable foods for burn patients, and by pasteurization of respiratory therapy equipment.

IV. *Streptococcus pyogenes* (see Upper Respiratory Tract Infections, I)

A. Impetigo

—is an easily spread exudative infection of the epidermis occurring primarily in children.

—may result in nephritis as a complication.

—should be treated with penicillin, and scratching should be prevented.

B. Cellulitis and erysipelas

—are initiated by infection through a small break in the skin.

—The term **cellulitis** applies if the lesion is confined; **erysipelas** applies if the lesion spreads, primarily through the lymphatics.

C. Fasciitis

—is a rapidly spreading, dangerous infection of the fascia.

—tends to occur in diabetic patients who are particularly susceptible.

—infections necessitate rapid surgical débridement of necrotic tissue followed by therapy with antibiotics.

V. *Bacteroides fragilis* (see Gastrointestinal Tract Infections, XI)

—causes cellulitis and necrotizing fasciitis, especially in diabetic patients, similar to group A streptococci.

—infection is treated with surgical débridement and drainage, followed by treatment with metronidazole.

VI. Other organisms

A. *Actinomyces israelii* (see Multisystem Infections, X)

—is a **gram-positive, anaerobic, filamentous bacterium** that causes a variety of soft tissue infections.

—is part of the **normal flora of gingival crevices and the female genital tract.**

—under conditions of tissue damage (lower tissue oxygenation), invades soft tissues and **bone and may disseminate (rarely) to the brain.**

B. Cutaneous diphtheria (see Upper Respiratory Tract Infections, III)

—occurs in tropics and hot arid regions.

—occurs as grayish skin ulcers started typically with an insect bite and perhaps superinfected by streptococci or *S aureus*.

—rarely results in toxic damage to heart or nerves but may spread to other persons, causing **pharyngeal diphtheria.**

EYE AND EAR INFECTIONS

I. *Chlamydia trachomatis*

A. General characteristics (see Genitourinary Tract Infections, VII)

B. Attributes of pathogenicity. Some toxic effects of antigens kill host cells.

C. Clinical diseases

1. Subtypes A–C

—cause a **chronic keratoconjunctivitis (trachoma)** that can progress to conjunctival and corneal scarring and blindness.

—are frequently accompanied by a concomitant secondary bacterial infection.

—cause neonatal pneumonia.

2. Subtypes D–K

—can be self-inoculated from genital secretions into the eye, resulting in an inclusion conjunctivitis.

D. Laboratory diagnosis is similar to that for genital infections with this agent.

E. Control. Treatment is with doxycycline or erythromycin.

II. *Neisseria gonorrhoeae* (see Genitourinary Tract Infections, V)

—causes **gonococcal ophthalmia.**
—is generally apparent in the **first 5 days of life;** most often seen in babies born at home without medical care and prophylaxis.
—is a **hyperpurulent conjunctivitis.**
—is **rapidly destructive** and, if not treated promptly, leads to blindness.

III. *Haemophilus influenzae* (see Upper Respiratory Tract Infections, II)

—**biotype** *aegyptius* causes bacterial **"pinkeye."**
—is an epidemic, **purulent conjunctivitis.**
—occurs often in **school-age children** but also spreads to adults.

IV. *Streptococcus pneumoniae* (see Lower Respiratory Tract Infections, I)

—is the most common cause of otitis media in infants older than 2 months of age.
—is treated with penicillin, although there are resistant strains.

V. *Haemophilus influenzae*

—is the **second most common causative agent of otitis media** in children, after *S pneumoniae.*
—often **recurs,** probably due to **drug resistance.**
—is most commonly caused by nonencapsulated strains.

VI. *Pseudomonas aeruginosa*

—causes **otitis externa** ("swimmer's ear"), sometimes along with normal flora.
—causes **malignant otitis externa,** an invasive pseudomonad infection that is generally found **in diabetic patients** and may be **life threatening.**

MULTISYSTEM INFECTIONS

I. *Listeria monocytogenes*

A. General characteristics—*Listeria monocytogenes*

—is a **gram-positive, facultative-intracellular bacillus** that has tumbling motility at room temperature and is a psychrophile, even growing at refrigeration temperatures.

—exposure comes from **vertebrate feces** contaminating **dairy products, deli meats and cheeses, unheated hotdogs,** and **uncooked cabbage.**

B. Attributes of pathogenicity—*Listeria monocytogenes*

—is **intracellular** (i.e., within mononuclear phagocytes and epithelial cells).

—"reorganizes" host cell actin; the resulting **actin trails propel *Listeria* directly into other cells,** avoiding the extracellular environment.

—produces **listeriolysin O,** which facilitates the rapid **phagosomal egress of** *Listeria* **into the cytoplasm prior to phagosome–lysosome fusion,** allowing protected intracellular replication.

C. **Clinical disease**

1. **Infections in pregnant women** result in **flu-like symptoms with fever** and the potential of transplacental transfer of *Listeria* to the fetus; alternatively, *Listeria* in the feces may infect the neonate during birth.

2. **Granulomatosis infantiseptica** (from in utero infection) results in widely distributed abscesses and granulomas in the fetus. The fatality rate is 30%–100%.

3. **Meningoencephalitis** occurs in **neonates,** patients with malignancy, immunocompromised patients (particularly renal transplant patients), and adults older than 40 years of age. This disease has become the **most common meningitis to occur in immunocompromised patients** but is recognized also in patients with no known compromising conditions.

4. **Septicemia** occurs in the same population as for meningoencephalitis.

5. **Focal lesions** result from direct contact, generally as eye or skin lesions.

D. **Laboratory diagnosis**

1. **Identification—***L monocytogenes*

—is a gram-positive coccobacillus (intracellular and/or extracellular).

—is β-hemolytic on blood agar.

—has characteristic **"tumbling motility" in 25°C broth cultures.**

—is catalase positive; in addition, it does not produce H_2S on triple sugar iron medium.

2. **Clinical specimens**

—are obtained from CSF, blood, amniotic fluid from the newborn, or the genital tract of the mother.

—**cold enrichment** (storage of specimen at 4°C with weekly 37°C cultures) may be necessary **for fecal specimens** (the other organisms die at 4°C). **Selective media** have largely replaced this technique. Gene probe methods will replace culture.

E. **Control**

1. **Treatment**

a. Ampicillin (intravenous) is given perinatally to infected pregnant women.

b. The prognosis without treatment is poor, with a high fatality rate in newborns.

2. **Prevention**

a. The presence of *Listeria* in farm animal feces and its subsequent survival in the environment and entry into processed meats and dairy products means there is a relatively high risk of exposure. This is of concern mainly for pregnant women and immunocompromised patients.

b. Pasteurization kills *Listeria* in milk. Pregnant women and immunocompromised patients should avoid raw cabbage and heat all processed meats before eating.

II. *Yersinia pestis*

A. General characteristics—*Yersinia pestis*

—is a **gram-negative Enterobacteriaceae** (oxidase negative, catalase positive, fermenter of glucose) and a **nonfermenter of lactose.**

—is the causative agent of **plague,** one of the most devastating diseases in humans. It is rapidly progressive and still has a death rate of approximately 20%.

—is endemic in the United States in the southwestern desert in wild rodents and langomorphs (e.g., ground squirrels, rats, rabbits, mice, prairie dogs) and is **spread to humans by flea bite.**

B. Attributes of pathogenicity

1. **Coagulase** plays a role in transmission.

2. **F1 protein** capsule is the major virulence factor inhibiting phagocytosis.

3. **V and W surface antigens** are also considered virulence factors.

4. **Endotoxin** plays a role in the peripheral vascular collapse and disseminated intravascular coagulopathy seen in plague.

5. *Y pestis* **is a facultative intracellular organism.**

6. *Yersinia* **outer membrane proteins** play a variety of roles.

C. Clinical disease

1. **Bubonic plague** begins as a **flea bite** with regional lymph node swelling caused by infection, necrosis, and suppuration to produce a bubo.

2. **Fever, buboes, and conjunctivitis** are the hallmark symptoms. The organism may **spread to the lungs (through pulmonary emboli)** to produce pneumonia (5% of cases), which is highly contagious.

3. **Pneumonic plague** occurs with respiratory exposure to *Y pestis.* This is a rapidly necrotic pneumonia, with death occurring within days.

D. Laboratory diagnosis

1. Cultures are hazardous; the organism grows on common laboratory media (e.g., MacConkey agar). The laboratory should be warned if *Y pestis* is suspected.

2. Distinctive **bipolar staining (Wayson's stain** or Gram stain) gives a **safety-pin appearance** under microscopy.

3. Immunofluorescence test (reference laboratory) gives a rapid diagnosis.

E. Control

1. **Treatment** is with streptomycin.

2. **Prevention** is with vaccine for individuals at high risk.

III. *Borrelia burgdorferi*

A. General characteristics—*Borrelia burgdorferi*

—is a **large, motile spirochete that causes Lyme disease.**

—is carried by *Ixodes* ticks:

1. *Ixodes scapularis* (formerly *Ixodes dammini*) in the northeastern and central United States

2. *Ixodes pacificus* in the northwestern United States

3. Tick larvae feed on the **white-footed mouse,** the most important source of *B burgdorferi,* before developing into nymphs. Adults feed on **deer,** which are important to its life cycle.

—usually infects people by **nymph**-stage *Ixodes* ticks biting from **May to September.**

B. Classification—*Borrelia burgdorferi*

—is taxonomically related to *Treponema;* there are some parallels between syphilis and Lyme disease in terms of spread, stages, and crossing of both the placenta and the blood–brain barrier.

—is related to *Borrelia recurrentis* (louse-borne) and the other *Borrelia* species (tick-borne), which cause relapsing fever. *B burgdorferi* shares with them the tendency for **antigenic variation.**

C. Attributes of pathogenicity include:

—production of blebs containing DNA and surrounded by a cell envelope containing antigens, peptidoglycan, and an outer membrane

—invasiveness and sequestration in immunologically privileged sites

D. Clinical disease—Lyme disease

—is a **blood stream infection** that seeds other tissues, especially the brain, heart, and joints.

1. **Stage 1.** The hallmark is **erythema (chronicum) migrans (EM),** an annular lesion with a rashy border and central clearing that spreads out from the site of the tick bite. It may enlarge to several inches in diameter, and additional EMs may appear. **Malaise, fatigue, headache, fever, chills, stiff neck, aches, and pains occur for several weeks.**

2. **Stage 2. Neural and cardiac problems** arise, including meningitis, cranial neuropathy (most commonly **Bell's palsy**), radiculoneuropathy, and some cardiac dysfunction; follows stage 1 by weeks to months.

3. **Stage 3. Joint problems** occur, especially in large joints, producing oligoarthritis. Intermittent bouts of arthritis may recur for 3–7 years. Neural dysfunction may lead to dementia and paralysis; it follows stage 1 by months to years.

E. Laboratory diagnosis—identification

1. The organism can be cultured on special media and may be seen in skin biopsy with Giemsa stain; however, the diagnosis is confirmed most frequently by **serology.**

2. The key to diagnosis is recognition of clinical manifestations along with tick bite. (Tick attachment, particularly of the nymph stage, may be missed by patients because the **ticks inject an antihistamine, anesthetic, and anticoagulant.**) EM may be missing in 25% of cases.

3. Several **antibody (both IgM and IgG) tests** are available [immunofluorescence assay (IFA), ELISA, and Western blot] but may be falsely negative in serious infection; they are negative early in infection and may remain negative if the patient is promptly treated with antibiotics.

4. **Lyme urine antigen capture tests** identify antigens.

5. **PCR** is being used on joint fluid and CSF to detect the presence of an organism's DNA.

F. **Control**

1. **Treatment**

a. For primary infection, therapy is with **doxycycline,** amoxicillin, or cefuroxime.

b. For carditis and meningitis, therapy is with ceftriaxone.

c. For arthritis, treatment is with doxycycline or amoxicillin.

2. **Prevention**

a. **Endemic areas** for Lyme disease are the northeastern and north central United States.

b. The highest incidence of Lyme disease correlates with tick season (summer). Prevent tick bites and remove ticks carefully without squeezing the body.

c. A human vaccine is available that contains OspA, an outer surface protein that is present on the *B burgdorferi* envelope in the tick. Because ticks do not have intestinal proteases, human anti-OspA (in the human blood meal) should damage the *Borrelia* in the ticks.

IV. *Ehrlichia*

—is **tick-borne.**

—is a rickettsia that causes human disease endemic to the United States.

—enters monocytes or granulocytes (depending on the species) by *Ehrlichia*-induced phagocytosis and replicates in phagosomes.

—causes **fever, myalgia, headache, malaise, leukopenia,** and **thrombocytopenia,** but **no rash.** There have been some fatalities. (It appears similar to Rocky Mountain spotted fever but without the rash.)

—may appear as **mulberry-like structures (morulae)** in infected cells.

—infection is treated with doxycycline.

V. *Rickettsia rickettsii*

A. **General characteristics—*Rickettsia rickettsii***

—is a weakly staining, gram-negative, **obligate intracellular bacterium** with a specific predilection for endothelial cells of capillaries.

—causes a **zoonotic** disease in which ticks are vectors of human disease. *R rickettsii* has dogs and rodents as its primary reservoir.

—induces **variable clinical manifestations,** ranging from benign and self-limiting to highly fulminant, which is highly fatal.

B. **Classification—*Rickettsia rickettsii***

—is related to less common organisms.

—is listed by disease and symptomatology in Table 3-8.

C. **Attributes of pathogenicity—*Rickettsia rickettsii***

—takes up intracellular (cytoplasmic) residence in endothelial cells of the vascular system.

—has an endotoxin.

D. **Clinical disease**

1. **Multisystemic diseases** of endothelial cells occur, resulting in hyperplasia, thrombus formation, inhibited blood supply, angiitis, and peripheral vasculitis.

2. **General rickettsial manifestations** involve **abrupt onset** of high fever, chills, headache (severe, frontal, unremitting), and myalgias; a few days later, hemorrhagic rash, stupor, delirium, and shock develop.

3. **Rocky Mountain spotted fever** (*R rickettsii,* carried by ticks) initially causes a rash on the extremities, which spreads to the trunk. The fatality rate varies from 20%–30%.

E. **Laboratory diagnosis**

1. **Identification**

—depends heavily on clinical manifestations, especially rash and abrupt onset of fever, headache, and chills with recent exposure to ticks.

—may be determined by comparing acute and convalescent sera measure-

Table 3-8. Important Rickettsial Diseases

Group	Disease	Organism	Spread	Clinical Presentation
Typhus	Epidemic	*Rickettsia prowazeckii*	Lice	Trunk rash, progressing to extremities, gangrene, shock, kidney, heart
	Epidemic	*Rickettsia typhi*	Rat fleas	Trunk rash, progressing to extremities (less severe than epidemic typhus)
Spotted fever	Rocky Mountain spotted fever	*Rickettsia rickettsii*	Ticks	Rash on extremities, progressing to trunk, fulminant vasculitis
	Rickettsialpox	*Rickettsia akari*	Mites	Rash similar to chickenpox (benign course), adenopathy, eschars
Q fever		*Coxiella burnetii*	Dust	Pneumonitis without rash; atypical pneumonia with hepatitis
Cat scratch fever		*Rochalimea henselae*	Cat scratches	Skin, eye rashes, temporary blindness

ments, using agglutination reactions and cross-reacting *Proteus* antigens, immunofluorescence reactions, and complement fixation tests.

   2. **Clinical specimens** for antibody detection are obtained from blood.

F. **Control**

  1. **Treatment**

    a. Doxycycline is the drug of choice.

    b. **Chloramphenicol** should be used if there is no time to differentiate between Rocky Mountain spotted fever and infection with *N meningitidis*.

    c. If Rocky Mountain spotted fever is suspected, treatment should be initiated immediately.

    d. The patient should continue the prescribed regimen of antibiotics. (After the rash disappears, patients tend to discontinue treatment.)

    e. Treatment failures are expected.

  2. **Prevention**

    a. Vectors should be avoided.

    b. The **endemic area** in the United States for Rocky Mountain spotted fever is primarily in the Appalachian states.

VI. *Coxiella burnetii*

A. **General characteristics—*Coxiella burnetii***

—is a genus of Rickettsiaceae and therefore a gram-negative, obligate intracellular organism that replicates in the cytoplasm.

—grows to high titers in infected pregnant animals.

—is transmitted by aerosols to humans from animals (cattle, goats, and sheep).

—is not transferred from person to person.

B. **Attributes of pathogenicity** include:

—a desiccation-resistant form

—intracellular replication

—endotoxin

—phase variation in surface polysaccharide

C. **Clinical manifestations** include:

—fever, chills, headache, but no rash

—interstitial pneumonia that may be mild

—hepatosplenomegaly with abnormal liver enzymes

—complications of myocarditis, pericarditis, endocarditis, or encephalitis

D. **Laboratory diagnosis** is by establishing an increasing complement fixation titer or by IFA or ELISA.

E. **Treatment** is with doxycycline.

VII. *Francisella tularensis* (Table 3-9)

A. General characteristics—*Francisella tularensis*

—causes a **zoonotic** disease, seen mainly in rabbits and rodents, that can be transmitted to humans through **ingestion or handling of infected animals** or through the **bites of ticks,** deer flies, black flies, mosquitoes, mites, or lice.

—is the **gram-negative bacterium** causing **tularemia** (also called deer fly fever or rabbit fever).

B. Attributes of pathogenicity. *Francisella* takes up **intracellular residence** within fixed macrophages of the reticuloendothelial system and within mononuclear phagocytes.

C. Clinical disease

1. Initial manifestations include **abrupt onset of fever, headache, and regional (painful) adenopathy;** back pain, anorexia, chills, sweats, and prostration follow. The fatality rate is 1%.

2. **Tularemia** is characterized by macrophage infiltration, **granulomas, and necrosis of infected tissues.** Regional lymph nodes become infected and suppurate. Spread to the lungs, liver, and spleen is common.

3. Manifestations vary according to the site of organism entry. Forms include **ulceroglandular tularemia** (the most common manifestation), oculoglandular, pneumonic, and typhoidal tularemia.

D. Laboratory diagnosis is most commonly made by immunofluorescent stain of biopsy specimen or serology; culture is hazardous.

E. Treatment is with **streptomycin.**

VIII. *Brucella* (see Table 3-9)

A. General characteristics—*Brucella*

Table 3-9. Important Bacterial Zoonoses

Organism	Spread to Humans	Site of Infection	Most Prominent Clinical Problem
Listeria monocytogenes	Birds, fish, mammals, food	Mononuclear phagocytes	Granulomas, especially in newborns and compromised adults
Yersinia pestis	Rat fleas	Monocytes	Vascular collapse; disseminated intravascular coagulation
Francisella tularensis	Rabbits, rodents	Mononuclear phagocytes	Granulomas; necrosis
Brucella species	Livestock	Reticuloendothelial system	Granulomas (generalized symptoms)
Bacillus anthracis	Sheep, cattle	Generalized toxemia	Necrosis, shock, respiratory distress

—is a **gram-negative bacillus.**

—is zoonotic, with most human infections occurring in livestock farmers, veterinarians, and meat processors.

B. Classification. Three species of the genus cause human **brucellosis:**

—*Brucella suis* (swine)

—*Brucella melitensis* (goats)

—*Brucella abortus* (cattle)

C. Attributes of pathogenicity

1. **Intracellular multiplication** occurs in **macrophages** of the reticuloendothelial system.

2. Initial exposure leads to phagocytosis by neutrophils, which carry organisms to the lymph nodes, spleen, bone marrow, and liver, with ensuing infection of these tissues.

D. Clinical disease

1. Organisms localize and cause **granulomas** in the spleen, liver, bone marrow, and lymph nodes.

2. The patient may have **intermittent fever** and nondescript findings, including **profound muscle weakness, chills, sweats, anorexia, headache, backache, depression** (prevalent in chronic disease), and **nervousness.**

3. Two types of infection occur:
    a. **Acute infection,** with **relapses and fever**
    b. **Chronic infection,** with protracted weakness, depression, arthralgias, and myalgias lasting more than 12 months

E. Laboratory diagnosis is by **culture and serology.**

F. Control

1. **Treatment**
    a. **Tetracycline** and **streptomycin** are given for 3–6 weeks.
    b. The infection is hard to eradicate because of its intracellular residence, so as many as 25% of patients relapse.

2. **Prevention** is by routine pasteurization of milk and bovine vaccination programs. Farmers, veterinarians, and meat processors are still at risk.

IX. *Bacillus anthracis*

A. General characteristics—*Bacillus anthracis*

—causes anthrax, a disease especially prevalent in goats, sheep, and cattle.

—is a **spore former.** Spores play an important role in transmission; they can survive in soil or on the skin of animals for years. Spores are either traumatically implanted or inhaled by humans and then taken up by macrophages and transported to regional lymph nodes. The spores germinate into vegetative cells.

B. **Attributes of pathogenicity**—*Bacillus anthracis* **vegetative cells**

—possess an antiphagocytic **capsule that is unique because it is polypeptide** instead of polysaccharide.

—produce a **tripartite protein exotoxin** consisting of **protective antigen (PA), lethal factor (LF),** and **edema factor (EF)**. PA serves as B component, triggering the internalization of either LF or EF. **EF is a calmodulin-activated adenylate cyclase. LF kills cells.**

C. **Clinical disease** depends on the route of spore entry.

1. **Cutaneous anthrax** (95% of anthrax cases in the United States) results from entry of spores into a cut or an abrasion (especially on the hands, forearms, or head).
   a. The **early papular lesion** develops into a **vesicular lesion filled with blood or clear fluid** that, due to cell death, develops **central necrosis (black eschar) with an erythematous raised margin.**
   b. The fatality rate is 10%.
2. **Pulmonary anthrax** (known as wool sorters' disease) occurs in 5% of anthrax cases and results from entry of spores into the lungs.
   a. This disease form is characterized by abrupt onset of high fever, malaise, cough, myalgias, **marked hemorrhagic necrosis of the lymph nodes,** respiratory distress, and cyanosis.
   b. The fatality rate is 50%.

D. **Laboratory diagnosis**

1. Visualization of the organism in cutaneous lesions or blood shows **large, gram-positive rods; spores are absent.**
2. Culture **aerobically** on blood agar.
3. Toxicity is demonstrated by injecting *B anthracis* into mice; death occurs in a few days, with large numbers of bacilli in the blood.
4. Rapid identification is available from reference laboratories.

E. **Control**

1. **Treatment** of anthrax is with **intravenous penicillin.**
2. **Prevention of anthrax**
   a. Infected animals should be killed and buried deeply. Vaccinate animals where outbreaks have occurred.
   b. Gas sterilize commercial wool, hair, and hides from endemic areas.
   c. Vaccinate at-risk users (anthrax lab workers, farmers, animal processors, military). The last reported case in the United States was in 1992.

X. *Actinomyces*

A. **General characteristics**—*Actinomyces*

—is a **non–acid-fast,** gram-positive bacterium.

—is **anaerobic.**

—may **branch in tissues** and convert to rod forms.

—is found as a commensal organism in the **gingival crevices** and **female genital tract.**

—causes **chronic granulomatous infections,** mainly of the soft tissues (although it also invades bone), with swelling and a tendency to form **sinus tracts** to the surface; exudate from these sinus tracts contains hard microcolonies called **granules.** *Actinomyces* **has little respect for anatomic barriers.**

B. **Classification.** The organism is related to the mycobacteria and belongs to the Actinomycetes.

C. **Attributes of pathogenicity.** The organism grows contiguously in tissues with reduced oxygenation.

D. **Clinical disease**

1. **Cervicofacial actinomycosis** (lumpy jaw) most commonly begins after dental work is performed.

2. **Thoracic actinomycosis** may involve the lungs and ribs.

3. **Abdominal actinomycosis** starts in the ileocecal region and frequently produces sinus tracts to the skin surface.

4. **Mycetoma** is an infection of the limb, with swelling, sinus tract formation, and granules.

E. **Laboratory diagnosis** is by Gram stain of granules and anaerobic culture.

F. **Control. Treatment** commonly involves penicillin and surgical drainage of necrotic tissues.

XI. *Staphylococcus aureus* (see Skin and Soft Tissue Infections, I)

—is a **catalase-positive, coagulase-positive, gram-positive coccus.**

A. **Clinical disease—toxic shock syndrome**

1. **TSST-1 circulates from the nidus of infection** (e.g., tampon or surgical infection). **TSST-1**

—is a **superantigen.**

—**reduces liver clearance of endogenous endotoxin** (from gram-negative organism in the body's normal flora), triggering shock and other symptoms.

2. Symptoms include **high fever, diarrhea, collapse of peripheral circulation, hypotensive shock, scarlatiniform rash with desquamation of palms and soles.**

3. Toxic shock syndrome may be associated with menstruating women using tampons, but it also occurs in other individuals, including patients with surgical packing.

B. **Control**

1. **Treatment** is with antibiotics and supportive care.

2. **Prevention,** in menstruating women, is by careful use of "super tampons."

XII. *Staphylococcus aureus* (see Skin and Soft Tissue Infections, I)—Osteomyelitis

—*S aureus* is the **major causative agent of hematogenously acquired osteomyelitis** in adults and children with no underlying trauma or disease. (***Salmonella* is most common in sickle cell disease.**)

—Disease is characterized by pain and fever; there may be overlying erythema and swelling.

XIII. Other Infections

A. ***Haemophilus influenzae* arthritis or osteomyelitis**

—is generally caused by type b strains in children younger than 2 years of age who have **not been vaccinated.**

B. ***Yersinia enterocolitica***

—is a **gram-negative Enterobacteriaceae** (oxidase negative, catalase positive, fermenter of glucose, nonfermenter of lactose).

—may have a **zoonotic reservoir.**

—may be transmitted in humans by the **fecal–oral** route.

—grows in the cold.

1. **Clinical disease**
   a. **Enterocolitis** occurs as **fever, diarrhea, and abdominal pain, resembling appendicitis;** symptoms include **invasive infection-producing mesenteric lymphadenitis, terminal ileitis, septicemia,** and, generally in adults, **reactive arthritis.**
   b. **Septicemia** is associated with blood transfusions. (Low numbers of bacteria replicate in the cold storage of blood.)
2. **Control.** The disease is generally self-limiting.

Table 3-10. Properties of Bacterial Pathogens

Bacterium	Distinguishing Characteristics	Diseases
Actinomyces	Anaerobe, branching rod "Sulfur" granular microcolonies Contiguous growth through anatomic barriers Cervicofacial, thoracic, and abdominal lesions	Actinomycosis
Bacillus anthracis	Potent exotoxin Capsular polypeptide inhibits phagocytosis Spore transmission	Cutaneous anthrax Pulmonary anthrax
Bacteroides fragilis	Non–spore-forming pleomorphic anaerobe Mixed infections Capsulated Possesses a β-lactamase Wound débridement important	Brain abscess Gastrointestinal abscess Cellulitis Pelvic inflammatory disease

(cont.)

Table 3-10. Properties of Bacterial Pathogens (*Continued*)

Bacterium	Distinguishing Characteristics	Diseases
Bordetella pertussis	Paroxysmal cough due to toxin Attaches via pili Component of DPT vaccine	Whooping cough
Borrelia burgdorferi	*Ixodes* transmission Corkscrew-shaped motile spirochete	Lyme disease
Campylobacter jejuni	Comma-shaped rod A frequent cause of diarrhea Enterotoxin Neutrophils and blood in stool	Gastroenteritis
Chlamydia pneumoniae	Obligate intracellular parasite Elementary and reticular body Divides by binary fission	Pneumonia
Chlamydia psittaci	Zoonotic (birds, parrots) Sudden onset	Respiratory disease
Chlamydia trachomatis	As for *C pneumoniae* 15 Serotypes	Chronic keratocon-junctivitis (subtypes A–C) Sexually transmitted infection (D–K) Lymphogranuloma venereum (L sub type) Arthritis, pelvic inflammatory disease
Clostridium botulinum	Spore-forming anaerobe Exotoxin acting at myoneural junction Suppresses acetylcholine release by peripheral nerves Produces flaccid muscle paralysis Caused by ingestion of preformed toxin or by ingestion of spores by infants	Botulism
Clostridium difficile	Spore-forming anaerobe Part of normal gastrointestinal flora Activated by antibiotic disruption of other flora Secrete an enterotoxin and cytotoxin	Gastroenteritis Pseudomembranous colitis
Clostridium perfringens	Spore-forming anaerobe Spores introduced by severe trauma Possesses an α-toxin (lecithinase)	Gas gangrene Food poisoning Soft tissue cellulitis
Corynebacterium diphtheriae	Phage-induced A/B exotoxin Lysogenic conversion Fragment A inhibits EF-2	Pharyngeal diphtheria Cutaneous diphtheria
Coxiella burnetii	Intracellular bacterium (rickettsia) Dust and tick transmitted Absence of rash	Q fever Pneumonitis
Ehrlichia	Tick-transmitted zoonosis Strict intracellular pathogen (WBC) Belong to family Rickettsiaceae	Ehrlichiosis
Enterococcus	Formely group D streptococci Most are α- or γ-hemolytic	Urinary tract infection Endocarditis

(cont.)

Table 3-10. Properties of Bacterial Pathogens (*Continued*)

Bacterium	Distinguishing Characteristics	Diseases
	Antibiotic resistance is a problem β-Lactamase Nosocomial opportunist	
Escherichia coli	Enterotoxigenic: heat-labile toxin stimulates adenylate cyclase similar to cholera toxin; heat-stable toxin activates guanylate cyclase Enteropathogenic: adherence to enterocytes→ infantile diarrhea Enterohemorrhagic: Shiga-like verotoxin→ bloody diarrhea (serotype 0157) Enteroinvasive: properties similar to shigellosis All strains possess endotoxin	Genitourinary tract infections Gastroenteritis Septic shock Neonatal meningitis
Fusobacterium nucleatum	Polymorphic, slender filaments Oral anaerobe Synergizes with *Borrelia vincentii*	Vincent's angina Brain abscess Head, neck, chest infections
Haemophilus aegyptius	Antiphagocytic polysaccharide capsule	Conjunctivitis (pinkeye)
Haemophilus influenzae	Antiphagocytic polysaccharide capsule Pyrogenic IgAase Grow on chocolate agar or with X and V factors Epiglottis requires a tracheotomy	Genitourinary infections Meningitis (to 6 years old) Epiglottitis
Helicobacter pylori	Curved rod Produces a potent urease and cytotoxin Treat with bismuth salts, metronidazole, and antibiotic	Gastric and peptic ulcers Increases risk for gastric adenocarcinoma
Legionella pneumophila	Aquaphile–inhalation transmission Association with amoeba Possesses a cytotoxin and endotoxin β-Lactamase Stains with Dieterle silver stain; no Gram stain Requires cysteine and iron for growth Intracellular parasite	Legionnaires' disease (pneumonia)
Listeria monocytogenes	Animal reservoir Infects monocytes (monocytosis) Hemolysin destroys vesicular membranes	*Granulomas* Abscesses Meningitis (newborns)
Mycobacterium avium-intracellulare	Group of acid-fast organisms Drug resistance Common infection in AIDS; noncontagious	Pulmonary disease
Mycobacterium tuberculosis	Peptidoglycan—arabinogalactam cell wall Mycolic acids require acid-fast stain Cord factor (trehalose mycolate) induces granuloma Purified protein derivative skin test Becoming isoniazid and rifampin resistant Bacille Calmette Guérin vaccine	Tuberculosis Granulomas

(*cont.*)

Table 3-10. Properties of Bacterial Pathogens (*Continued*)

Bacterium	Distinguishing Characteristics	Diseases
Mycoplasma pneumoniae	Lacks a cell wall Smallest extracellular bacterium; not an L form Mucosal tissue tropism Requires cholesterol	Primary atypical pneumonia
Neisseria gonorrhoeae	Intracellular gram-negative diplococcus Produces an IgAase and a penicillinase plasmid Purulent exudate Requires chocolate agar (Thayer-Martin) Oxidase positive	Urethritis Pelvic inflammatory disease Conjunctivitis in newborns
Neisseria meningitidis	Antiphagocytic capsule Endotoxin (lipopolysaccharide) IgAase Vasculitic purpura Headache and stiff neck are common	Meningococcemia Waterhouse-Fridericksen syndrome
Nocardia	Aerobic soil bacterium Inhalation transmission	Pulmonary infections
Prevotella melaninogenica	Aerobic black colonies on agar Found in mouth, gastrointestinal and genitourinary tracts Putrid sputum Débride and drain lesion Formerly in genus *Bacteroides*	Lung abscesses Female genitourinary infections
Proteus mirabilis	Highly motile Produces urease	Pneumonia Nosocomial infections
Pseudomonas aeruginosa	Glycocalyx slime layer Pyocyanin–blue-green pigment Exotoxin similar in action to diphtheria Endotoxin (lipopolysaccharide)	Burn infections Cystic fibrosis infections Septic shock
Rickettsia rickettsii	Tick transmission Intracellular dwelling bacterium	Rocky Mountain spotted fever
Salmonella	Wide host range; except *S typhosa* Many serotypes Intracellular multiplication Can invade blood stream Endotoxin lipopolysaccharide Enterotoxin	Enterocolitis Septicemia Enteric fever (typhoid)
Shigella	No known animal reservoir Pathogenic in small numbers Perpetuation by small numbers Perpetuation by human carriers Possesses an endotoxin and an exotoxin Stools can contain mucus, pus, and blood Blood stream invasion is rare Culture on differential and selective media Only *Shigella sonnei* ferments lactose	Shigellosis
Staphylococcus aureus	Grape-like cluster morphology Antibiotic resistance Catalase and coagulase positive Enterotoxin Short incubation period (hours)	Local abscesses Impetigo Food poisoning

(cont.)

Table 3-10. Properties of Bacterial Pathogens (*Continued*)

Bacterium	Distinguishing Characteristics	Diseases
Staphylococcus epidermidis	Slime layer Instrument contamination Noninvasive nosocomial infections	Urinary tract infections Endocarditis
Staphylococcus saprophyticus	Noninvasive nosocomial infections	Urinary tract infections
Streptococcus agalactiae	Group B Can be part of normal vaginal and oral flora Capsule Inhibits complement	Neonatal sepsis (early and late onset) Meningitis
Streptococcus pneumoniae	α-Hemolytic Large antiphagocytic capsule Diplococcus Sensitive to bile and optochin Quellung reaction Vaccine contains 23 capsular serotypes Anticapsular antibody is protective Differentiates from *S viridans*	Pneumonia Otitis media Septicemia
Streptococcus pyogenes	Group A M protein; (more than 80 types); anti-phagocytic β-Hemolytic Sensitive to bacitracin Erythrogenic exotoxins	Pharyngitis Scarlet fever Rheumatic fever Acute glomerulo-nephritis Impetigo Cellulits–erysipelas Endocarditis
Treponema pallidum	Spirochete Unable to be cultured Immunosuppressive Darkfield microscopy examination Serologic tests	Syphilis, 1°, 2°, 3°
Vibrio cholerae	Comma-shaped morphology A/B enterotoxin overproduces cAMP Vomiting and rice-water diarrhea Must replace copious fluid loss	Cholera
Viridans streptococci	Noninvasive opportunist in normal oral flora α-Hemolytic Differentiate from *S pneumoniae* because the *S viridans* are bile insoluble and not inhibited by optochin	Endocarditis Dental caries
Yersinia pestis	Zoonotic disease (rats and fleas) Intracellular multiplication Fever, conjunctivitis, regional buboes	Bubonic plague Pneumonic plague Yersiniosis

AIDS = acquired immunodeficiency syndrome; cAMP = cyclic adenosine monophosphate; DTP = diphtheria and tetanus toxoids and pertussis; EF-2 = elongation factor 2.

IMPORTANT MICROBIAL MEDIA AND TESTS USED IN THE IDENTIFICATION OF BACTERIA (SEE COLOR PLATE)

Review Test

1. Which of the following organisms is anaerobic?

(A) *Nocardia*
(B) *Actinomyces*
(C) Mycobacteria

2. Which of the following organisms spreads through inhalation of infected dust?

(A) *Rickettsia akari*
(B) *Rickettsia typhi*
(C) *Rickettsia rickettsii*
(D) *Coxiella burnetii*
(E) All of the above

3. All of the following statements about clinical manifestations of *Haemophilus influenzae* are correct EXCEPT

(A) acute bacterial epiglottitis is a mild disease in children.
(B) severe central nervous system deficits occur in one-third of recovered meningitis patients.
(C) pus production is typical.
(D) during viral influenza outbreaks, incidence of *H influenzae* increases.
(E) pneumonia is a complication usually seen in children or the aged.

4. A 22-year-old cystic fibrosis patient presents because of fever and increasing dyspnea. A gram-negative organism is found in unusually high numbers in the mucus. Which virulence factor is most important in colonization and maintenance of the organism in the lungs?

(A) Exotoxin A
(B) Pyocyanin (blue-green pigment)
(C) Polysaccharide slime
(D) Endotoxin

5. Exotoxin A most closely resembles the action of which of the following?

(A) Heat-labile (LT) *Escherichia coli*
(B) Shiga toxin
(C) Diphtheria toxin
(D) *Vibrio cholerae* toxin
(E) Verotoxin

6. Of the following components of *Mycobacterium tuberculosis*, which one promotes intracellular survival by inhibiting phagosome–lysosome fusion?

(A) Cord factor
(B) Mycolic acid
(C) Purified protein derivative (PPD)
(D) Sulfatides
(E) Wax D

7. What is the most likely causative agent of gastroenteritis starting on day 5 of clindamycin treatment?

(A) *Clostridium perfringens*
(B) *Clostridium difficile*
(C) *Pseudomonas aeruginosa*
(D) *Shigella sonnei*

8. Which of the following organisms causes a relatively mild form of gastroenteritis?

(A) *Vibrio cholerae*
(B) *Vibrio parahaemolyticus*
(C) *Salmonella typhi*
(D) *Shigella sonnei*

9. Yersinia pestis may be transferred by:

(A) *Dermacentor* tick bit.
(B) Human body louse bite.
(C) *Ixodes* tick bite.
(D) Respiratory droplets.

10. Which of the following staphylococcal organisms causes subacute bacterial endocarditis that occurs 2 months or more after heart surgery?

(A) *Staphylococcus aureus*
(B) *Staphylococcus epidermidis*
(C) *Staphylococcus haemolyticus*
(D) *Staphylococcus saprophyticus*

11. Which of the following statements about clinical manifestations of clostridial infections is correct?

(A) *Clostridium perfringens* does not infect nontraumatized tissues due to the high oxidation–reduction potential (E_h) of normal tissue.
(B) Infant botulism results from ingestion of preformed toxins in contaminated food.
(C) Tetanus causes death from cardiac dysfunction.
(D) The anaerobic cellulitis produced by *C perfringens* spreads to surrounding healthy tissues.
(E) *Clostridium difficile* produces a mild gastroenteritis.

12. Which of the following statements about *Streptococcus pneumoniae* is true?

(A) It secretes an enterotoxin.
(B) It contains an endotoxin.
(C) It possesses both an enterotoxin and endotoxin.
(D) It possesses neither an enterotoxin nor an endotoxin.

13. Which of the following organisms grows in 40% bile?

(A) *Enterococcus faecalis*
(B) *Streptococcus pneumoniae*
(C) Group B streptococci
(D) Viridans streptococci

14. Which of the following statements about treatment of clostridial infections is correct?

(A) Anaerobic cellulitis may require amputation or skin grafting.
(B) Clostridial food poisoning is severe, and patients infected with either *Clostridium perfringens* or *Clostridium botulinum* frequently require hospitalization.
(C) Infant botulism should be treated with antibiotics to eradicate the organism.
(D) Antitoxins must be administered as soon as clostridial infection is suspected.
(E) Patients with anaerobic cellulitis should be given antitoxin and antibiotics.

15. All of the following are characteristics of *Salmonella typhimurium* EXCEPT

(A) it has a multianimal reservoir.
(B) it is one of the most common causes of enterocolitis.
(C) it ferments lactose.
(D) it is a common contaminant of poultry.
(E) it is a gram-negative, motile, endotoxin-bearing rod.

16. Which of the following is a characteristic of *Bacteroides fragilis*?

(A) Colonies have a distinctive black appearance.
(B) Organisms are susceptible to penicillin.
(C) Organisms possess a β-lactamase.
(D) Organisms are rarely found in the gastrointestinal tract.

17. Which of the following group A streptococcal diseases is highly communicable in infants?

(A) Impetigo
(B) Scarlet fever
(C) Rheumatic fever
(D) Cellulitis

18. Which of the following conditions is necessary for effective diagnosis of anaerobic infections?

(A) Streaking on eosin-methylene blue (EMB) agar
(B) Rapid transport of culture to the laboratory
(C) Assay for superoxide dismutase
(D) Sputum sampling

19. Which of the following organisms is partially acid-fast and filamentous?

(A) *Nocardia*
(B) *Actinomyces*
(C) Mycobacteria

20. All of the following statements about *Mycoplasma pneumoniae* infections are true EXCEPT

(A) Eaton agent causes primary atypical pneumonia.
(B) *M pneumoniae* produces surface mucous membrane infections that do not disseminate to other tissues.
(C) *M pneumoniae* is a slow-growing organism that requires 1–3 weeks to culture in the laboratory.
(D) serologic tests for *M pneumoniae* involve complement fixation or cold agglutination.
(E) incidence of *M pneumoniae* is highest in elderly persons.

21. Which one of the following statements concerning *Vibrio cholerae* infections is correct?

(A) Death occurs in 2–4 weeks from exhaustion and respiratory failure.
(B) The disease is marked by organism invasion and hemorrhagic necrosis of the small intestine.
(C) Most pathology is attributable to a protein exotoxin.
(D) *V cholerae* produces an acute febrile disease with meningitis.
(E) There is no need to hospitalize patients with *V cholerae* infections. Organisms in stools are not contagious because the organism is sensitive to acid pH.

22. Which of the following organisms causes septicemic disease?

(A) *Vibrio cholerae*
(B) *Vibrio parahaemolyticus*
(C) *Salmonella typhi*
(D) *Shigella sonnei*

23. Which of the following statements about Lyme disease and its clinical manifestations is correct?

(A) It is characterized by a rash throughout the trunk and extremities.
(B) The three stages of the disorder are distinctive and do not overlap.
(C) It is caused by *Borrelia burgdorferi*.
(D) Manifestations of stage 3 may appear within 4 weeks of the initial infection.

24. Which of the following organisms is characterized by abrupt onset of fever, chills, and unremitting headache?

(A) *Rickettsia akari*
(B) *Rickettsia typhi*
(C) *Rickettsia rickettsii*
(D) *Coxiella burnetii*
(E) All of the above

25. Which of the following organisms causes neonatal sepsis?

(A) *Enterococcus faecalis*
(B) *Streptococcus pneumoniae*
(C) Group B streptococci
(D) Viridans streptococci

26. Which of the following organisms causes relapsing fever and is transmitted by lice or ticks?

(A) *Treponema*
(B) *Borrelia*
(C) *Leptospira*

27. All of the following statements are true of staphylococcal and *Neisseria* infections EXCEPT

(A) pus production is a helpful diagnostic aid.
(B) localized infections may disseminate and cause severe clinical problems.
(C) both types of organisms cause urinary tract infections.
(D) Gram stain of clinical specimens is an important diagnostic aid.
(E) they both produce an enzyme that degrades IgA (IgAase).

28. Which of the following statements about congenital syphilis is correct?

(A) Syphilis serology test should be performed in the first and third trimesters of pregnancy.
(B) Clinical manifestations are generally mild.
(C) Newborns are infected only when they pass through the infected birth canal.
(D) Specimens should be cultured on blood agar.

29. Of the following components of *Mycobacterium tuberculosis,* which one is used for skin testing?

(A) Cord factor
(B) Mycolic acid
(C) Purified protein derivative (PPD)
(D) Sulfatides
(E) Wax D

30. A patient has a gastric ulcer not induced by nonsteroidal anti-inflammatory agents. Which characteristic appears to play a central role in the ability of the organism to colonize the stomach?

(A) Phospholipase C production
(B) Urease production
(C) Microaerophilic lifestyle
(D) O antigens
(E) Motility

31. Which of the following statements about mycobacterial disease is correct?

(A) Nontuberculous mycobacterial disease is as contagious as tuberculosis.
(B) Tuberculosis is caused by *Mycobacterium tuberculosis,* and nontuberculous disease is caused by other mycobacteria, including *Mycobacterium bovis, Mycobacterium kansasii,* and *Mycobacterium avium-intracellulare.*
(C) Water is a source of exposure to nontuberculous mycobacteria.
(D) Only nontuberculous disease is seen with great frequency in patients with acquired immunodeficiency syndrome (AIDS).
(E) *M tuberculosis* is the only acid-fast mycobacterium.

32. Which of the following organisms is zoonotic and can be spread to humans by arthropod vectors?

(A) *Rickettsia akari*
(B) *Rickettsia typhi*
(C) *Rickettsia rickettsii*
(D) *Coxiella burnetii*
(E) All of the above

33. All of the following are characteristics of *Legionella* EXCEPT

(A) it is associated with water.
(B) it causes granulomatous lung infection.
(C) it is weakly gram-negative.
(D) it is a facultative, intracellular parasite.
(E) it is catalase positive.

34. Which of the following organisms grows contiguously in tissues with no respect to anatomic barriers?

(A) *Actinomyces israelii*
(B) *Mycobacterium leprae*
(C) *Mycobacterium kansasii*
(D) *Mycobacterium tuberculosis*

35. Which of the following organisms is generally rod-shaped and acid-fast?

(A) *Nocardia*
(B) *Actinomyces*
(C) Mycobacteria

36. The Ghon complex, a lesion in the lung and regional lymph nodes, is found in

(A) actinomycotic mycetoma.
(B) tuberculoid leprosy.
(C) primary tuberculosis.
(D) cervical facial actinomycosis.
(E) soft tissue infections caused by *Mycobacterium marinum.*

37. Which of the following organisms has diverse animal reservoirs?

(A) *Vibrio cholerae*
(B) *Vibrio parahaemolyticus*
(C) *Salmonella typhi*
(D) *Shigella sonnei*

38. Which of the following organisms causes acute icteric disease with protean manifestations?

(A) *Treponema*
(B) *Borrelia*
(C) *Leptospira*

39. Which statement about the two major forms of leprosy (tuberculoid and lepromatous) is correct?

(A) Tuberculoid leprosy is the hardest to treat due to poor cell-mediated immunity.
(B) In either extreme form of leprosy, the lepromin test will be positive.
(C) Diagnostic work-up on the patient should include a physical examination, skin test, and cultures.
(D) Biopsy sample of lesions from a lepromatous leprosy patient generally contains many *Mycobacterium leprae.*
(E) Lepromatous leprosy patients usually have few lesions.

40. All of the following statements about non–spore-forming anaerobes are correct EXCEPT

(A) they are pleomorphic and can be either gram-negative or gram-positive.
(B) they are a common cause of intra-abdominal infections.
(C) they usually are found in mixed infections.
(D) they represent a minority of the total fecal flora.
(E) they include the *Fusobacterium* genus found in the oral cavity.

41. Which of the following statements about *Pseudomonas aeruginosa* is true?

(A) It secretes an enterotoxin.
(B) It contains an endotoxin.
(C) It possesses both an enterotoxin and endotoxin.
(D) It possesses neither an enterotoxin nor an endotoxin.

42. Which one of the following statements about *Francisella tularensis* infections and their treatment is correct?

(A) Culture of the suspected infection by the hospital laboratory is important.
(B) An effective vaccine is available, but only for use in high-risk groups.
(C) *F tularensis* causes a noninvasive focal skin infection.
(D) Relapses do not occur after treatment.
(E) The hallmark of *F tularensis* infection is regional buboes.

43. Of the following components of *Mycobacterium tuberculosis,* which one is responsible for the acid-fast property of the organism?

(A) Cord factor
(B) Mycolic acid
(C) Purified protein derivative (PPD)
(D) Sulfatides
(E) Wax D

44. Which of the following statements about *Brucella* infections is true?

(A) *Brucella suis* is the human pathogen; *Brucella melitensis* and *Brucella abortus* cause infections in animals only.
(B) *Brucella* infection produces profound muscle weakness along with other relatively nondescript manifestations.
(C) *Brucella* infection is a zoonotic disease spread to humans primarily by rat fleas.
(D) Untreated infections are self-limiting and resolve in 2 weeks.
(E) *Brucella* is an extracellular parasite.

45. Which of the following organisms presents with an initial rash on the extremities that spreads to the trunk?

(A) *Rickettsia akari*
(B) *Rickettsia typhi*
(C) *Rickettsia rickettsii*
(D) *Coxiella burnetii*
(E) All of the above

46. Which of the following statements about anthrax infections is correct?

(A) The early cutaneous form may mimic a staphylococcal furuncle or insect bite.
(B) Pulmonary and gastrointestinal anthrax tend to be chronic, with frequent treatment failure.
(C) Spores are routinely observed in lesion aspirates.
(D) The capsule is a long-chain polysaccharide.
(E) Primary animal reservoirs are rabbits and other rodents.

47. All of the following statements about *Campylobacter* infections are correct EXCEPT

(A) sepsis is a problem in debilitated patients with *Campylobacter fetus* species infection.
(B) human infections with *Campylobacter jejuni* are rare relative to *Salmonella* and *Shigella* infections.
(C) *C jejuni* infection is usually self-limiting.
(D) *C jejuni* clinical specimens should be incubated at 42°C.

48. Which of the following group A streptococcal diseases is characterized by rash due to erythrogenic toxins?

(A) Impetigo
(B) Scarlet fever
(C) Rheumatic fever
(D) Cellulitis

49. Which of the following is a virulence factor for *Streptococcus pneumoniae*?

(A) C-reactive protein
(B) Bacitracin
(C) Endotoxic lipopolysaccharide
(D) Capsular polysaccharide

50. All of the following are characteristics of group A streptococci EXCEPT

(A) they are part of the normal intestinal flora.
(B) they attach to epithelial cells via fimbriae containing lipoteichoic acid.
(C) they are rarely resistant to penicillin.
(D) they produce β-hemolysis with streptolysin S.

51. Which one of the following statements about laboratory diagnosis of diphtheria is correct?

(A) Organisms are delicate and survive poorly outside the host.
(B) It is sufficient to identify *Corynebacterium diphtheriae* in the isolate.
(C) Organisms are impossible to identify by Gram stain because of their small size.
(D) Culture on Löffler's medium or tellurite medium should reveal characteristic Chinese letter formation.
(E) Organisms are coagulase positive.

52. Which of the following statements about laboratory diagnosis of whooping cough is correct?

(A) Lymphocyte numbers are greatly decreased.
(B) Cough plate is the method of choice to isolate organisms from the patient.
(C) The clinical specimen should be plated on Bordet-Gengou agar.
(D) The best chance to isolate the organism is during the paroxysmal stage.
(E) The causative organism is a gram-positive rod.

53. Which of the following statements about *Shigella dysenteriae* is true?

(A) It secretes an enterotoxin.
(B) It contains an endotoxin.
(C) It possesses both an enterotoxin and endotoxin.
(D) It possesses neither an enterotoxin nor an endotoxin.

54. Which of the following organisms is an obligate intracellular bacterium with predilection for multiplication within capillary endothelial cells?

(A) *Rickettsia akari*
(B) *Rickettsia typhi*
(C) *Rickettsia rickettsii*
(D) *Coxiella burnetii*
(E) All of the above

55. All of the following are characteristics of Enterobacteriaceae EXCEPT

(A) they are a common cause of hospital-acquired infections.
(B) they are usually noninvasive and are part of the normal intestinal flora.
(C) some can produce both endotoxins and exotoxins.
(D) they have a short incubation period (several hours), leading to gastrointestinal disturbances.
(E) they ferment glucose.

56. Which of the following organisms invades mucosal epithelial cells?

(A) *Vibrio cholerae*
(B) *Vibrio parahaemolyticus*
(C) *Salmonella typhi*
(D) *Shigella sonnei*

57. A 54-year-old man develops a pyogenic infection along the suture line after knee surgery. The laboratory gives a preliminary report of a β-hemolytic, catalase-positive, coagulase-positive, gram-positive coccus. The most likely causative agent is

(A) *Moraxella catarrhalis*
(B) *Staphylococcus aureus*
(C) *Staphylococcus epidermidis*
(D) *Streptococcus agalactiae*
(E) *Streptococcus pyogenes*

58. Which of the following statements about treatment and prevention of *Haemophilus* is correct?

(A) Give rifampin to index case of *Haemophilus influenzae* meningitis and to family members to eradicate the carrier state.
(B) Bacterial pinkeye is treated with intravenous ampicillin.
(C) Soft chancre is poorly contagious, and asymptomatic sexual partners need not be treated.
(D) The capsule is a highly effective vaccine in a target population of children 3 months to 6 years of age.
(E) Meningitis patients should be treated for 14 days with oral antibiotics.

59. Which of the following statements about *Salmonella typhimurium* is true?

(A) It secretes an enterotoxin.
(B) It contains an endotoxin.
(C) It possesses both an enterotoxin and endotoxin.
(D) It possesses neither an enterotoxin nor an endotoxin.

60. Which of the following organisms causes pneumonitis resembling atypical pneumonia?

(A) *Rickettsia akari*
(B) *Rickettsia typhi*
(C) *Rickettsia rickettsii*
(D) *Coxiella burnetii*
(E) All of the above

61. All of the following statements about the incidence of bacterial shock are correct EXCEPT

(A) it is usually a hospital-induced syndrome.
(B) it can occur after catheterization.
(C) it is reversible by penicillin.
(D) mortality is dependent on admission prognosis.
(E) it is usually preceded by a fever spike.

Color Plate

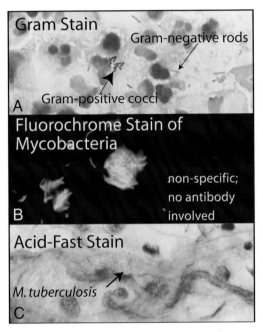

Gram Stain
Gram-negative rods
Gram-positive cocci
A

Fluorochrome Stain of Mycobacteria
non-specific; no antibody involved
B

Acid-Fast Stain
M. tuberculosis
C

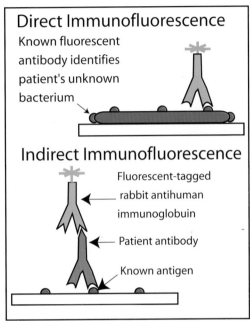

Direct Immunofluorescence
Known fluorescent antibody identifies patient's unknown bacterium

Indirect Immunofluorescence
Fluorescent-tagged rabbit antihuman immunoglobuin
Patient antibody
Known antigen

Color Plate 3-1. (*A*) **Gram stain.** On this Gram stain, both gram-positive (purple) diplococci and gram-negative (red) rods can be seen among the inflammatory cells. (*B*) **Fluorochrome stain.** The auramine binds nonspecifically to the waxy mycobacterial cell wall. Because there is no antibody involved in this binding, this is not a specific stain, but it is a sensitive screening test for sputa and is easy to read because of the contrast of the bound dye with everything else dark. A positive fluorochrome stain is confirmed by an acid-fast stain. (*C*) **Acid-fast stain.** Mycobacteria (acid-fast = red) are shown in this sputum. All of these images have been enlarged greater than is possible with the light or fluorescent microscope, making the images generally easier to read than on the actual microscope.

Color Plate 3-2. Immunofluorescent staining (also known as fluorescent antibody staining). With **direct immunofluorescence,** highly specific (depending on antibody choice) fluorescent staining can be achieved by conjugating fluorescent dye to specific antibody. For example, because *Bordetella pertussis* is often difficult to culture after the characteristic cough has been present for several days, a nasopharyngeal smear can be made and stained with tagged antibody. Thus, these gram-negative rods, which on a Gram stain would be confused with nonpathogenic normal flora, can be positively identified because of the specificity of the antibody–antigen combination. **Indirect immunofluorescence** uses fluorescent dye–tagged animal (e.g., rabbit) antibody to human immunoglobulins. This technique is used most commonly to detect the presence of a specific human antibody that has bound to its specific known antigen, which was fixed on a surface before incubation with the patient's serum; unbound antibody is washed away before applying the tagged rabbit antihuman antibody.

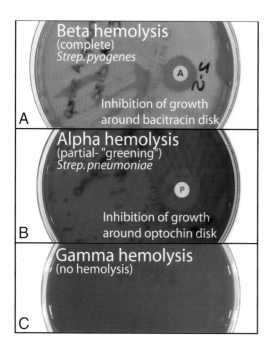

A

Beta hemolysis
(complete)
Strep. pyogenes

Inhibition of growth
around bacitracin disk

B

Alpha hemolysis
(partial- "greening")
Strep. pneumoniae

Inhibition of growth
around optochin disk

C

Gamma hemolysis
(no hemolysis)

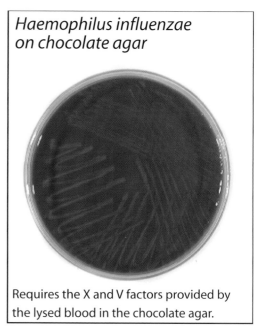

Haemophilus influenzae
on chocolate agar

Requires the X and V factors provided by
the lysed blood in the chocolate agar.

Color Plate 3-3. Examples of the different types of he-molysis. Note that the colonies on these plates do not show up well because transmitted light was used to show the hemolysis. (*A*) **Beta hemolysis** is **complete lysis** of the red blood cells, which results in a transparent area around the colony. (*B*) **Alpha hemolysis** is **partial hemolysis** of the red blood cells with a change in the color of hemoglobin, resulting in a translucent area with a **greenish coloration.** (*C*) **Gamma hemolysis** is **no hemolysis.**

Color Plate 3-4. Chocolate agar. Some organisms, such as *Haemophilus influenzae* and pathogenic *Neisseria,* will not grow on blood agar but will grow on agar that has lysed blood in the base. This agar is called chocolate agar despite the fact that there is no chocolate in it.

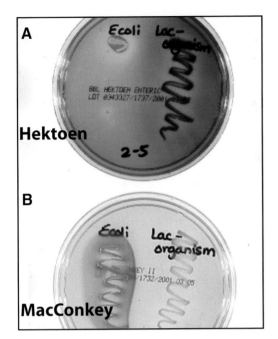

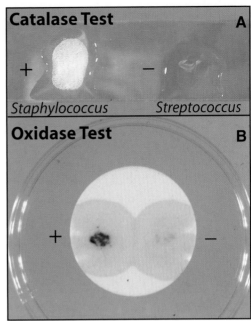

Color Plate 3-5. Differential media allow distinction of certain groups directly from the growth and substrate changes directly on a plate. Thus, on several of the enteric media, bacteria that ferment lactose can be distinguished from those that do not ferment lactose. (*A*) **Hektoen agar.** Lactose fermentation (here by *Escherichia coli*) produces acid, which turns the colonies and medium into colors in the yellow range. (*B*) **Mac-Conkey medium.** The pale straw color of the medium turns to red when the pH becomes acidic from the lactose fermentation products.

Color Plate 3-6. (*A*) **Catalase test.** Hydrogen peroxide is reacted with a small amount of the bacterial growth. The production of bubbles (oxygen) suggests that the organism produces catalase. The organism on the left side of the slide is positive, and the organism on the right side (hard to see because there are no bubbles) is negative. (*B*) **Oxidase test.** Test detects presence of cytochrome oxidase and is used largely for gram-negative bacteria. All Enterobacteriaceae are oxidase-negative. Most others are oxidase-positive.

Drug Susceptibility Testing

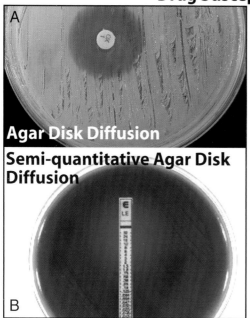

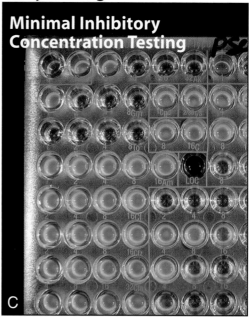

Color Plate 3-7. Drug susceptibility testing. (*A*) **Agar disk diffusion.** A disk with a known concentration of dried antibiotic is placed on the surface of an agar plate spread inoculated with the patient's bacterial isolate. After incubation, the diameter of the zone of inhibition determines if the isolate is susceptible, intermediate, or resistant to that antibiotic. This is a qualitative technique. (*B*) **Semiquantitative agar disk diffusion.** A sterile plastic "ruler" with a drop of dried antibiotic on the back is placed on a plate inoculated to create a lawn of bacteria. After the incubation, the zone of growth inhibition can be correlated with the expected minimal inhibitory concentration from reading the measurements on the ruler. The "ruler" is different for each antibiotic. (*C*) **Minimal inhibitory concentration.** Each well has a specific concentration of a single drug and the same approximate number of the patient's bacterial isolate. Drugs are tested in achievable concentration ranges in this test. Growth is measured by a variety of methods

62. Which one of the following statements about laboratory diagnosis of *Neisseria gonorrhoeae* is correct?

(A) Purulent discharge contains primarily neutrophils and intracellular diplococci.
(B) Asymptomatic patients are identified by culturing organisms from a clinical specimen with a lubricated swab.
(C) Purulent discharge contains only intracellular diplococci.
(D) Clinical specimens should be plated onto blood agar to determine type of hemolysis.
(E) In disseminated infections, organisms can be routinely isolated from skin lesions.

63. Which of the following organisms is a mite-borne agent causing a rash that may be confused with chickenpox?

(A) *Rickettsia akari*
(B) *Rickettsia typhi*
(C) *Rickettsia rickettsii*
(D) *Coxiella burnetii*
(E) All of the above

64. Which of the following organisms is zoonotic and is transmitted to humans primarily by contact with animal urine?

(A) *Treponema*
(B) *Borrelia*
(C) *Leptospira*

65. All of the following are characteristic of group B streptococci EXCEPT

(A) an effective vaccine incorporates proteinaceous capsular antigens.
(B) they are part of the normal vaginal flora.
(C) they are bacitracin-resistant.
(D) they agglutinate with *Streptococcus agalactiae* antiserum.
(E) they can cause neonatal sepsis and meningitis.

66. Which of the following statements about *Vibrio cholerae* is true?

(A) It secretes an enterotoxin.
(B) It contains an endotoxin.
(C) It possesses both an enterotoxin and endotoxin.
(D) It possesses neither an enterotoxin nor an endotoxin.

67. Which of the following organisms is a very slow grower?

(A) *Nocardia*
(B) *Actinomyces*
(C) Mycobacteria

68. All of the following statements about *Listeria monocytogenes* infection are correct EXCEPT

(A) abscesses and granulomas occur in many different tissues.
(B) laboratory isolation involves cold enrichment technique.
(C) neonatal infections have a poor prognosis.
(D) bacteria parasitize neutrophils and monocytes.
(E) neonatal infections occur only during passage through the infected birth canal.

69. Of the following components of *Mycobacterium tuberculosis,* which one interrupts mitochondrial function?

(A) Cord factor
(B) Mycolic acid
(C) Purified protein derivative (PPD)
(D) Sulfatides
(E) Wax D

70. Which of the following staphylococcal organisms causes urinary tract infections, primarily in adolescent females?

(A) *Staphylococcus aureus*
(B) *Staphylococcus epidermidis*
(C) *Staphylococcus haemolyticus*
(D) *Staphylococcus saprophyticus*

71. Which of the following group A streptococcal diseases causes skin infection capable of giving rise to a septicemia?

(A) Impetigo
(B) Scarlet fever
(C) Rheumatic fever
(D) Cellulitis

72. All of the following statements about *Yersinia pestis* infections are true EXCEPT

(A) wild rodents and their infected fleas are the primary reservoir.
(B) a key early manifestation is a slowly progressing malaise.
(C) the pneumonic form is far more contagious than the bubonic form.
(D) the bubonic form may progress to the pneumonic form.

73. Which of the following organisms is the most frequent cause of bacterial endocarditis?

(A) *Enterococcus faecalis*
(B) *Streptococcus pneumoniae*
(C) Group B streptococci
(D) Viridans streptococci

Answers and Explanations

1–B. Only *Actinomyces* is anaerobic; the rest are aerobic.

2–D. *Coxiella burnetii* is the only rickettsial disease that can be spread via dust particles. All other rickettsia rapidly die in the environment.

3–A. Epiglottitis is a medical emergency requiring hospitalization. It can be fatal in 24 hours. Severe central nervous system defects occur in one-third of meningitis patients. Pus production is diagnostic. Pneumonia occurs primarily in adults older than 50 years of age or in young children.

4–C. *Staphylococcus aureus* and *Pseudomonas aeruginosa* are two primary pulmonary colonizers that cause pneumonia in patients with cystic fibrosis. Of the two, *Pseudomonas* is gram-negative. Its slime material (alginate) produces the resistance to phagocytic killing and poor penetration of antibiotics to the site, which, in conjunction with the antibiotic resistance of *Pseudomonas,* make these serious infections.

5–C. Both *Pseudomonas* exotoxin A and *Corynebacterium diphtheriae* toxin inhibit protein synthesis through the inhibition of elongating factor (EF-2). Shiga toxin is a cytotoxin, enterotoxin, and neurotoxin. *Vibrio cholerae* enterotoxin and *Escherichia coli* labile toxin (LT) both result in increased cyclic adenosine monophosphate (cAMP).

6–D. Sulfatides decrease the ability of phagocytes to kill *Mycobacterium tuberculosis* by inhibiting phagosome–lysosome fusion.

7–B. *Clostridium difficile* has been shown to be the major causative agent of pseudomembranous colitis, which causes diarrhea most commonly starting after 3–4 days of antibiotic administration.

8–B. *Vibrio cholerae* causes classic cholera; *Vibrio parahaemolyticus,* in contrast, causes a relatively mild gastroenteritis.

9–D. Most transmission in the United States is from infected flea bite (a choice not given in the question.) The other route of transmission is through respiratory droplets from patients who have developed pneumonic emboli and pneumonia.

10–B. *Staphylococcus epidermidis* is ubiquitous as part of the normal flora. Organisms are introduced into the host during invasive procedures.

11–A. *Clostridium perfringens* requires a low oxidation–reduction potential (E_h) to reproduce and does not infect nontraumatized tissues with a high E_h. Infant botulism results from ingesting spores in food. Death from tetanus occurs as a result of exhaustion and respiratory failure. Anaerobic cellulitis does not spread to healthy tissues. Gastroenteritis caused by *Clostridium difficile* is severe.

12–D. The gram-positive organism *Streptococcus pneumoniae* contains neither an endotoxin nor an exotoxin; rather, it expresses its toxicity through sheer numbers.

13–A. Enterococci can be differentiated by their reactivity with group D antiserum, bacitracin resistance, and growth in 40% bile or pH 9.6.

14–D. Antitoxin should be administered as soon as clostridial infection is suspected, because once the toxin is bound, the antitoxin is ineffective. Myonecrosis caused by *Clostridium perfringens,* but not anaerobic cellulitis, may require amputation or skin grafting; treatment of anaerobic cellulitis involves only removal of necrotic tissue. Food poisoning due to *C perfringens* is self-limiting and does not require treatment. Antibiotic therapy should not be used to treat infant botulism, because the antibiotics rapidly kill the organisms, thereby releasing the toxin and increasing the severity of disease. Patients with cellulitis should be given antibiotics.

15–C. *Salmonella* species do not ferment lactose, although some species produce acid, gas, and hydrogen sulfide from glucose.

16–C. Most of the *Bacteroides* are resistant to tetracyclines, penicillin, and cephalosporins, possessing a β-lactamase. This organism is found mainly in the gut and the female genital tract. *Prevotella melaninogenicus* is the species possessing a black colonial pigment.

17–A. Impetigo causes local infection of superficial skin layers and is highly communicable in infants.

18–B. The culture should be transported to the laboratory immediately in an anaerobic transport tube, because oxygen is lethal to these organisms. These organisms do not grow on eosin-methylene blue (EMB) agar and do not contain superoxide dismutase. Sputum sampling is ineffective because normal flora interferes with interpretation.

19–A. *Nocardia* is a gram-positive, filamentous bacteria that is partially acid-fast.

20–E. The incidence of *Mycoplasma pneumoniae* is highest in the young (5–15 years of age), not in the elderly.

21–C. The disease is rapidly progressive and may be fatal in 2 days because of bacterial multiplication and shock. Organisms do not invade. Although *Vibrio cholerae* are sensitive to acid pH, the "rice-water" stools are highly contagious.

22–C. Septicemia due to *Salmonella* is a fulminant, sometimes fatal, extraintestinal disease; blood stream invasion by *Shigella* is rare.

23–C. The causative agent in Lyme disease is *Borrelia burgdorferi*. The three stages frequently overlap. Stage 3 manifestations are slow to develop and may not emerge until several months or years after the initial infection. The hallmark rash is circular, spreading out from the site of the tick bite.

24–E. Rickettsial diseases in general exhibit these three manifestations.

25–C. Group B streptococci cause neonatal sepsis in two forms: an early-onset form, occurring in infants from birth to 4 days old, and a late-onset form, occurring in infants from 7 days to 4 months old.

26–B. *Borrelia recurrentis* causes epidemic relapsing fever, which is transmitted by lice; other species cause tick-borne relapsing fever.

27–E. Only *Neisseria* possesses the ability to degrade the IgA antibody, which protects against invasion of the mucosal surfaces.

28–A. Serology should be evaluated in the first and third trimesters of pregnancy. The clinical manifestations of congenital syphilis are generally severe and may include abortion, stillbirth, or birth defects. *Treponema pallidum* readily penetrates the maternal–fetal barrier and can infect in utero. *T pallidum* cannot be grown in vitro.

29–C. Purified protein derivative (PPD) is used in skin testing for infection.

30–B. The major virulence factor of *Helicobacter pylori* appears to be the neutralizing ability of the urease.

31–C. The nontuberculous mycobacteria are not considered contagious; they are picked up from the environment (e.g., from surface water of lakes and some water supplies). Tuberculosis is caused by both *Mycobacterium tuberculosis* and *Mycobacterium bovis*. Both tuberculous and nontuberculous mycobacterial infections are seen in patients with acquired immunodeficiency syndrome (AIDS), and all *Mycobacteria* are acid-fast.

32–E. All of these organisms are associated with zoonosis spread to humans by arthropod vectors. *Coxiella burnetii* is usually transmitted by dust particles but can be transmitted by ticks.

33–B. *Legionella* causes a fibrinopurulent pneumonia, not a granulomatous pulmonary infection. It is a weakly gram-negative, facultative, intracellular parasite found in streams and air-conditioning cooling tanks and is both catalase and oxidase positive.

34-A. *Actinomyces israelii* grows contiguously in tissues, crossing anatomic barriers; thus, it often invades bone. *Mycobacterium tuberculosis* may be hematogenously spread to any tissue.

35-C. Mycobacteria are slender rods and are acid-fast.

36-C. The Ghon complex is the combination of the initial Ghon lesion at the site of *Mycobacterium tuberculosis* infection in the lung and involvement of the adjoining lymph node. This lesion heals after primary tuberculosis.

37-C. *Salmonella* is associated with intestinal tracts of humans, other animals, reptiles, amphibians, fish, and birds.

38-C. The acute icteric disease caused by *Leptospira* is characterized by abrupt onset of fever, chills, headache, myalgia, gastrointestinal upset, conjunctival suffusion, and aseptic meningitis.

39-D. Numerous *Mycobacterium leprae* organisms are found in the skin in lepromatous leprosy, and the patient has many skin lesions from failure of cell-mediated immunity to restrict infection. Lepromatous leprosy patients usually have a poor response to the lepromin skin test. Leprosy is diagnosed by cytologic findings and a lepromin skin test, not by culture, because the organism cannot be cultured in vitro.

40–D. The non–spore-forming anaerobes are present to the extent of 10^{11} organisms/g of stool, comprising approximately 99% of the normal fecal flora.

41–C. Many if not all gram-negative bacteria contain an endotoxin. In addition, many such as *Pseudomonas, Shigella, Salmonella,* and *Vibrio* also secrete an exotoxin.

42–B. A vaccine is recommended for high-risk groups, such as sheep handlers, fur trappers, and laboratory workers. This organism is highly contagious after in vitro growth and only specially equipped laboratories (not hospitals) should attempt to culture it. When *Francisella tularenis* is implanted into skin, it is carried to lymph nodes, where it replicates and causes ulceroglandular tularemia. These bacteria parasitize fixed macrophages and mononuclear phagocytes, and relapses may occur because of failure to eradicate intracellular organisms.

43–B. The long-chain fatty acids, or mycolic acids, confer acid-fastness to the organism.

44–B. Typically, the patient with *Brucella* infection has intermittent fever and nondescript findings, including profound muscle weakness. The infection is hard to eradicate; acute infections are marked by relapses. Chronic infection may last more than 12 months. All three species of *Brucella* are human pathogens. *Brucella* is spread to humans primarily by the handling of infected meat. The organism is an intracellular parasite of macrophages.

45–C. Rocky Mountain spotted fever rash characteristically appears initially on hands and feet.

46–A. The early cutaneous form of anthrax infection may mimic a staphylococcal furuncle (or boil) or insect bite. Pulmonary and gastrointestinal infections are rapidly fatal. Spores are never observed in lesions. The capsule of *Bacillus anthracis* is unique for bacteria in that it is a polypeptide of glutamic acid. Sheep and cattle are the usual sources of infection.

47–B. *Campylobacter jejuni* infections are at least as common as *Salmonella* and *Shigella* infections.

48–B. Scarlet fever is marked by a rash due to erythrogenic toxins.

49–D. Capsular polysaccharide is the virulence determinant. This organism does not have an endotoxin. C-reactive protein is an endogenous host factor in response to *Streptococcus pneumoniae*. Bacitracin is an antibiotic.

50–A. Group A streptococci are not part of the normal oral or intestinal flora. When present, antibiotic treatment should be begun.

51-D. Organisms are fairly resistant to environmental influences and can survive for weeks in dried pseudomembranes. Organisms can be routinely Gram stained but cannot be distinguished from normal oral flora diphtheoids. Therefore, it is important to demonstrate toxin production by the isolate. Only *Staphylococcus aureus* and *Yersinia pestis* are coagulase positive.

52-C. Lymphocytosis is prevalent. The nasopharyngeal swab is used to isolate organisms, which are plated on Bordet-Gengou agar. The organism is a gram-negative coccobacillus, most readily isolated during the catarrhal stage.

53–C. *Shigella dysenteriae* possesses an endotoxin and an enterotoxin.

54-E. All of these organisms are obligate intracellular bacteria with a predilection for multiplication within capillary endothelial cells.

55-D. One of the differentiating characteristics between gastrointestinal upsets caused by *Staphylococcus* or the Enterobacteriaceae is the shorter incubation period following infection by the staphylococci (approximately 6 hours versus 1–2 days for the enterics).

56-D. *Shigella* invades the intestinal epithelium, resulting in liquid stools containing mucus, pus, and occasionally blood.

57-B. In this list, only the streptococci and staphylococci are gram-positive. The streptococci are catalase negative and staphylococci are catalase positive. Of the two staphylococci, *Staphylococcus aureus* is the β-hemolytic, coagulase-positive one and thus the correct answer.

58-A. Meningitis is treated with intravenous antibiotics, but rifampin is still necessary to eliminate carriage. Bacterial pinkeye is relatively mild and can be treated with topical sulfonamides. Soft chancre is highly contagious and partners have to be treated. *Haemophilus* capsular vaccine is poorly immunogenic in the target population, especially in children 3 months to 2 years of age.

59-C. *Salmonella typhimurium* possesses an endotoxin and an enterotoxin.

60-D. *Coxiella burnetii;* only *Coxiella* causes a pneumonia.

61-C. Although penicillin may lower the number of bacteria, the endotoxin component responsible for shock is liberated and is unaffected by antibiotics.

62-A. Culturing organisms from a clinical specimen is the only method to diagnose gonorrhea in asymptomatic patients. Organisms should be cultured on Thayer-Martin agar in a candle jar. However, organisms are labile and will be killed by lubricants.

63-A. *Rickettsia akari* results in a vesicular rash typical of chickenpox, with the greatest concentration on the trunk. There is generally a smaller eschar at the site of the mite bite.

64-C. Leptospirosis infects humans through contact with the urine of wild rodents and domestic animals.

65-A. Group B streptococci have polysaccharide capsules, which are poorly antigenic in neonates and children.

66-C. *Vibrio cholerae* possesses both an enterotoxin and an endotoxin.

67–C. The mycobacteria are mostly very slow growers; *Mycobacterium leprae* cannot be cultured in vitro.

68-E. Neonatal infections can arise either from infection during delivery or from an in utero infection. In either case, the prognosis is poor.

69-A. Cord factor disrupts the mitochondrial membrane, ultimately interrupting mitochondrial function.

70-D. *Staphylococcus saprophyticus* is the etiologic agent in 10%–20% of primary urinary tract infections in young women.

71-D. Group A streptococci infection of the skin can invade and quickly traverse the lymphatics to the blood stream, giving rise to a potentially lethal septicemia.

72-B. Key early manifestations of *Yersinia pestis* infection are a sudden onset of fever, conjunctivitis, and regional bubo formation. No exotoxin has been described.

73-D. The viridans streptococci are the most frequent cause of bacterial endocarditis.

4

Virology

I. Nature of Animal Viruses

A. Virus particles

—are called **virions.**

—are composed of either RNA or DNA that is encased in a protein coat called a **capsid.**

—are either naked or enveloped, depending on whether the capsid is surrounded by a lipoprotein **envelope.**

—replicate only in living cells and therefore are **obligate intracellular parasites.**

—cannot be observed with a light microscope.

1. The viral genome

—may be single-stranded or double-stranded, linear or circular, and segmented or nonsegmented.

—is used as one criterion for viral classification.

—is associated with viral-specific enzymes, other proteins within the virion, or both.

2. The viral capsid

—is composed of structural units called **capsomers,** which are aggregates of **viral-specific polypeptides.**

—has a symmetry that is classified as **helical, icosahedral** (a 20-sided polygon), or **complex.**

—is used as a criterion for viral classification.

—serves four functions:

a. As protection of the viral genome

b. As the site of receptors necessary for naked viruses to initiate infection

c. As the stimulus for antibody production

d. As the site of antigenic determinants important in some serologic tests

3. The viral nucleocapsid

—refers to the capsid and enclosed viral genome.

—is identical to the virion in naked viruses.

4. The viral envelope

—surrounds the nucleocapsid of enveloped viruses.

—is composed of **viral-specific glycoproteins** and **host-cell–derived lipids and lipoproteins.**

—contains molecules that are necessary for enveloped viruses to initiate infection, act as a stimulus for antibody production, and serve as antigens in serologic tests.

—is the basis of either sensitivity of a virus.

B. Viral classification

—is based on chemical and physical properties of virions.

—has resulted in the classification of viruses into **major families,** which are further subdivided by physiochemical and serologic characteristics into **genera.**

C. DNA viruses (Table 4-1)

—contain double-stranded DNA (except for parvovirus).

—are naked viruses (except for herpesviruses, poxviruses, and hepadnaviruses).

—have icosahedral capsids and replicate in the nucleus (except for poxviruses).

Table 4-1. Virion and Nucleic Acid Structure of DNA Viruses

Virus Family	Prominent Examples	Virion Structure	Virion Polymerase	Capsid Symmetry	DNA Structure
Adenoviridae	Adenoviruses	Naked	No	Icosahedral	Linear, double-stranded
Herpesviridae	Herpes simplex virus Varicella-zoster virus Epstein-Barr virus Cytomegalovirus	Enveloped	No	Icosahedral	Linear, double-stranded
Poxviridae	Smallpox virus Vaccinia virus Molluscum contagiosum virus	Brick-shaped, enveloped	Yes	Complex	
Papovaviridae	Papillomaviruses Polyomaviruses	Naked	No	Icosahedral	Circular, double-stranded
Hepadnaviridae	Hepatitis B virus	Enveloped	Yes	Icosahedral	Circular, double-stranded
Parvoviridae	B19 virus	Naked	No	Icosahedral	Linear, single-stranded

D. RNA viruses (Tables 4-2 through 4-4)

—contain single-stranded RNA (except for reoviruses).

—are enveloped (except for caliciviruses, picornaviruses, and reoviruses).

—have helical capsids (except for picornaviruses, reoviruses, and togaviruses).

—are classified positive, negative, or ambisense depending on the ability of virion RNA to act as messenger RNA (mRNA) [see II C 1].

—replicate in the cytoplasm (except for orthomyxoviruses and retroviruses, which have both a cytoplasmic and a nuclear phase).

II. Viral Replication and Genetics

A. Viral replication

—occurs only in living cells.

Table 4-2. Virion and Nucleic Acid Structure of Positive-Sense RNA Viruses

Virus Family	Prominent Examples	Virion Structure	Virion Polymerase	Capsid Symmetry	RNA Structure
Caliciviridae	Norwalk agent	Naked	No	Icosahedral	Linear, single-stranded, non-segmented
Picornaviridae	Coxsackieviruses Echoviruses Enteroviruses Hepatitis A virus Polioviruses Rhinoviruses	Naked	No	Icosahedral	Linear, single-stranded, non-segmented
Flaviviridae	Dengue virus Hepatitis C virus St. Louis encephalitis virus Yellow fever virus	Enveloped	No	Icosahedral	Linear, single-stranded, non-segmented
Togaviridae	Eastern, Western, and Venezuelan equine encephalo-myelitis viruses Rubella virus	Enveloped	No	Icosahedral	Linear, single-stranded, non-segmented
Retroviridae	Human immuno-deficiency virus Leukemia viruses Sarcoma viruses	Enveloped	No*	Helical	Linear, single-stranded, nonseg-mented*
Coronaviridae	Coronaviruses	Enveloped	No	Helical	Linear, single-stranded, non-segmented

*Retroviruses are diploid and have a reverse transcriptase.

Table 4-3. Virion and Nucleic Acid Structure of Negative-Sense RNA Viruses

Virus Family	Prominent Examples	Virion Structure	Virion Polymerase	Capsid Symmetry	RNA Structure
Paramyxoviridae	Mumps virus Measles virus Parainfluenza virus Respiratory syncytial virus	Enveloped	Yes	Helical	Linear, single-stranded, nonsegmented
Rhabdoviridae	Rabies virus Vesicular stomatitis virus	Enveloped	Yes	Helical	Linear, single-stranded, nonsegmented
Filoviridae	Ebola virus Marburg virus	Enveloped	Yes	Helical	Linear, single-stranded, nonsegmented
Orthomyxoviridae	Influenza viruses	Enveloped	Yes	Helical	Linear, single-stranded, eight segments
Bunyaviridae	California encephalitis virus Hantavirus	Enveloped	Yes	Helical	Circular, single-stranded, three segments
Delta virus	Hepatitis delta virus	Naked	No	Helical	Circular, single-stranded

—involves many host-cell enzymes and functions.

—may be incomplete in some cells (**abortive infection**) and yield **defective particles** (lack a functional replication gene) in some cells.

—may lead to the death of the host cell (**virulent viruses**) or may occur without apparent damage to the host cell (**moderate viruses**).

—is similar for all viruses in a specific family.

Table 4-4. Virion and Nucleic Acid Structure of Other RNA Viruses

Virus Family	Prominent Examples	Virion Structure	Virion Polymerase	Capsid Symmetry	RNA Structure
Arenaviridae	Lassa fever virus Lymphocytic choriomeningitis virus	Enveloped	Yes	Helical	Circular, single-stranded, two segments (one negative sense and one ambi-sense)
Reoviridae	Colorado tick fever virus Reoviruses Rotaviruses	Naked	Yes	Icosahedral	Linear, double-stranded, 10–11 segments

1. **Replication process**

   —has a sequential pattern that includes the following steps:

   a. Attachment

   b. Penetration

   c. Uncoating of the viral genome

   d. Synthesis of early proteins involved in genome replication

   e. Synthesis of late proteins (structural components of the virion)

   f. Assembly

   g. Release

2. **Plaques and pocks**

   —are focal areas of viral-induced cytopathology observed in tissue culture cells, monolayers, and membranes of embryonated eggs.

   —are counted after application of serial dilutions of a virus suspension to susceptible cells to quantitate the infectious virions present.

3. **One-step multiplication curves**

   —are plots of time after infection versus the number of viral plaques or pocks.

   —show that viruses have an **eclipse period** (the time from the start of infection to the first appearance of intracellular infectious virus) and a **latent period** (the time from the start of infection to the first appearance of extracellular virus).

   —indicate that viruses take a much longer time (hours or days) to replicate than phage.

4. **Attachment**

   —involves the interaction of viral receptors and specific host-cell receptor sites.

   —plays an important role in viral pathogenesis, determining **viral cell trophism.**

   —may be inhibited by antibodies (neutralizing antibodies) against viral receptors or cellular receptor sites.

5. **Penetration**

   —can occur by a cellular mechanism called **receptor-mediated endocytosis,** which is referred to as **viropexis** when viruses are involved.

   —can involve the fusion of the virus envelope with the plasma membrane of the host cell.

6. **Uncoating**

   —refers to the separation of the capsid from the viral genome.

   —results in the loss of virion infectivity.

7. **Budding**

   —is the process by which enveloped viruses obtain their envelope.

   —is preceded by the insertion of virus-specific glycoproteins into the membranes of a host cell.

—occurs most frequently at the plasma membrane, but also occurs at other membranes.

—confers infectivity to enveloped viruses.

B. DNA viruses (see Table 4-1)

1. Transcription

—occurs by host-cell, DNA-dependent RNA polymerases (except for virion-associated RNA polymerase of poxviruses).

—results in transcripts that must have a poly A tail and methylated cap added before translation.

—occurs in a specific temporal pattern, such as immediate early, delayed early, and late mRNA transcription.

—may be followed by **posttranscriptional processing** of primary mRNA transcripts (late adenovirus transcripts).

—occurs in the nucleus (except for poxviruses).

2. Translation

—occurs on cytoplasmic polysomes.

—is followed by transport of newly synthesized proteins to the nucleus (except for poxviruses).

3. Genome replication

—is **semiconservative.**

—is performed by a DNA-dependent DNA polymerase, which may be supplied by the host cell (adenoviruses) or may be virus specific (herpesviruses).

—occurs after the synthesis of the early proteins.

4. Assembly

—occurs in the nucleus (except for poxviruses).

—is frequently an inefficient process that leads to accumulation of viral proteins that may participate in the formation of **inclusion bodies** (focal accumulations of virion or viral gene products).

C. RNA viruses (see Tables 4-2 through 4-4)

1. The viral genome

—may be single-stranded or double-stranded and segmented or nonsegmented.

—may have **messenger (positive-sense) polarity** if it is single-stranded and able to act as mRNA (picornaviruses and retroviruses).

—may have **antimessenger (negative-sense) polarity** if it is single-stranded and complementary to mRNA (orthomyxoviruses and paramyxoviruses).

—is **ambisense** if it is single-stranded with segments of messenger polarity and segments of antimessenger polarity.

2. Transcription

—involves an RNA-dependent RNA polymerase for all viruses, except retroviruses, which use a host-cell, DNA-dependent RNA polymerase.

—involves a virion-associated enzyme (transcriptase) with negative-sense viruses.

3. Translation

—occurs on cytoplasmic polysomes.

—may result in the synthesis of a large polyprotein that is subsequently cleaved (in **posttranslational processing**) into individual viral polypeptides (picornaviruses and retroviruses).

4. Genome replication

—occurs in the cytoplasm (except for orthomyxoviruses and retroviruses).

—is performed by a viral-specific **replicase enzyme** (except for retroviruses).

—involves a replicative intermediate RNA structure for all single-stranded RNA genomes.

—is asymmetric and conservative for double-stranded RNA genomes.

D. Genetics

1. Phenotypic mixing

—occurs when pairs of related viruses with similar but distinct surface antigens infect the same cell.

—results when surface antigens from two related viruses enclose the genome of one of the viruses.

2. Phenotypic masking (transcapsidation)

—occurs when pairs or related viruses infect the same cell.

—results when the genome of one virus is surrounded by the capsid or capsid and envelope of the other virus.

3. Complementation

—can occur when two mutants of the same virus or, less frequently, two mutants of different large DNA viruses, infect the same cell.

—results when one mutant virus supplies an enzyme or factor that the other mutant lacks.

4. Genetic reassortment

—can occur when two strains of mutants of a segmented RNA virus infect a cell.

—results in a stable change in the viral genome.

5. Viral vectors

—can be constructed with recombinant DNA technology and allow gene transfer into cells.

—are usually defective viruses that cannot replicate but can infect cells.

—have been used for the production of some vaccines (e.g., hepatitis B vaccine).

III. Viral Pathogenesis

A. General characteristics—viral pathogenesis

—is the process of disease production following infection.

—may lead to **clinical** or **subclinical** (asymptomatic) disease.

—is the result of several viral and host factors.

1. Viral entry into a host

—occurs most often through the mucosa of the respiratory tract.

—may occur through the mucosa of the gastrointestinal or genitourinary tract.

—can be accomplished by direct virus injection into the blood stream via a needle or an insect bite.

2. Asymptomatic viral disease

—may also be called **subclinical infection** because no clinical symptoms are evident.

—occurs with most viral infections.

—can stimulate humoral and cellular immunity.

3. Clinical viral disease

—frequently depends on the size of the viral inoculum.

—does not always follow infection and therefore is not an accurate index of viral infection.

—results from direct or indirect viral effects (e.g., viral-induced cytolysis, immunologic attack on infected cells), which lead to physiologic changes in infected tissues.

—is much less common than inapparent infection.

—is associated with a particular **target organ** for a specific virus.

B. Viral aspects of pathogenesis

1. Viral surface receptors

—interact with cellular receptor sites to initiate infection.

—may react with specific antibodies (neutralizing antibodies) and become incapable of interaction with cellular receptor sites.

—can be inactivated by pH, enzymes, and other host biochemical factors.

2. Viral virulence

—refers to the ability of a particular viral strain to cause disease.

—is genetically determined.

—is a composite of all the factors that allow a virus to overcome host defense mechanisms and damage its target organ.

—is decreased with **attenuated strains** of virus.

C. Cellular aspects of pathogenesis

1. Cellular receptor sites

—interact with virion receptors to initiate infection.

—help determine **cell trophism** of viruses.

—may be determined by the differentiation stage of a cell.

2. Cell trophism

—refers to the propensity of a virus to infect and replicate in a cell.

—is largely determined by the interaction of virus receptors and cellular receptor sites and the ability of the cell to provide other components (e.g., substrates and enzymes) essential for viral replication.

3. Target organ

—refers to that organ responsible for the major clinical signs of a viral infection.

—is largely determined by viral virulence and cell trophism.

4. Cellular responses to viral infection

—result in clinical disease.

—may be inapparent or may include:

a. Cytopathic effects

b. Cytolysis

c. Inclusion body formation

d. Chromosomal aberrations

e. Transformation

f. Interferon (IFN) synthesis

5. Cytopathogenic effects

—include inhibition of host-cell macromolecular biosynthesis, alterations of the plasma membrane and lysosomes, and development of **inclusion bodies.**

—may occur without the production of infectious virus progeny.

—may aid in identification of certain viruses (e.g., polykaryocyte formation by measles virus).

D. Types of infections

1. Inapparent infections

—occur when too few cells are infected to cause clinical symptoms.

—are synonymous with **subclinical disease.**

—can result in sufficient antibody stimulation to cause immunity from further infections.

—occur frequently when the virus inoculum is small.

—occur when the virus does not reach its target organ.

2. Acute infections

—occur when clinical manifestations of disease are observed for a short time (days to weeks) after a short incubation period.

—have recoveries associated with elimination of the virus from the body.

—are classified as **localized** or **disseminated,** depending on whether the virus has traveled from its site of implantation to its target organ.

—may lead to **persistent** or **latent** infections.

3. Persistent infections

—are associated with the continuing presence of the infectious virus in the body for an extended, perhaps lifelong, period.

—may or may not involve clinical symptoms.

—may involve infected individuals known as **carriers.**

—provide constant viral antigenic stimulation that leads to high antibody titers for some antigens.

4. Latent infections

—occur when the infecting virus persists in the body in a noninfectious form that can periodically reactivate to an infectious virus and produce clinical disease.

—are synonymous with **recurrent disease.**

—produce antibody stimulus only during the initial (**primary**) infection and during recurrent episodes.

—can have subclinical reactivations.

—are difficult to detect in cells because viral antigen production is not detected and cytopathology is not observed during "silent" periods.

5. Slow infections

—have a **prolonged incubation** period lasting months or years.

—do not cause clinical symptoms during incubation.

—produce some infectious viruses during incubation.

—are most often associated with **chronic, progressive, fatal viral diseases of the central nervous system (CNS),** such as kuru and Creutzfeldt-Jakob disease.

E. Patterns of acute disease

1. Localized disease

—occurs when viral multiplication and cell damage remain localized to the site of viral entry into the body.

—has a short incubation time.

—may have systemic clinical features (e.g., fever).

—is not associated with pronounced viremia (virions in the blood).

—occurs in the **respiratory tract** (influenza, rhinovirus), **alimentary tract** (picornaviruses, rotaviruses), **genitourinary tract** (papillomavirus), and the **eye** (adenovirus).

—can spread over the surface of the body to other areas where it causes another localized infection (picornavirus-induced conjunctivitis).

—induces a much weaker immune response than disseminated infections.

2. Disseminated infections

a. General characteristics—disseminated infections

—involve the spread of virus from its entry site to a target organ.

—involve a **primary viremia** and perhaps a **secondary viremia.**

—involve moderate incubation times (e.g., weeks).

—have main clinical symptoms that are associated with infection of one target organ, although infection of other organs is involved.

  —generate a substantial immune response that frequently confers lifelong immunity to the host.

  —allow more time for the host's immune system to eliminate the viral infection.

 b. Viral dissemination

  —is a major feature of disseminated infections.

  —may involve virus travel in other cells (red blood cells and mononuclear peripheral white blood cells), the plasma, extracellular spaces, and nerve fibers.

  —is prevented by viral-specific cytotoxic cells and neutralizing antibodies.

3. Congenital infections

 —are viral infections of a fetus.

 —result from maternal viremia.

 —lead to **maldeveloped organs.**

 —are serious because of the immaturity of the fetal immune system, the placental barrier to maternal immunity, and the undifferentiated state and rapid multiplication of fetal cells.

IV. Host Defenses to Viruses

A. Host defense mechanisms

 —are responsible for the self-limiting nature of most viral infections.

 —have immune and nonimmune aspects.

 —operate during all stages of a viral infection.

 —may contribute to the clinical pattern of disease (immunopathology).

B. Nonimmune defenses

1. Innate immunity

 —includes **anatomic barriers** (dead cells of the epidermis) and **chemical barriers** (mucous layers) that limit contact of the virus with susceptible cells.

 —includes the complex parameters associated with the **age and physiologic status** of the host.

2. Cellular resistance

 —involves **nonpermissive cells,** which lack factors necessary for virus replication.

 —involves **lack of receptor sites** for virus on cells.

3. Inflammation

 —limits the spread of virus from an infection site.

 —results in unfavorable environmental conditions for viral replication (e.g., antiviral substances, low pH, elevated temperatures).

4. IFN

—is a host-specific, viral-induced glycoprotein that inhibits viral replication (see Chapter 7, VII B 3, Table 7-2).

—is not viral specific, but is fairly species specific.

—is the **first viral-induced defense mechanism** at the primary site of infection.

C. Humoral immunity

—involves the production of antibodies against viral-specific antigen by **B lymphocytes.**

—is the defense mechanism most important to cytolytic viral infections accompanied by viremia and viral infections of epithelial surfaces.

—involves both **virus-neutralizing antibodies** and **nonneutralizing antibodies.**

1. Neutralizing antibodies

—inhibit the ability of a virus to replicate.

—can inhibit viral attachment, penetration, or uncoating or all three processes.

—can induce lesions in the viral envelope, with the aid of complement.

—are most protective if they are present at the time of infection or during viremia.

2. Nonneutralizing antibodies

—enhance viral degradation.

—act as opsonins to enhance phagocytosis of virions.

D. Cell-mediated immunity

—involves cytotoxic **T lymphocytes,** antibody-dependent cell-mediated cytotoxicity, natural killer cells, and activated macrophages.

—involves soluble factors from T lymphocytes (**lymphokines**) and macrophages (**monokines**) that regulate cellular immune responses.

—is the defense mechanism most important to noncytolytic infection in which the membrane of the virus-infected cell is antigenically altered by the virus.

E. Viral-induced immunopathology

—can contribute to the disease process.

—can result from various immunologic interactions, including immediate hypersensitivity, antibody–antigen complexes [as in hepatitis B virus (HBV)], and tissue damage due to cytotoxic cells or antibody and complement.

—is frequently observed in **persistent viral infections.**

F. Viral-induced immunosuppression

—results when infecting viruses alter the immune responsiveness or decrease the numbers of lymphocytes.

—can occur during cytolytic or noncytolytic infection.

—is frequently observed as a **transient consequence** of disseminated viral infections that involve lymphocyte infection by the virus.

V. Immunotherapy, Antivirals, and Interferon (IFN)

A. Immunotherapy

1. **Virus vaccines** (Table 4-5)

   —lead to **active immunization.**

   —are effective in preventing infections caused by viruses with few antigenic types.

   —may use **live virus, killed virus, virion subunits, viral polypeptides,** or **viral DNA.**

   a. **Live virus vaccines**

      —use **attenuated virus strains** that are relatively avirulent.

      —have advantages of administration in a single dose by the natural route of infection and the ability to induce a wide spectrum of antibodies and cytotoxic cells.

      —have the disadvantages of a limited shelf life, possible reversion to virulence, and possible production of persistent infection.

      —include vaccines for **measles, mumps, rubella, chickenpox, polio (Sabin vaccine), yellow fever,** and some **adenovirus strains.**

Table 4-5. Viral Immunotherapy

Virus	Passive Immunization*	Active Immunization (Vaccines)		
		Live Strain	Killed	Subunit
Adenovirus	No	Yes (military use)	No Havrix	No
Hepatitis A virus	Yes	No	VAQTA	No
Hepatitis B virus	Yes	No	No	Engerix-B or Recombivax-HB
Influenza virus	No	No	Yes	Yes
Measles virus	Yes	Enders	No	No
Mumps virus	No	Jeryl Lynn	No	No
Poliovirus	No	Sabin†	Salk	No
Rabies virus	Yes	No	Yes (Human diploid cell)	No
Respiratory syncytial virus	Yes	No	No	No
Rotavirus	No	Yes‡	No	No
Rubella	No	RA 27/3	No	No
Smallpox (variola) virus	No	Vaccinia	No	No
Varicella-zoster virus	Yes	Oka	No	No
Yellow fever virus	No	17D	No	No

*Commercial preparations available
†No longer recommended
‡Not approved for infants

b. Killed virus vaccines

—are prepared from whole virions by **heat** or **chemical inactivation** of infectivity.

—are injected into the body and stimulate antibodies only to surface antigens of the virus.

—have the advantage of easy combination into **polyvalent vaccines** (vaccines containing virions from several virus strains).

—have the disadvantages of lack of development of secretory immunoglobulin A (IgA), need for boosters, poor cell-mediated response, and possible hypersensitivity reactions.

—include vaccines for **poliovirus (Salk vaccine), rabies, influenza, and hepatitis A virus (HAV).**

c. Virion subunit vaccines

—are purified proteins (viral receptors) obtained from virions.

—have the same advantages and disadvantages as killed vaccines.

—are available for **adenovirus.**

d. Viral polypeptides

—are **polypeptide sequences of virion receptors** that have been synthesized or result from the purification of proteins made from cloned genes.

—have the same advantages and disadvantages as killed vaccines.

—are used in a vaccine for **HBV.**

e. DNA vaccines

—are plasmid DNA expression vectors containing **specific viral genes** (usually envelope genes).

—elicit both humoral and cell-mediated immune responses.

—are being evaluated for human use to protect against **human immunodeficiency virus (HIV)** and **influenza viruses.**

2. Passive immunization (see Table 4-5)

—is acquired by injection of pooled human plasma or γ-globulin fractions from immune individuals into high-risk individuals.

—is valuable in prevention of some viral diseases but has little value after disease onset.

—is used to prevent **rubella, measles, mumps, HAV, HBV, rabies, and varicella-zoster virus (VZV) infections.**

B. Antiviral agents (Tables 4-6 through 4-8)

1. General characteristics—antiviral agents

—must selectively inhibit viral replication without affecting the viability or normal functions of the host cell (**selective toxicity**).

—inhibit the viral nucleic acid replication process, the penetration and uncoating process, or specific viral enzyme function.

—are available for few viral infections.

2. Inhibitors of herpesviruses

Table 4-6. Licensed Antiviral Drugs in Current Use–Inhibitors of Herpesviruses

Drug	Administration Route	Mechanism of Action	Indications
Acyclovir	Topical or oral	Inhibits HSV and VZV DNA synthesis	Primary genital herpes (HSV), encephalitis, and keratitis Primary varicella infections Localized or ophthalmic zoster HSV and VZV in immunocompromised or transplant patients
Cidofovir	Parenteral	Inhibits CMV DNA synthesis	CMV retinitis in AIDS patients
Famciclovir	Oral	Inhibits HSV and VZV DNA synthesis	Zoster
Foscarnet	Parenteral	Inhibits herpesvirus DNA polymerase	Acyclovir-resistant HSV and VZV infections Ganciclovir-resistant CMV retinitis
Ganciclovir	Oral or parenteral	Inhibits herpesvirus DNA synthesis	CMV retinitis Disseminated CMV infection of immunocompromised or AIDS patients Prophylaxis for disseminated CMV infections in transplant patients
Trifluridine	Topical	Inhibits herpesvirus DNA polymerase	HSV keratoconjunctivitis
Vidarabine	Topical or parenteral	Inhibits herpesvirus DNA polymerase	HSV keratitis and encephalitis (acyclovir is the drug of choice)

AIDS = acquired immunodeficiency syndrome; CMV = cytomegalovirus; HSV = herpes simplex virus; VZV = varicella-zoster virus.

Table 4-7. Licensed Antiviral Drugs in Current Use–Inhibitors of Human Immunodeficiency Virus (HIV)

Drug	Administration Route	Mechanism of Action	Indications
Amprenavir	Oral	Inhibits HIV protease	AIDS, HIV infection
Delavirdine	Oral	Inhibits HIV reverse transcriptase (non-nucleoside)	AIDS, HIV infection
Didanosine	Oral	Inhibits HIV reverse transcriptase	AIDS, HIV infection
Efavirenz	Oral	Inhibits HIV reverse transcriptase (non-nucleoside)	AIDS, HIV infection
Indinavir	Oral	Inhibits HIV protease	AIDS, HIV infection
Lamivudine	Oral	Inhibits HIV reverse transcriptase	AIDS, HIV infection
Nevirapine	Oral	Inhibits HIV reverse transcriptase (non-nucleoside)	AIDS, HIV infection
Ritonavir	Oral	Inhibits HIV protease	AIDS, HIV infection
Saquinavir	Oral	Inhibits HIV protease	AIDS, HIV infection
Starudine	Oral	Inhibits HIV reverse transcriptase	AIDS, HIV infection
Zalcitabine	Oral	Inhibits HIV reverse transcriptase	AIDS, HIV infection
Zidovudine	Oral	Inhibits HIV reverse transcriptase	AIDS, HIV infection

AIDS = acquired immunodeficiency syndrome.

Table 4-8. Licensed Antiviral Drugs in Current Use–Inhibitors of Other Viruses

Drug	Administration Route	Mechanism of Action	Indications
Amantadine	Oral	Inhibits influenza A virus penetration or uncoating	Prophylaxis for influenza A virus
Interferon-α	Parenteral	Induces antiviral proteins	Chronic hepatitis B and hepatitis C virus infections
Oseltamivir	Oral	Inhibits influenza A and B virus neuraminidase	Influenza A and B virus infections
Ribavirin	Oral or inhalation	Inhibits nucleic acid polymerases	Severe Rous sarcoma virus infection Lassa fever
Rimantadine	Oral	Inhibits influenza virus penetration or uncoating	Prophylaxis for influenza A virus
Zanamivir	Inhalation	Inhibits influenza A and B virus neuraminidase	Influenza A and B virus infections

    —are mostly nucleoside analogues (except for foscarnet) that must be phosphorylated by viral enzymes before they become effective.

    —inhibit viral replication by inhibiting DNA synthesis.

    —are effective only against replicating virus, not latent virus.

  3. Inhibitors of retroviruses

    —are used mostly for HIV infections.

    —consist of nucleoside and nonnucleoside reverse transcriptase inhibitors and viral protease inhibitors.

    —do not eradicate HIV infection, but when used in combination (**HAART: highly active antiretroviral therapies**) can decrease viral replication, improve immunologic status, and prolong life.

    —may be active against nonretroviruses with reverse transcriptases (e.g., HBV).

  4. Inhibitors of other viruses

    —affect viral-specific enzymes, affect the process of virus penetration or uncoating, or induce antiviral proteins in the infected cell.

    —are active against influenza A and B viruses, some hepatitis viruses, and respiratory syncytial virus.

C. Interferons (IFNs)

    —are host-coded proteins, or **glycoproteins,** produced in response to viruses, synthetic nucleotides, and foreign cells.

    —are **host specific** but not viral specific.

    —are divided into three groups or families: **IFN-α, IFN-β,** and **IFN-γ;** IFN-α (Intron-A) is licensed for treatment of chronic HBV and hepatitis C virus (HCV) infections and can produce adverse effects at high doses or with chronic therapy.

    —are produced in and secreted from virus-infected cells.

—bind to cell-surface receptors and **induce antiviral proteins,** including a **protein kinase and 2,5 A synthetase** (which synthesizes an oligoadenylic acid), leading to the destruction of viral mRNA.

—have toxic side effects, including bone marrow suppression.

VI. Diagnostic Virology

A. Laboratory viral diagnosis

—involves one of three basic approaches: **virus isolation; direct demonstration** of virus, viral nucleic acid, or antigens in clinical specimens; or **serologic testing** of viral-specific antibodies.

—is frequently not necessary because the clinical symptoms of a virus are often distinctive.

—begins with identification of the most likely viruses based on clinical symptoms and the patient's history.

—is often not possible during the first few days after infection.

B. Virus isolation

1. General characteristics—virus isolation

—depends on virus replication in susceptible cells.

—may involve tissue culture cells, embryonated eggs, or animal hosts.

—requires proper collection and preservation of specimens.

—is best accomplished during the onset and acute phase of disease.

2. Viral replication

—may be detected in live infected tissue culture cells by observing a characteristic **cytopathogenic effect** (CPE), such as polykaryocyte formation or hemadsorption (adhesion of red blood cells to infected cells).

—may be observed in fixed infected tissue culture cells by observing characteristic **inclusion bodies** (Table 4-9) or performing immunohistochemical staining of **viral antigens.**

Table 4-9. Viral Inclusion Bodies

Virus	Inclusion Site	Staining Properties	Inclusion Name
Adenovirus	Nucleus	B	. . .
Cytomegalovirus	Nucleus	B	Owl's eye
Herpes simplex virus	Nucleus	A	Cowdry type A
Measles virus	Both	A	. . .
Poxvirus	Cytoplasm	A	Guarnieri bodies (smallpox)
			Molluscum bodies (molluscum contagiosum)
Rabies virus	Cytoplasm	A	Negri body
Reovirus	Cytoplasm	A	. . .
Rubella virus	Cytoplasm	A	. . .

A = acidophilic; B = basophilic.

—is detected in embryonated egg by pock formation and in animals by the development of clinical symptoms.

C. Direct examination of clinical specimens

—may be done on sections of tissue biopsies, tissue imprints or smears, blood, cerebrospinal fluid, urine, throat swabs, feces, or saliva.

—should be performed only on those specimens likely to contain the virus (e.g., throat swabs for respiratory tract infection).

—involves one of the following **assays** for virus detection: **viral-induced CPE, immunohistochemical staining, nucleic acid hybridization, or solid-phase immunoassay.**

1. Immunohistochemical staining

—uses fixed or fresh specimens and **chemically labeled (fluorescein) or enzymatically labeled (peroxidase) antibodies** to detect viral antigens.

—may use impression slides made from specific tissues.

—may involve either a **direct or an indirect staining method.**

2. Nucleic acid hybridization

—involves the **detection of viral DNA or RNA sequences** in nucleic acid extracted from specimens.

—may use **polymerase chain reaction** (PCR) techniques to amplify viral genes.

—may involve **dot blot** hybridization techniques that usually use single-stranded, complementary **nucleic acid probes.**

—is highly sensitive and specific.

—is a popular technique for identifying adenovirus in nasopharyngeal washings, cytomegalovirus (CMV) in urine, and HIV in the blood of seronegative individuals.

3. Solid-phase immunoassays

—are highly sensitive, specific assays used to detect **viral antigens.**

—use specific viral antibodies and radioimmunoassay **(RIA)** or enzyme-linked immunosorbent assay **(ELISA)** techniques.

—are popular for the detection of rotavirus and HAV in feces.

D. Serologic tests

—are used to determine the titer of specific antiviral antibodies.

—are helpful in diagnostic virology if paired blood samples are taken (one sample at the onset and one sample during the recovery phase of the illness).

—must show at least a fourfold increase in titer between the samples to indicate a current infection.

—may be diagnostic without the use of paired samples if significant levels of IgM antiviral antibodies are obtained.

—include virus neutralization, complement fixation, hemagglutination inhibition tests, and solid-phase immunoassays.

1. Virus neutralization tests

—are based on the principle that certain antiviral antibodies will neutralize the CPE of the virus.

—involve incubations of constant amounts of virus with decreasing amounts of serum added to susceptible cells.

—are expensive to perform and must be standardized for each virus.

2. Hemagglutination inhibition tests

—are based on the principle that antihemagglutinin antibodies in serum will inhibit viral agglutination of erythrocytes.

—can be performed only on viruses with hemagglutinins on their surface (influenza, measles).

—involve careful standardization of erythrocytes and viral hemagglutinin preparations.

3. Solid-phase immunoassays

—are highly sensitive and specific assays used to detect **specific viral antibodies.**

—use viral antigens in RIA and ELISA protocols.

—are several hundred times more sensitive than other serologic tests.

VII. DNA Viruses (Table 4-10)

A. Human adenoviruses

—are naked viruses with an icosahedral nucleocapsid composed of **hexons, pentons,** and **fibers.**

—have **toxic activity** associated with pentons and **hemagglutinating activity** associated with pentons and fibers.

—contain **double-stranded DNA** that **replicates asymmetrically.**

—replicate in the nucleus of epithelial cells.

—cause localized infections of the eye, respiratory tract, gastrointestinal tract, and urinary bladder.

—frequently cause subclinical infections.

—can cause tumors in other animals because **EIA and EIB gene products bind to cellular tumor suppressor proteins p110^{Rb} and p53.**

1. Classification—human adenoviruses

—are classified into seven groups (A through G) based on DNA homology.

a. Group A adenoviruses

—do not cause a specific clinical disease in humans.

—induce **tumors** in newborn hamsters.

b. Group B adenoviruses

Table 4-10. Properties of DNA Viruses

Virus Family	Virus Name	Unique Genes or Gene Products	Associated Acute Diseases	Associated Chronic or Persistent Diseases	Diagnostic Methods
Adenoviridae	Groups A–F adenoviruses	E1A E1B genes, hexons, pentons, fibers	Acute respiratory infection Keratoconjunctivitis Gastroenteritis (infants)	Lymphoid tissue	Virus isolation Serology
Hepadnaviridae	Hepatitis B virus	HB_sAg (Australian ag) HB_cAg (core ags) HB_eAg Reverse transcriptase	Serum hepatitis	Hepatitis	ELISA test for antibodies and antigen
Herpesviridae	Herpes simplex virus type 1	...	Gingivostomatitis Cold sores Keratoconjunctivitis Encephalitis	Cold sores	Tzanck smear Cowdry type A inclusion Virus isolation
	Herpes simplex virus type 2	...	Genital herpes	Genital herpes	Tzanck smear Cowdry type A inclusion Virus isolation
	Varicella-zoster virus	...	Chickenpox Reye's syndrome	Shingles	Tzanck smear
	Cytomegalovirus	...	Congenital CID Heterophil-negative mononucleosis	Retinitis or pneumonia in immunocompromised patients	Owl's eye inclusion Virus isolation

	Virus	Antigen	Disease		Diagnosis
	Epstein-Barr virus	Early antigen, Epstein-Barr nuclear antigen, Viral capsid antigen, Lymphocyte-determined membrane antigen	Infectious mononucleosis, Chronic fatigue syndrome	...	Atypical lymphocytes (Downey cells) mononucleosis spot test
	Human herpes virus type 6	...	Exanthem subitum (roseola)	...	...
	Human herpes virus type 8	...	...	Kaposi's sarcoma	...
Papovaviridae	Human papilloma virus	E6 and E7	Warts, Laryngeal papillomas	...	Keilocytotic cells FA or IP staining
	Polyomaviruses (BK, JC, and SV40)	Tumor antigens (7)	...	PML (JC virus), Urethral stenosis, hemorrhagic cystitis in immunocompromised patients (BK virus)	Pap smear or urinary sediment for viral inclusions FA or IP staining
Parvoviridae	B19 virus	...	Erythema infectiosum (fifth disease)	...	ELISA test for IgM antibody
Poxviridae	Variola virus	...	Smallpox (extinct)	...	...
	Orf virus	...	Orf	...	...
	Cowpox virus	...	Cowpox	...	...
	Molluscum contagiosum virus	...	Molluscum contagiosum	...	Molluscum inclusion bodies

CID = cytomegalic inclusion disease; ELISA = enzyme-linked immunosorbent assay; FA = fluorescent antibody; HB_cAg = hepatitis B core antigen; HB_eAg = hepatitis B e antigen; HB_sAg = hepatitis B surface (Australia) antigen; IP = immunoperoxidase; PML = progressive multifocal leukoencephalopathy; SV40 = simian virus 40; Pap = Papanicolaou.

—cause acute respiratory disease, pharyngoconjunctival fever, and hemorrhagic cystitis.

—can cause epidemics in military recruits (adenovirus type 7).

c. Group C adenoviruses

—cause approximately 5% of acute respiratory diseases in young children.

—cause latent infections in the tonsils, adenoids, and other lymphatic tissue.

d. Group D adenoviruses

—are associated with sporadic and epidemic keratoconjunctivitis.

—cause **pinkeye** (adenovirus type 8).

e. Group E adenoviruses

—are associated with acute respiratory disease accompanied by fever and with epidemic keratoconjunctivitis in military recruits.

f. Groups F and G adenoviruses

—cause gastroenteritis.

2. Adenovirus vaccines

—are used by the military for protection against type 4 (group E) and type 7 (group B) adenoviruses.

—may be of the **subunit (hexons and fibers) type** or the **live virus type.**

3. Diagnosis of adenovirus infections

—may be made by observing an increase in neutralizing antibody titer.

—may be made by virus isolation from the eyes, throat, or urine.

—may involve ELISA procedures on fecal specimens from patients with gastrointestinal infections.

B. Hepadnaviruses

—have a complex virion structure that includes an envelope.

—have **circular, double-stranded DNA** containing **single-strand breaks,** a primer protein, and a viral-specific DNA polymerase associated with the DNA.

—need a viral-coded reverse transcriptase to replicate because the virion DNA is synthesized from an RNA template.

—have their **DNA integrated into cellular DNA** during replication.

—cause liver disease as indicated by their names: human HBV, woodchuck hepatitis virus, and duck hepatitis virus.

1. HBV

—causes **serum hepatitis** and frequently causes subclinical infections.

—has a special name given to its virion—the **Dane particle.**

—is associated with specific antigens: a surface antigen (**HBsAg or Australia antigen**) and core-associated antigens (**HBcAg** and **HBeAg**).

—has a viral-encoded reverse transcriptase involved in viral DNA replication.

—has been implicated in **hepatocellular carcinoma.**

2. **Serum hepatitis**

—has a long incubation period (50–180 days).

—involves antigen–antibody complexes.

—is usually contracted through a parenteral route.

—can be transmitted by blood products if HBeAg is present.

—can progress to a **chronic carrier state** with or without clinical symptoms.

—is a potential high risk for the staff of hemodialysis units and healthcare workers exposed to fresh blood.

—may be acute or chronic depending on the amount of HBeAg and HBsAg and of anti-HBs and anti-HBc, as determined by ELISA tests (Table 4-11).

—may be treated prophylactically by **passive immunization** with hepatitis B immune globulin (HBIG) or HBsAg vaccine produced from particles in healthy carriers or from recombinant DNA techniques.

—may use IFN-α alone or in combination with ribavirin to treat chronic cases.

C. **Herpesviruses**

—are enveloped viruses with an **icosahedral nucleocapsid** containing **double-stranded DNA.**

—have linear DNA that consists of a short (18%) component and a long (82%) component, which are covalently linked and contain unique sequences flanked by inverted repeats.

—have a **tegument,** or fibrous material, between the nucleocapsid and envelope.

—replicate in the nucleus of the host cell.

—have **oncogenic potential.**

—can cause **latent infections** as well as **acute infections.**

—are classified into subfamilies: **alphaherpesviruses** [e.g., herpes simplex virus (HSV) types 1 and 2 and VZV], **betaherpesviruses** (e.g., CMV), and **gammaherpesviruses** [e.g., Epstein-Barr virus (EBV)].

1. **HSV types 1 and 2**

—have approximately 50% DNA sequence homology.

Table 4-11. Serologic Test Results in Three Stages of Hepatitis B Virus Infection

Test	Acute Disease	Complete Recovery	Chronic Disease
HBsAg	Positive	Negative	Positive
HbsAb	Negative	Positive	Negative
HBAb*	Positive	Positive	Positive

*IgM is found in the acute stage; IgG is found in subsequent stages.

—produce both **common antigens** and **type-specific antigens.**

—replicate by the regulated temporal synthesis of classes of proteins (alpha, beta, and gamma).

—produce a virus-specific DNA polymerase and thymidine kinase, which are necessary for replication.

—can cause transformation of hamster cells.

—are frequently **latent in neurons.**

—can produce distinctive cytopathology (cell rounding and **polykaryocyte formation**) or inclusion bodies (**Cowdry type A inclusions**) in infected cells.

—are treated clinically by acyclovir, famciclovir, trifluridine, and vidarabine.

a. **HSV-1 disease**

—may involve a primary infection (e.g., gingivostomatitis) or a recurrent infection (e.g., cold sores).

—is usually clinically inapparent as a primary disease.

—usually presents as a **lip, skin, or eye lesion.**

—can progress to a severe, fatal encephalitis.

—may be diagnosed by **Tzanck smear** for rapid identification when skin lesions are involved.

—may be diagnosed by virus isolation or serologic testing involving neutralization or complement fixation tests or ELISA procedures.

—cannot be treated prophylactically by vaccine.

b. **HSV-2 disease**

—may involve a primary or recurrent infection.

—affects the **genital or lip area.**

—is most frequently transmitted sexually.

—includes **neonatal herpes,** a severe generalized disease of the newborn caused by virus infection during passage through an infected birth canal.

—may be diagnosed and treated as described for HSV-1.

—may include cervical and vulvar carcinoma (viral nonstructural antigens have been found in biopsy specimens).

2. **VZV**

—causes an acute primary disease (chickenpox) and a recurrent disease (zoster).

—is **latent in neurons.**

a. **Varicella (chickenpox)**

—is a mild, highly infectious, generalized disease usually affecting children.

—is characterized clinically by vesicles on the skin and mucous membranes.

—may be diagnosed by **Tzanck smear** or **fluorescent antibody staining** of viral antigens in scrapings; **virus isolation** also is possible.

—may be prevented by a live, attenuated vaccine containing the **Oka virus strain.**

—may be treated prophylactically in immunocompromised children by giving varicella-zoster immune globulin.

b. Zoster

—is a reactivated virus infection in adults.

—is characterized by severe pain and the presence of vesicles in a specific area of the skin or mucosa supplied with nerves from one ganglia.

—can disseminate in immunocompromised individuals.

—is also called **shingles.**

—may be treated with famciclovir.

3. CMV

—replicates more slowly and is more cell-associated than HSV.

—replicates only in human fibroblasts.

—can transform hamster and human cells in vitro.

—causes an acute primary infection and a latent infection that is reactivated to clinical disease only during immunosuppression.

—may be treated with ganciclovir.

a. Clinical manifestations

(1) CMV most commonly causes **inapparent disease** in children and adults, but can cause an **infectious mononucleosis-like disease.**

(2) Retinitis and **pulmonary disease** may occur in immunosuppressed individuals.

(3) Cytomegalic inclusion disease

—is a **generalized infection of infants,** with a distinct clinical syndrome that includes jaundice with hepatosplenomegaly, thrombocytopenic purpura, pneumonitis, and CNS damage.

—is caused by intrauterine (congenital) or early postnatal infection.

—may cause fetal death.

b. Diagnosis

(1) CMV forms owl's eye inclusions in cells found in urinary sediments of infected individuals.

(2) CMV can be isolated from the saliva and urine.

(3) Cytomegalic inclusion disease can be diagnosed by virus isolation from urine or peripheral blood leukocytes, serologic tests, and new **DNA hybridization tests** involving extraction of viral DNA from urine specimens.

4. EBV

—infects and can transform human B lymphocytes.

—use complement receptor 3 (CD-21 or CR2) as the cellular receptor.

—produces several distinct antigens, including latent membrane proteins (LMPs), nuclear antigens (EBNAs), early antigens (EAs), a membrane antigen (MA), and a viral capsid antigen (VCA).

—usually causes clinically inapparent infections, but may cause **infectious mononucleosis** and is associated with **Burkitt's lymphoma** and **nasopharyngeal carcinoma.**

a. **Infectious mononucleosis**

—is a disease of children and young adults (sometimes called **kissing disease**), characterized by fever and enlarged lymph nodes and spleen.

—is associated with the production of **atypical lymphocytes** and IgM **heterophil antibodies** (antibodies detected using antigens from a source different than the one used to induce them) identified by the **mononucleosis spot test.**

—can also be diagnosed by serologic tests involving indirect immunofluorescence procedures on fixed EBV-producing cells or ELISA tests.

b. **Burkitt's lymphoma and nasopharyngeal carcinoma**

—result in increased antibody titers to EBV.

—have cells that express EBNAs and LMPs and carry multiple copies of viral DNA.

5. **Human herpesvirus type 6**

—infects and establishes latent infection of the T lymphocyte.

—causes a common **exanthem disease** of children (roseola or exanthem subitum) and mononucleosis.

6. **Human herpesvirus type 8 (Kaposi's sarcoma-associated herpesvirus)**

—is associated with Kaposi's sarcoma.

—is linked to some acquired immunodeficiency syndrome (AIDS)-associated B-cell lymphomas.

—is implicated in multiple myeloma.

D. **Parvoviruses**

1. **General characteristics—parvoviruses**

—are small, naked viruses with **icosahedral nucleocapsids.**

—contain **single-stranded DNA** and replicate in the nucleus.

—include **human parvovirus** (B19) and **adenoassociated virus,** a defective virus of the *Dependovirus* genus that requires adenovirus to replicate.

2. **Human parvovirus**

—enters the body through the respiratory tract and infects and lyses progenitor erythroid cells.

—causes **febrile illness** in blood recipients, **aplastic crises** in patients with hemolytic anemias, and **erythema infectiosum** (fifth disease) in healthy individuals.

E. **Papovaviruses**

—are naked viruses with an **icosahedral nucleocapsid** that contains **double-stranded, circular DNA.**

—replicate in the nucleus of the cell.

—produce **latent and chronic infections** in their natural host.

—can induce tumors in some animals (see XII B).

—include the animal viruses papillomavirus, polyomavirus, and simian virus 40 (SV40).

1. **Human papillomavirus**

   —replicates in epithelial cells of the skin.

   —forms **keilocytotic (vacuolated) cells** during replication.

   —is directly transferred from person to person.

   —causes **common warts or plantar warts (types 1 through 4), genital warts (types 6 and 11), and laryngeal papillomas.**

   —has been associated with **benign cervical tumors and vulvar and penile cancers (types 16 and 18).**

2. **Human polyomaviruses**

   —include the **JC virus** (isolated from patients with progressive multifocal leukoencephalopathy).

   —include the **BK virus,** which latently infects the kidney but can cause urinary tract infections in immunocompromised persons.

   —are detected by virus isolation from urine (BK virus), Papanicolaou smear of urinary sediment cells, or fluorescent antibody or immunoperoxidase staining of tissues on cells.

F. **Poxviruses**

   —have a complex brick-shaped virion that consists of an outer envelope enclosing a core containing **linear, double-stranded DNA** and two **lateral bodies.**

   —have more than 100 structural polypeptides, including many enzymes and a **transcriptional system** associated with the virion.

   —replicate in the cytoplasm of the cell.

   —are unique because **de novo formation of the viral membrane** is required for replication.

   —have **posttranslational cleavage** of proteins as part of their replication process.

   —produce eosinophilic inclusion bodies called **Guarnieri bodies** and membrane **hemagglutinins** in infected cells.

   —share a common nucleoprotein (NP) antigen in their inner core.

   —may be inhibited by rifampin (which blocks envelope formation) and methisazone (which interferes with late proteins and assembly).

   —include the human viruses (**vaccinia, variola,** and **molluscum contagiosum**) and the animal viruses [**cowpox virus, paravaccinia virus** (in cows), and **orf virus** (in sheep)]; the animal viruses can cause highly localized occupational infections (usually of the finger).

1. **Variola virus**

—causes **smallpox,** a generalized viral infection that presumably has been eradicated by a World Health Organization vaccine program.

—grows on the chorioallantoic membrane of eggs, where it forms **pocks,** focal areas of viral-induced cellular necrosis.

—was treated prophylactically with methisazone and by vaccination with the vaccinia virus.

2. Vaccinia virus

—is the variant of variola virus that generally produces only a mild disease and is used as the **immunogen in smallpox vaccination.**

—causes **postvaccinal encephalitis** in a minority (three per one million) of vaccinated persons.

—produces a 140-residue polypeptide closely related to epidermal growth factor.

—is being studied as a possible **immunizing vector** containing foreign genes for polypeptides, which would elicit neutralizing antibodies for other viruses (e.g., HSV types 1 and 2).

3. Molluscum contagiosum virus

—infects epithelial cells, where it causes a localized disease that usually resolves spontaneously in several months but may persist for 1–2 years.

—causes small, **wart-like lesions** on the face, arms, back, buttocks, and genitals.

—is transmitted by direct or indirect contact.

—can cause a sexually transmitted disease with papular lesions that can ulcerate and mimic genital herpes.

—forms characteristic eosinophilic inclusion bodies in infected cells.

VIII. Positive-Sense RNA Viruses (Table 4-12)

A. Coronaviruses

—are enveloped viruses with a **helical nucleocapsid** that contains **single-stranded RNA** with **positive (messenger) polarity.**

—have distinctive club-shaped surface projections that give the appearance of a **solar corona** to the virion.

—replicate in the cytoplasm and bind to cytoplasmic vesicles; no viral antigens appear on the surface of the infected cell.

—produce the **common cold** in adults (the second most frequent cause) and are implicated in **infant gastroenteritis.**

—usually are not diagnosed in the laboratory, although complement fixation and neutralization tests are available.

—are represented in humans by **prototype strains 229E and OC43.**

—are represented in mice by **mouse hepatitis virus,** which causes a

Table 4-12. Properties of Positive-Sense RNA Viruses

Virus Family	Virus Name	Unique Genes or Gene Products	Associated Acute Diseases	Associated Chronic or Persistent Diseases	Diagnostic Methods
Coronaviridae	Coronaviruses	...	Colds (adults) Gastroenteritis (infants)	...	...
Flaviviridae	Dengue (arbovirus)	...	Break bone fever Hemorrhagic fever	...	...
	Hepatitis C virus	...	Post-transfusion hepatitis	Hepatitis	ELISA test for IgM
	Yellow fever virus (arbovirus)	...	Yellow fever	...	Councilman bodies
	St. Louis encephalitis virus (arbovirus)	...	Encephalitis, frequent inapparent disease	...	...
	West Nile virus (arbovirus)	...	Encephalitis	...	...
Picornaviridae	Enteroviruses Poliovirus	...	Inapparent to mild febrile illness (abortive polio-myelitis) to paralytic poliomyelitis	...	Virus isolation
	Coxsackie A viruses	...	Herpangina Hand-foot-and-mouth disease Common cold Aseptic meningitis	...	Occasional rashes Virus isolation
	Coxsackie B viruses	...	Myocarditis Pericarditis Pleurodynia (Bornholm disease) Common cold Aseptic meningitis Juvenile diabetes (B4)	...	Occasional rashes Virus isolation

(cont.)

Table 4-12. Properties of Positive-Sense RNA Viruses (*Continued*)

Virus Family	Virus Name	Unique Genes or Gene Products	Associated Acute Diseases	Associated Chronic or Persistent Diseases	Diagnostic Methods
	Echoviruses	...	Aseptic meningitis Common cold Infantile diarrhea Hemorrhagic conjunctivitis	...	Frequent rashes Virus isolation
	Hepatitis A virus	...	Infectious hepatitis	...	ELISA test for IgM
	Rhinovirus	...	Common cold	...	...
Retroviridae	Human immunodeficiency viruses 1 and 2	Regulatory proteins: TAT, REV, and NEF Envelope glycoproteins: gp41 and gp120 Core proteins: p18, p24, and reverse transcriptase (RT) Regulatory genes: TRE and RRE	Inapparent disease or flu-like syndrome	AIDS AIDS dementia	Syncytia formation ELISA for p24 Western blot
	Human T-cell leukemia viruses types 1 and 2	Regulatory proteins: TAX and REX	Adult acute T-cell lymphocytic leukemia; some hairy cell leukemias	...	
Togaviridae	Alphaviruses Eastern equine encephalomyelitis virus (arbovirus) Western equine encephalomyelitis virus (arbovirus)	...	Severe encephalitis	...	
	Rubiviruses Rubella	...	Encephalitis (usually inapparent disease)	...	
			German measles Congenital rubella syndrome	...	Rash ELISA: IgM for recent infection, IgG for protection
Caliciviridae	Norwalk agent	...	Epidemic gastroenteritis	...	RIA serology

ELISA = enzyme-linked immunosorbent assay; RIA = radioimmunoassay; AIDS = acquired immunodeficiency syndrome.

chronic demyelinating disease used as a model for multiple sclerosis in humans.

B. Flaviviruses

—are enveloped viruses with a **single-stranded, positive-sense RNA** and no discernible capsid structure.

—replicate in the cytoplasm of the cell, where their RNA is translated into a large polyprotein that is subsequently cleaved (by posttranslational cleavage) into individual proteins.

—bud into the endoplasmic reticulum.

1. Dengue virus

—is an **arbovirus** transmitted from monkeys to humans by mosquitoes.

—causes characteristic skin lesions as well as fever and muscle and joint pain.

—may be fatal if hemorrhages are associated with the infection.

—is sometimes called **break bone fever.**

2. HCV

—is also known as **non-A, non-B hepatitis virus.**

—infects the body after parenteral entry, causing hepatitis after a 14- to 20-day incubation period.

—causes 90% of blood transfusion–associated or blood product administration–associated hepatitis.

—can cause **chronic infections;** therefore, individuals with the virus are in a **carrier state.**

—is diagnosed by ELISA for the antigen.

3. St. Louis encephalitis virus

—is an **arbovirus** with a mosquito vector that transfers the virus from wild birds to humans.

—usually causes inapparent infections but may produce encephalitis.

4. Yellow fever virus

—is an **arbovirus** that is usually transferred from monkeys to humans by mosquitoes.

—is a **biphasic disease** with clinical signs involving the vascular endothelium during initial virus replication and involving the liver during later replication.

—can be diagnosed by eosinophilic hyaline masses called **Councilman bodies** in the cytoplasm of infected liver cells.

—does not occur after immunization with the **attenuated vaccine strains 17D and Dakar.**

—can cause **chronic infections;** therefore, individuals with the virus are in a **carrier state.**

5. West Nile virus

—is an arbovirus that is transferred from a bird reservoir to humans by a mosquito vector.

—causes an encephalitis that is most serious for those older than 50 years of age.

C. Picornaviruses

—are small, naked viruses with an **icosahedral nucleocapsid** that contains **single-stranded, positive-sense RNA covalently linked to a small protein** (VPg in poliovirus).

—replicate in the cytoplasm of the cell, where their RNA is translated into a large polyprotein that is subsequently cleaved (**posttranslational cleavage**).

—modify their capsid proteins while in the assembled capsid.

—have cytopathic effects that include the formation of virus crystals in the cytoplasm of infected cells.

—are frequently cytolytic to infected cells.

—are classified as enteroviruses or rhinoviruses.

1. Enteroviruses

—cause a variety of human diseases involving infections of the alimentary tract.

—are stable at acidic pH (3–5).

—include the polioviruses, coxsackie A and B viruses, echoviruses, enteroviruses, and HAV.

—that have been isolated since 1969 are classified simply as enteroviruses and given a serotype number instead of being classified as either coxsackieviruses or echoviruses.

a. Poliovirus infections

—are usually subclinical but can occur as **mild illness, aseptic meningitis,** or an acute disease of the CNS (**poliomyelitis**) in which spinal cord motor neurons (anterior horn cells) are killed and flaccid paralysis results.

—are caused by **three serotypes** of virus.

—can occur in epidemics.

—begin in the oropharynx and intestine but can travel inside axons to the spinal cord.

—are controlled by immunization with a **killed trivalent vaccine** (Salk vaccine); a live attenuated trivalent vaccine (Sabin vaccine) is no longer recommended.

—are diagnosed serologically by a complement fixation test or by virus isolation from the throat (early in illness) or feces (later in illness).

b. Coxsackievirus infections

—are caused by 29 serotypes of viruses divided into two groups based on the type of paralysis observed after inoculation into mice; group A viruses cause flaccid paralysis, whereas group B viruses cause spastic paralysis.

—are the most common cause of **viral heart disease** (type B).

—tend to occur in the summer and early fall.

—can be diagnosed by virus isolation from throat washings, stools, or both or from serologic tests using specific viral antigen if a particular virus strain is suspected.

—are associated with various diseases:

(1) Herpangina (group B)

(2) Hand-foot-and-mouth disease (group A)

(3) Hemorrhagic conjunctivitis (group A)

(4) Pleurodynia, myocarditis, pericarditis, and meningoencephalitis (group B)

(5) Aseptic meningitis and colds (groups A and B)

c. **Echovirus infections**

—are caused by more than 30 serotypes of viruses that initially infect the human small intestine but cause diseases ranging from common colds and fevers (with or without rashes) to aseptic meningitis and acute hemorrhagic conjunctivitis.

—may be diagnosed by virus isolation from the throat or stools; however, this is done only in summer outbreaks of **aseptic meningitis or febrile illness with rash.**

d. **Enterovirus infections**

—are associated with various respiratory tract infections, CNS disease (enterovirus type 71), and acute hemorrhagic conjunctivitis (enterovirus type 70).

e. **HAV infections**

—are caused by an enterovirus that could be called **enterovirus type 72.**

—are called **infectious hepatitis.**

—are distinguished from HBV infections by their abrupt onset, relatively short incubation period (15–45 days), and transfer by the fecal–oral route.

—are acute infections that can occur in epidemics.

—may be treated prophylactically by immune human globulin or prevented by immunization with **killed virus vaccine (Havrix or VAQTA).**

—are diagnosed serologically by increases in IgM detected by an ELISA test.

2. **Rhinoviruses**

—cause localized upper respiratory tract infections.

—are the most frequent cause of the **common cold.**

—exist in more than **100 serotypes.**

—are acid-labile.

D. **Retroviruses**

—are enveloped viruses that probably have an **icosahedral capsid** surrounding a **helical nucleocapsid,** which contains an inverted dimer of **linear, single-stranded, positive-sense RNA** (diploid genome).

—are divided morphologically into four types (A, B, C, and D).

—are classified into three groups: **lentiviruses** (visna and maedi viruses of sheep, **HIV**), **spumaviruses,** and **oncoviruses** (types B, C, and D RNA tumor viruses).

—have a virion-associated reverse transcriptase (which makes DNA copies from RNA) and replicate in the nucleus.

—need host-cell transfer RNA to interact with reverse transcriptase before the reverse transcriptase complex can bind to RNA and initiate DNA synthesis.

—have three distinctive genes: *gag* **(structural proteins),** *pol* **(reverse transcriptase),** and *env* **(envelope glycoproteins),** which are flanked by **long terminal repeat sequences** with regulatory functions.

—use posttranslational cleavage processes during the synthesis of Gag and Env gene products.

—cause mostly "slow" diseases of animals and various cancers (see XII), except for HIV, which causes AIDS.

1. **HIV**
   a. **General characteristics—HIV**
      —is a member of the lentivirus subfamily.
      —initiates infection by interaction of an envelope glycoprotein (gp120) with the cellular T4 (CD4) lymphocyte surface receptor.
      —synthesizes core proteins (p18, p24, and RT) and transregulatory proteins (TAT, REV, and NEF).
      —has regulatory genes (TRE and RRE).
      —infects and **kills T helper cells,** resulting in **depression of both humoral and cell-mediated immunity.**
      —travels throughout the body, particularly in macrophages.
      —induces a distinctive CPE called **giant-cell (syncytia) formation.**
   b. **AIDS**
      —results from suppression of the immune system.
      —is characterized by unusual cancers (e.g., Kaposi's sarcoma), severe opportunistic infections (e.g., *Pneumocystis carinii,* CMV), or, frequently, **AIDS dementia complex.**
      —is a high-risk disease for homosexuals, bisexual men, and intravenous drug users.
      —does not always occur in persons who are seropositive for HIV.
      —is diagnosed by clinical symptoms and serologic assays, including ELISA and Western blot tests.
      —is directed with combination therapy using two nucleoside analogues and a protease inhibitor or two nucleoside analogues and a nonnucleoside inhibitor (**HAART: highly active antiretroviral therapies**).

2. Endogenous type C retroviruses

—are viruses of type C RNA tumor virus morphology (see XII C 2).

—have a provirus that is a constant part of the genome of an organism and whose expression is regulated by the host cell.

—are transmitted genetically to all offspring.

—are not pathogenic for their hosts.

—are frequently induced to replicate when cells are placed in tissue culture.

—are called **ecotrophic** if they multiply in cells of the species in which they were induced, **xenotrophic** if they cannot infect cells from the species in which they were induced but infect other species, and **amphotrophic** if they grow in cells of the species from which they were induced as well as in cells from other species.

E. Togaviruses

—are enveloped viruses with an **icosahedral nucleocapsid** containing **single-stranded, positive-sense RNA.**

—have **hemagglutinins** associated with their envelope.

—replicate in the cytoplasm and posttranslationally process the polyproteins they synthesize.

—cause generalized infections.

—are divided into four groups of which two (alphaviruses and rubiviruses) are human pathogens.

1. Alphaviruses

—bud from the cell surface.

—are **arboviruses** with mosquito vectors and animal reservoirs.

—produce encephalitis or moderate systemic disease following the bite of a mosquito that has fed on an animal viral reservoir.

—lead to more serious encephalitis than do flaviviruses.

—are diagnosed by serologic tests, usually ELISA for IgM, because virus isolation is difficult.

—include **eastern equine encephalomyelitis virus, western equine encephalomyelitis virus,** and **Venezuelan equine encephalomyelitis virus.**

2. Rubiviruses

a. General characteristics—rubiviruses

—bud into the endoplasmic reticulum and the cell surface.

—include **rubella virus.**

b. Rubella virus infections

—cause **German measles,** a systemic infection characterized by lymphadenopathy and morbilliform rash.

—are often subclinical in adults.

—can produce **congenital infections,** which can cause serious damage to the infected fetus during the first 10 weeks of pregnancy and lead to rubella syndrome.

—are difficult to diagnose clinically but can be diagnosed by serologic tests for IgM antibodies, including hemagglutination inhibition or ELISA.

—can be prevented by immunization with the **live attenuated vaccine strains HPV77** or **RA 27/3.**

F. Norwalk virus

—is most likely a member of the **Caliciviridae** family.

—is a naked virus with an **icosahedral nucleocapsid** containing **single-stranded, positive-sense RNA.**

—replicates in the cytoplasm.

—causes **epidemic gastroenteritis.**

—has never been grown in tissue culture.

—may be demonstrated by a RIA blocking test or immune adherence methods.

IX. Negative-Sense RNA Viruses (Table 4-13)

A. Bunyaviruses

1. General characteristics—bunyaviruses

—are enveloped viruses with **three circular helical nucleocapsids,** each containing a unique piece of **single-stranded, negative-polarity RNA** (L, M, and S segments), viral nucleoprotein, and transcriptase enzyme.

—replicate with cytoplasm and bud from the **membranes of the Golgi apparatus.**

—can interact with viruses that are closely related serologically to produce **recombinant viruses by genetic reassortment.**

—are arboviruses that have rodent hosts and infect humans during an arthropod bite.

—produce mosquito-borne encephalitis (**California** and **La Crosse encephalitis viruses**), sandfly- and mosquito-borne fever (**sandfly fever virus** and **Rift Valley fever virus**), rodent-borne hemorrhagic fever (**Hantaan virus**), or respiratory distress syndrome (**Hantavirus**).

2. Bunyavirus encephalitis

—is caused by the California and La Crosse viruses, which occur mainly in the Mississippi and Ohio River valleys.

—has a small forest rodent reservoir for the virus and a mosquito vector.

—is usually mild (sometimes causing only meningitis), with an excellent prognosis and rare sequelae.

3. Hantavirus pulmonary syndrome

Table 4-13. Properties of Negative-Sense RNA Viruses

Virus Family	Virus Name	Unique Genes or Gene Products	Associated Acute Diseases	Associated Chronic or Persistent Diseases	Diagnostic Methods
Bunyaviridae	California encephalitis virus (arbovirus) La Crosse encephalitis virus (arbovirus) Hantavirus	...	Mild febrile illness Encephalitis Severe respiratory distress	...	Serology
Orthomyxoviridae	Influenza A, B, and C viruses	Hemagglutinin neuraminidase Nucleoprotein Matrix protein	Influenza Reye's syndrome (type B virus)	...	Clinical manisfestations Virus isolation
Paramyxoviridae	Newcastle disease virus	Hemagglutinin only	Mild conjunctivitis (poultry workers)	...	
	Measles virus	Fusion factor Matrix protein	Measles Giant-cell pneumonia Encephalitis	SSPE	Koplik's spots Warthin-Finkeldey cells ELISA for IgM
	Mumps virus	Hemagglutinin neuraminidase Fusion factor Matrix protein	Mumps Orchitis Aseptic meningitis	...	Clinical manifestations
	Parainfluenza virus (types 1–4)	Hemagglutinin neuraminidase Fusion factor Matrix protein	Croup (types 1–3) Pharyngitis Upper and lower respiratory tract infections	...	IF of respiratory secretions Virus isolation
	Respiratory syncytial virus	Fusion factor Matrix factor	Bronchiolitis and pneumonia in infants Nosocomial infections Colds in adults	...	Viral antigen in nasal washing by FA
Rhabdoviridae	Rabies Vesicular stomatitis virus	...	Rabies Foot-and-mouth disease in cattle	...	Negri bodies FA staining of tissue sections

ELISA = enzyme-linked immunosorbent assay; FA = fluorescent antibody; IF = immunofluorescence; SSPE = subacute sclerosing panencephalitis.

—is caused by inhaling Hantavirus contained in dried deer mouse saliva, urine, or feces.

—may evolve to a fatal disease (> 50%) characterized by respiratory insufficiency.

B. Orthomyxoviruses

—are enveloped, spherical, or filamentous viruses with **eight helical nucleocapsids** containing a unique **single-stranded, negative-sense RNA.**

—have a **hemagglutinin (H),** a **neuraminidase (N),** and a **matrix protein (M)** associated with the envelope, a **transcriptase (P)** that is associated with the nucleocapsid, and an **NP** associated with the RNA.

—form **defective interfering (DI) particles** that lack a segment of RNA necessary for productive replication.

—are assembled in the cytoplasm but depend on host nuclear functions, including RNA polymerase II, for transcription.

—are **influenza viruses** and are classified as type A, B, or C, depending on a nucleocapsid antigen.

—have the capacity to undergo **genetic reassortment** due to the segmented nature of the genome.

—do not replicate well in tissue culture and are grown in animals or embryonated eggs.

—are designated by the nomenclature, which indicates virus type, species isolated from (unless human), site of isolation, strain number, year of isolation, and hemagglutinin and neuraminidase subtype; for example, A/swine/New Jersey/8/76 (H1N1) and A/Phillippines/2/82 (H3N2).

1. Glycoproteins

a. Influenza virus hemagglutinin

—is an envelope glycoprotein containing a **virus receptor** that binds to the cellular receptor site.

—agglutinates many species of red blood cells.

—induces neutralizing antibodies.

—has **fusion activity** that allows the virion envelope to fuse with the host-cell plasma membranes.

—is responsible for influenza epidemics when it changes antigenically.

—undergoes frequent minor mutations that result in antigenic changes leading to **antigenic drift.**

—undergoes **antigenic shift** when major antigenic changes follow reassortment between the hemagglutinin-coding RNA segments of animal or human viruses.

b. Influenza virus neuraminidase

—is an envelope glycoprotein that removes terminal sialic acid residues from oligosaccharide chains.

—is involved in the **release of virions** from infected cells.

—can undergo antigenic shift and drift mutations; however, epidemics do not result from these changes.

2. Influenza

—is a localized infection of the respiratory tract.

—is usually not serious, except in the elderly or in patients with a secondary bacterial pneumonia.

—is associated with Guillain-Barré syndrome (influenza virus types A and B) and Reye's syndrome (influenza virus type B).

—can be diagnosed by virus isolation or a hemagglutination inhibition serologic test.

—may result in pandemics due to reassortment of the hemagglutinin.

—may be treated prophylactically with amantadine or rimantadine if type A virus is involved or with a polyvalent killed vaccine containing the prevailing type A and type B strains.

—may be treated with **oseltamivir** or **zanamivir** (neuraminidase inhibitors) [types A and B] or amantadine or rimantidine (type A only).

—may be prevented by active immunization with a polyvalent killed (Fluzone), split (Flushield), or subunit (Fluvirus) vaccine.

C. Paramyxoviruses

—are spherical, enveloped viruses with a **single helical nucleocapsid** containing **single-stranded, negative-sense RNA.**

—have a **hemagglutinin-neuraminidase** (HN), a **fusion protein** (F), and a **matrix protein** (M) associated with the envelope and a nucleocapsid-associated **transcriptase** (P).

—replicate in the cytoplasm of the cell.

—form **DI particles** by segment deletions within the genome.

—form **heteroploid particles** (two nucleocapsids from unrelated paramyxoviruses in the same envelope) or **polyploid particles** (multiple copies of the same nucleocapsid in a large envelope).

—cause acute and persistent infections.

—are divided into three genera on the basis of chemical and biologic properties: **paramyxoviruses** (parainfluenza and mumps viruses), **morbilliviruses** (measles virus), and **pneumoviruses** (respiratory syncytial virus).

—exist in few antigenic types.

1. Glycoproteins

a. Paramyxovirus hemagglutinin–neuraminidase

—is a large surface glycoprotein with both **hemagglutinating** and **neuraminidase activity,** except in measles virus, which lacks neuraminidase activity, and in respiratory syncytial virus, in which both activities have been lost.

—is responsible for **virus adsorption.**

—stimulates the production of neutralizing antibodies.

b. Paramyxovirus fusion protein

—is a surface glycoprotein with **fusion and hemolysin activities,** except in respiratory syncytial virus, in which hemolysis activity is lost.

—is responsible for **virus penetration** into the cell.

—is composed of two subunits, F_1 and F_2, formed by proteolytic cleavage of precursor F_0 by a host enzyme.

2. Parainfluenza virus infections

—are caused by **parainfluenza type 1 virus (Sendai virus).**

—cause a variety of upper and lower respiratory tract illnesses, usually occurring in the fall and winter.

—cause **croup** (parainfluenza type 2 virus) in infants.

—can be diagnosed using hemagglutination inhibition or complement fixation tests.

3. Mumps virus infections

—are frequently subclinical and occur in winter or early spring.

—result in generalized disease characterized by enlargement of one or both parotid glands.

—may affect the testes and ovaries, causing swelling and pain.

—cause 10%–15% of aseptic meningitis cases.

—are most frequently diagnosed by clinical observation, although the virus can be isolated from the saliva, cerebrospinal fluid, or urine.

—are inhibited by a **live attenuated vaccine** containing the Jeryl Lynn strain of virus (usually included with live attenuated measles and rubella virus strains).

4. Measles virus infections

—cause an acute generalized disease characterized by a maculopapular rash, fever, respiratory distress, and **Koplik's spots** on the buccal mucosa.

—can produce **Warthin-Finkeldey cells** (large multinuclear cells) in nasal secretions.

—can progress to **encephalomyelitis** (in 1 of every 1000 cases) or **giant-cell pneumonia.**

—cause temporary depression of cell-mediated immunity (due to viral infection of lymphocytes), which sometimes leads to secondary bacterial infections.

—can produce **subacute sclerosing panencephalitis,** a slowly progressive, degenerative neurologic disease of children and young adults.

—can be prevented by a **live attenuated measles vaccine** (Moraten strain) that is part of the trivalent (measles, mumps, and rubella) vaccine given to children.

5. Respiratory syncytial virus infections

—are localized virus infections that are most often confined to the upper respiratory tract but can involve the lower respiratory tract.

—are the major cause of **serious bronchiolitis** and **pneumonia** in infants.

—may be treated with ribavirin if infection is severe.

—may have an immediate hypersensitivity component.

—are caused by an extremely labile virus that produces a characteristic **syncytial effect (cell fusion)** in infected cells.

—may be rapidly diagnosed by a direct immunofluorescent test on exfoliated cells in nasopharyngeal smears.

—may be diagnosed by demonstration of viral antigens in nasal washings by fluorescent antibody or immunohistochemical techniques.

6. Newcastle disease virus infections

—are caused by a paramyxovirus that is a natural respiratory tract pathogen of birds, particularly chickens.

—occur as an **occupational disease** of poultry workers.

—are observed clinically as a **mild conjunctivitis** without corneal involvement.

D. Rhabdoviruses

—are enveloped, **bullet-shaped** viruses with a **helical nucleocapsid** containing **single-stranded, negative-sense RNA.**

—have a virion-associated transcriptase and replicate in the cytoplasm.

—generate deletion mutants that form **DI particles.**

—establish persistent infections in cell cultures.

—are represented by the human pathogen **rabies virus** and the bovine pathogen **vesicular stomatitis virus.**

1. Rabies virus

—produces specific cytoplasmic inclusion bodies, called **Negri bodies,** in infected cells.

—can travel throughout the nervous system in nerve fibers.

—has a predilection for the hippocampus (Ammon's horn cells).

—is called **street virus** if it is freshly isolated and **fixed virus** if it is serially passaged in a rabbit brain so that it no longer multiplies in extraneural tissue.

—produces disease after inoculation by an animal bite or, occasionally, by inhalation.

—causes fatal disease unless the infected person previously received immunization or receives postexposure prophylaxis consisting of passive immunization with human rabies immune globulin and immunization with a vaccine.

—is identified in suspected tissues by a direct immunofluorescence test.

—is grown in rabbit brain (**Semple's vaccine**), embryonated eggs (**duck embryo vaccine**), or W1-38 cells (**human diploid cell vaccine**) before inactivation and use as a vaccine.

—has been attenuated by growth in a chick embryo for use as an animal, not human, vaccine (**Flury's vaccine**).

2. Vesicular stomatitis virus

—causes foot-and-mouth disease in cattle.

—is well known for its ability to produce DI particles and persistent infections.

E. Marburg and Ebola viruses

—belong to a virus family called **Filoviridae.**

—are enveloped viruses with a **helical nucleocapsid** containing **single-stranded, negative-sense RNA.**

—cause **African hemorrhagic fevers,** which often lead to death.

X. Other RNA Viruses (Table 4-14)

A. Arenaviruses

—are enveloped viruses with **two string-of-beads nucleocapsids,** each containing a unique **single-stranded, circular RNA.**

—have one molecule of genomic RNA (L, or large) with negative polarity and one molecule (S, or short) that is **ambisense** (i.e., has both a negative and a positive sense).

—replicate in the cytoplasm and have **host-cell ribosomes** in their virion.

—infect mice, rats, or both as their natural hosts.

—are initially passed from rodents to humans but can be transferred by direct human contact.

—cause highly contagious hemorrhagic fevers (**Junin, Machupo,** and **Lassa viruses**) that are not endemic to the United States and meningitis or flu-like illness (**lymphocytic choriomeningitis virus**) that is endemic.

B. Reoviruses

—are naked viruses with a **double-shelled** (outer shell and core) **icosahedral capsid** containing **10 or 11 segments of double-stranded RNA.**

—replicate in the cytoplasm.

—have a core-associated transcriptase.

—are classified into three groups: reoviruses, rotaviruses, and orbiviruses.

1. Reoviruses

—have **10 segments of double-stranded RNA.**

—have an **outer shell–associated hemagglutinin** (σ 1) that agglutinates human or bovine erythrocytes; is the **viral receptor,** therefore determining tissue trophism; and is the determinant for the three serotypes of reoviruses.

Table 4-14. Properties of Other RNA Viruses

Virus Family	Virus Name	Unique Genes or Gene Products	Acute Diseases	Chronic or Persistent Diseases	Diagnostic Methods
Arenaviridae	Junin, Machupo, and Lassa viruses	…	Hemorrhagic fevers	…	…
	Lymphocytic choriomeningitis virus	…	Flu-like illness	…	…
Reoviridae	Reoviruses	σ-Hemagglutinin	Mild upper respiratory infections	…	…
			Gastroenteritis		
	Colorado tick fever virus (arbovirus)	…	Colorado tick fever	…	FA staining of erythrocytes
	Rotaviruses	…	Infantile diarrhea		Enzyme immunoassay for viral antigen in stool
			Gastroenteritis in children		
Unknown	Delta agent	Delta antigen	Hepatitis	Hepatitis	ELISA for IgM

ELISA = enzyme-linked immunosorbent assay; FA = fluorescent antibody.

—form distinctive eosinophilic inclusion bodies.

—replicate their RNA **conservatively,** not semiconservatively.

—produce **minor upper respiratory tract infections** and **gastrointestinal disease,** but also are frequently recovered from healthy people.

—are diagnosed by a complement fixation test and serotyped by hemagglutination inhibition assays.

—may be isolated from feces and throat washings.

2. Rotaviruses

—have **11 segments of double-stranded RNA.**

—exist in at least four serotypes, with type A being involved in most human infections.

—cause **infantile diarrhea** and are the most common cause of **gastroenteritis in children.**

—are frequent causes of **nosocomial infections.**

—may be prevented by an attenuated vaccine (Rotashield) that is currently recommended only for adults.

—are diagnosed by demonstrating virus in the stool or by serologic tests, particularly ELISA.

3. Orbiviruses

—have **10 segments of double-stranded RNA.**

—infect insects, which transfer the virus to humans.

—cause mild fevers in humans.

—are represented by **Colorado tick fever virus,** which is carried by the wood tick *Dermacentor andersoni.*

C. Hepatitis D virus (delta-associated virus)

—is a virus with **circular, single-stranded RNA** molecules (viroid-like) and an **internal core δ** antigen surrounded by an **HBV envelope.**

—is **defective** and can replicate only in the presence of HBV.

—is associated with both acute and chronic hepatitis and always with HBV.

—causes more severe hepatitis than does HBV alone.

—may be diagnosed serologically with an ELISA test.

XI. Slow Viruses and Prions

A. Subacute sclerosing panencephalitis virus

—is a variant or close relative of measles virus.

—causes **subacute sclerosing panencephalitis,** a rare, fatal, slowly progressive demyelinating CNS disease of teenagers and young adults.

—may result from improper synthesis or processing of the matrix (M) viral protein.

B. JC virus

—is a papovavirus that frequently infects humans but rarely produces disease unless the host is immunosuppressed.

—has been isolated from patients with **progressive multifocal leukoencephalopathy,** a rare CNS disease.

—causes demyelination by infecting and killing oligodendrocytes.

C. Animal lentiviruses

—are retroviruses that cause slow, generalized infections of sheep (**visna** and **progressive pneumonia virus**) and goats (**caprine arthritis virus**).

—produce minimal amounts of infectious virus in their hosts.

—undergo considerable **antigenic variation** in their host due to mutations in envelope glycoproteins.

D. Prions

—are not viruses but are proteinaceous material lacking nucleic acid.

—are associated with several degenerative CNS diseases (**subacute spongiform virus encephalopathies**): kuru and Creutzfeldt-Jakob disease of humans, scrapie of sheep, bovine spongiform encephalopathy (or mad cow disease), and transmissible encephalopathy of mink.

—have a **prion protein (PrP)** that is associated with their infectivity but is encoded by a cellular gene.

XII. Oncogenic Viruses (Table 4-15)

A. General characteristics—oncogenic viruses

—are classified as DNA or RNA tumor viruses.

—produce tumors when they infect appropriate animals.

—transform infected cells by altering cell growth, cell surface antigens, and biochemical processes.

—introduce "transforming" genes or induce expression of quiescent cellular genes, which results in the synthesis of one or more transforming proteins.

—form **proviruses** (viral genomes integrated into host-cell chromosomes).

B. DNA tumor viruses

—cause **transformation** in **nonpermissive cells** (infected cells that do not support total virus replication).

—include human papillomaviruses: adenoviruses, HBV, EBV, molluscum contagiosum virus, JC and BK viruses, and possibly HSV-2.

—include animal viruses: chicken **Marek's disease virus** (a herpesvirus), mouse **polyomavirus** (a papovavirus), and monkey **SV40 virus** (a papovavirus).

Table 4-15. Oncogenic Viruses

Virus	Proteins or Process Implicated in Transformation	Associated Disease
DNA tumor viruses		
Simian virus 40	Large tumor antigen	Hamster sarcomas
Polyoma viruses (JC and BK viruses)	Tumor antigen	Hamster brain tumors
Human papillomaviruses types 16 and 18	E6 and E7 protein	Cervical dysplasia and neoplasia
Adenovirus (types 12, 18, and 31)	E1A and E1B	Hamster sarcomas
Epstein-Barr virus	EBNA and LMP proteins	Burkitt's lymphoma Nasopharyngeal carcinoma
Hepatitis B virus	X protein	Primary hepatocellular carcinoma
Molluscum contagiosum virus	. . .	Benign skin lesions
Herpes simplex virus type 2	. . .	Cervical carcinoma
RNA tumor viruses		
Human T-cell leukemia virus type 1	Transactivating gene products (e.g., TAX)	Adult acute T-cell lymphocytic leukemia
Human T-cell leukemia virus type 2	. . .	Atypical hairy cell leukemia
Oncovirus type B (mouse mammary tumor virus)	Proximal activation of growth genes	Mouse adenocarcinoma and mammary cancers
Oncoviruses type C (avian and murine sarcoma and leukemia viruses)	Oncogenes, insertional mutagenesis, or proximal activation of growth genes	Avian and murine sarcomas and leukemias

EBNA = Epstein-Barr nuclear antigen; LMP = latent membrane proteins.

—have protein products (e.g., adenovirus, papillomavirus, and polyomavirus) that interact with cellular **tumor suppressor gene** or **antioncogene** products that suppress oncogene expression.

1. **SV40 virus**

—undergoes productive replication in monkey cells but transforms non-permissive hamster and mouse cells.

—synthesizes an early protein called **large tumor (T) antigen,** which associates with two antioncogene proteins, p53 and p110^{Rb}, and the retinoblastoma gene product, and establishes and maintains **SV40-induced transformation.**

—synthesizes two other tumor antigens, middle T and small T antigens.

2. **Polyomavirus**

—grows permissively in mouse cells but transforms nonpermissive hamster and rat cells.

—synthesizes a **transforming large T antigen.**

3. **Human adenovirus**

—may be highly oncogenic (types 12, 18, and 31) or weakly oncogenic (types 3, 7, 14, 16, and 21) when injected into hamsters.

—synthesizes an **E1A** protein that binds to cellular p53 and **E1B** protein that binds to cellular p110^{Rb} if highly oncogenic.

4. Human papillomavirus

—may have a strong association (types 16 and 18) or a moderate association (types 31, 33, 35, 45, 51, 52, and 56) with cervical carcinoma.

—synthesizes an **E6 protein** that binds to cellular p53 and **E7 protein** that binds to cellular p110^{Rb}.

5. EBV

—is a cofactor in the etiology of **Burkitt's lymphoma** and **nasopharyngeal carcinoma.**

—can immortalize and transform B lymphocytes due to specific EBNA and LMP proteins.

6. HBV

—is associated with primary hepatocellular carcinoma.

—synthesizes an X protein, which binds to cellular p53.

C. RNA tumor viruses

—are **retroviruses** (oncovirus group).

—infect permissive cells but transform rather than kill.

—cause tumors of the reticuloendothelial and hematopoietic systems (leukemias), connective tissues (sarcomas), or mammary glands.

—are also called **oncornaviruses.**

1. Type B tumor viruses

—have an eccentric electron-dense core structure in their virion.

—are best exemplified by **mouse mammary tumor virus,** also called **Bittner virus.**

2. Type C tumor viruses

—have electron-dense cores in the center of the virion.

—include most RNA tumor viruses.

—are classified as nondefective or defective based on replicative ability.

—contain a cellular-derived **oncogene** (which codes for a cancer-inducing product) as well as **virogenes** (*gag, pol,* and *env*); however, a few nondefective murine leukosis viruses (AKR and Moloney viruses) lack oncogenes.

a. Oncogenes

—are genes that cause cancer.

—have copies in viruses (**v-*onc***) and cells (**c-*onc*** or **proto-oncogene**).

—are "switched off" or down-regulated in normal cells by antioncogene proteins (e.g., p53 and p110^{Rb}).

—have products that are essential to normal cell function or development.

—may code for proteins, which can be:

      (1) Tyrosine protein kinases (*src* gene-Rous sarcoma virus, ab1 gene-Abelson leukemia virus)

      (2) Guanine-nucleotide–binding proteins (Ha-*ras*-Harvey sarcoma virus)

      (3) Chromatin-binding proteins (*myc*-MC29 myclocytomatosis virus and *fos*-FBJ osteosarcoma virus)

      (4) Cellular surface receptors such as epidermal growth factor receptor (*erb*-B product of avian erythroblastosis virus)

      (5) Cellular growth factors such as platelet-derived growth factor (SIS gene product of simian sarcoma virus)

  b. Nondefective viruses

    —have all their virogenes and can therefore replicate themselves.

    —have high oncogenic potential if they also contain an oncogene (e.g., **Rous chicken sarcoma virus**).

    —have low oncogenic potential if they do not have an oncogene [e.g., **AKR** and **Moloney murine leukemia viruses** and **human T-cell leukemia viruses (HTLV) I and II**].

  c. Defective viruses

    —have a virogene or part of a virogene replaced by an oncogene.

    —need **helper viruses** to provide missing virogene products for replication.

    —have high oncogenic potential, for example, murine sarcoma viruses (**Kirsten** and **Harvey viruses**) and murine leukemia viruses (**Friend** and **Abelson viruses**).

  d. HTLV

    —are nondefective, exogenous retroviruses.

    —replicate and transform T4 antigen-positive cells.

    —produce giant multinucleated cells.

    —have no identifiable oncogene.

    —are associated with human adult acute T-cell lymphocytic leukemia and tropical spastic paraparesis (HTLV-1) and some forms of hairy cell leukemia virus (HTLV-2).

Review Test

1. Which of the following statements about clinical viral disease is true?

(A) It is most frequently due to toxin production.
(B) It usually follows viral infection.
(C) It can result without infection of host cells.
(D) It is associated with target organs in most disseminated viral infections.

2. The eclipse period of a one-step viral multiplication curve is defined as the period of time between the

(A) uncoating and assembly of the virus.
(B) start of the infection and the first appearance of extracellular virus.
(C) start of the infection and the first appearance of intracellular virus.
(D) start of the infection and uncoating of the virus.

3. Which of the following is the most frequent cause of blood transfusion–associated hepatitis?

(A) Hepatitis A virus
(B) Hepatitis B virus
(C) Hepatitis C virus
(D) Hepatitis D virus

4. Anti–viral capsid antigen (VCA) antibodies are found in

(A) cytomegalovirus infections.
(B) Epstein-Barr virus infections.
(C) herpes simplex virus infections.
(D) varicella-zoster virus infections

5. Passive immunization is available for protection from

(A) influenza A virus.
(B) hepatitis A virus.
(C) parainfluenza type 2 virus.
(D) rubella virus.

6. Linear, single-stranded DNA is the genetic material of

(A) caliciviruses.
(B) flaviviruses.
(C) papovaviruses.
(D) parvoviruses.

7. Infantile diarrhea is usually attributable to

(A) adenovirus.
(B) coronavirus.
(C) Norwalk virus.
(D) rotavirus.

8. Which of the following is an RNA virus that has a nuclear phase to its replication process?

(A) Coronavirus
(B) Rhabdovirus
(C) Retrovirus
(D) Togavirus

9. Negri bodies are associated with

(A) cytomegalovirus infections.
(B) herpes simplex virus infections.
(C) rabies virus infections.
(D) rubella virus infections.

10. Persistent virus infections

(A) are usually confined to the initial site of infection.
(B) are preceded by acute clinical disease.
(C) elicit a poor antibody response.
(D) may involve infected carrier individuals.

11. Which of the following is an example of a killed virus vaccine?

(A) Jeryl Lynn mumps vaccine
(B) Enders measles vaccine
(C) Salk poliovirus vaccine
(D) Oka varicella-zoster vaccine

12. Which of the following is the first viral-induced defense mechanism in a nonimmune individual?

(A) Generation of cytotoxic T lymphocytes
(B) Production of interferon
(C) Synthesis of lymphokines
(D) Synthesis of neutralizing antibodies

13. Localized viral disease

(A) is a major feature of congenital viral infections.
(B) is associated with a pronounced viremia.
(C) can be associated with carrier individuals.
(D) may have systemic clinical features such as fever.

14. Viral-induced heart disease is most frequently associated with

(A) arenavirus infections.
(B) coxsackievirus infections.
(C) echovirus infections.
(D) enterovirus infections.

15. Where are viral oncogenes found?

(A) JC virus
(B) Human T-cell lymphotrophic virus type I
(C) Rous sarcoma virus
(D) Simian virus 40

16. Dane particles are associated with

(A) hepatitis A virus.
(B) hepatitis B virus.
(C) hepatitis C virus.
(D) hepatitis E virus.

17. Which of the following terms refers to the exchange of homologous segments of RNA between two different influenza type A viruses?

(A) Complementation
(B) Genetic reassortment
(C) Phenotypic masking
(D) Phenotypic mixing

18. Which of the following is a virus that may cause a winter illness characterized by red blood cells in the cerebrospinal fluid and temporal lobe dysfunction?

(A) Coxsackie A virus
(B) Herpes simplex virus
(C) Poliovirus
(D) Western equine encephalomyelitis virus

19. Subacute sclerosing panencephalitis is a slowly progressive, degenerative neurologic disease associated with

(A) herpes simplex virus infection.
(B) measles virus infection.
(C) mumps virus infection.
(D) varicella-zoster virus infection.

20. Which of the following is a virus infection involving the presence of a noninfectious form of the virus?

(A) Abortive
(B) Latent
(C) Persistent
(D) Subclinical

21. The nanogram level of antigen in serum is detected by

(A) dot blot tests.
(B) enzyme-linked immunosorbent assay.
(C) fluorescent antibody staining.
(D) protein–protein hybridization tests.

22. Which of the following is a virus that infects and lyses progenitor erythroid cells causing aplastic crises in patients with hemolytic anemia?

(A) California encephalitis virus
(B) Epstein-Barr virus
(C) Parvovirus B19
(D) Yellow fever virus

23. Which of the following is a viral protein that is thought to induce tumors by binding to a cellular tumor suppressor protein?

(A) Adenovirus E1A
(B) Epstein-Barr nuclear antigen proteins
(C) Hepatitis B virus e protein
(D) Human immunodeficiency virus *gag* protein

24. Viruses whose genomes have messenger (positive-sense) polarity are

(A) adenoviruses
(B) papovaviruses
(C) paramyxoviruses
(D) polioviruses

25. Antiviral nucleoside analogues

(A) are effective only against replicating viruses.
(B) include foscarnet.
(C) inhibit replicases.
(D) may block viral penetration.

26. A commercial vaccine consisting of virion subunits prepared by recombinant technology exists for

(A) hepatitis B virus.
(B) rabies virus.
(C) rotavirus.
(D) varicella-zoster virus.

27. Which of the following causes a nosocomial infection with the potential to cause serious respiratory disease in an infant pediatric ward?

(A) Adenovirus
(B) Picornavirus
(C) Coxsackie A virus
(D) Respiratory syncytial virus

Answers and Explanations

1–D. Many viral infections are asymptomatic or subclinical. Clinical disease, however, is often associated with viral replication in target organs during disseminated viral infections.

2–C. The period of time between the adsorption and penetration of the virus until the first appearance of intracellular virus is the eclipse phase.

3–C. Hepatitis can be transmitted by both the oral and parenteral routes; hepatitis C virus is the virus most associated with hepatitis following the transfusion of blood products.

4–B. Antibodies to the viral capsid antigen (VCA) are important in identifying Epstein-Barr virus infections.

5–B. A commercially available human immune globulin preparation is available for pre- and postexposure prophylaxis for hepatitis A virus.

6–D. Parvoviruses have linear, single-stranded DNA while papovaviruses have circular, double-stranded DNA. Caliciviruses and flaviviruses are RNA viruses.

7–D. Although adenoviruses, Norwalk virus, and rotaviruses can cause diarrhea, infantile diarrhea is usually caused by rotaviruses.

8–C. The reverse transcriptase of retroviruses makes a DNA copy of the genomic RNA. This DNA must be integrated into the host-cell DNA in the nucleus for the remaining steps in the replication process to occur.

9–C. Negri bodies are intracytoplasmic inclusion bodies found in rabies virus–infected neurons and are important in the diagnosis of infected animals.

10–D. Some persistent virus infections, such as serum hepatitis caused by hepatitis B virus, involve carrier individuals who may or may not have clinical signs of the disease.

11–C. Although many of the childhood vaccines like measles, mumps, and chickenpox contain live, attenuated virus, the Salk poliovirus vaccine contains killed virus.

12–B. The production of interferons that induce the synthesis of antiviral replication proteins in neighboring cells occurs before the appearance of any other viral-induced immune defense mechanisms.

13–D. Although localized infections are not associated with pronounced viremia, they can have clinical features similar to viremic systemic infections.

14–B. Coxsackie B viruses are cardiotrophic and infect myocytes.

15–C. Viral oncogenes are found in many RNA tumor viruses. Both Rous sarcoma virus and human T-cell lymphotrophic virus type I are RNA tumor viruses, but only Rous sarcoma virus carries an oncogene (v-*src*).

16–B. The spherical virion of hepatitis B virus is called the Dane particle.

17–B. Genetic reassortment is the name given to the process whereby homologous pieces of RNA are exchanged between two different strains of influenza viruses replicating in the same cell.

18–B. Herpes simplex virus causes an encephalitis that localizes within the temporal lobe; western equine encephalomyelitis virus requires a mosquito vector and would not be observed during the winter months.

19–B. Subacute sclerosing panencephalitis is a late (10 or more years) complication of measles caused by a defective virus variant of the original infecting measles virus.

20–B. Some viruses, such as herpes simplex virus, can exist as noninfectious forms in the same cells of the body and later convert (reactivate) to infectious forms that cause disease.

21–B. Enzyme-linked immunosorbent assay (ELISA) is the most sensitive method of detecting antigens in the serum.

22–C. The target cells of human parvovirus B19 are progenitor erythroid cells; infections in patients with hemolytic anemia can be serious.

23–A. In permissive cells, adenovirus E1A protein is involved in the replication process, but in nonpermissive cells it can bind to cellular tumor suppressor protein p110^{Rb} and inactivate its normal cellular function, which results in cellular transformation.

24–D. The genetic material of poliovirus is single-stranded RNA, which can be translated into a large polyprotein that is subsequently cleaved into the individual viral proteins.

25–A. Nucleoside analogues inhibit viral replication by inhibiting viral DNA synthesis or function; they do not affect RNA replicases or block penetration.

26–A. Both the Recombivax-HB and Engerix-B vaccines for protection from hepatitis B virus contain the virus surface antigen prepared from yeast using recombinant DNA technology.

27–D. Respiratory syncytial virus is a serious respiratory disease pathogen for infants and has been associated with hospital-acquired (nosocomial) infections.

5

Mycology

I. Fungi

—are **eukaryotic.**

—are commonly called **yeasts, molds,** and **mushrooms.**

—have a complex cell wall.

—reproduce typically by asexual and sexual mechanisms.

A. Fungal cell wall

—protects cells from osmotic shock and determines shape.

—is composed primarily of polysaccharides, notably **chitin,** but also **glucans** and **mannans.**

—is **antigenic.**

B. Fungal cell membrane

—has a typical eukaryotic **bilayered** membrane.

—has **ergosterol** as the **dominant sterol** rather than cholesterol, which is an **important difference targeted by imidazoles and polyene antifungals.**

C. Fungal cellular components

—include eukaryotic **nuclei, mitochondria,** and numerous **vacuoles.**

—do not include chloroplasts.

D. Fungal forms

1. Hyphae

—are **filamentous subunits of molds and mushrooms.**

—**may lack septa (cross-walls);** these forms are referred to as **nonseptate, aseptate** (without regularly occurring cross-walls), or **coenocytic** (multinucleate) [Figure 5-1*A*].

—**may be septate** (see Figure 5-1*B*).

—may be **dematiaceous (dark colored) or hyaline (colorless).**

—**grow apically.** A mass (or **colony**) of hyphae is a **mycelium;** an **organized body** of hyphae is a **fruiting body** (e.g., a mushroom).

2. Yeasts

—are **single-celled** fungi, generally round to oval shaped (see Figure 5-1*D*).

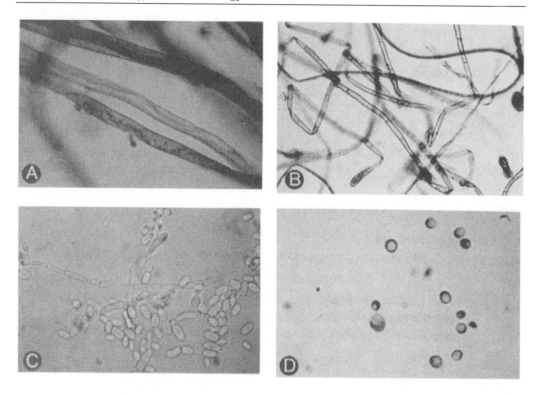

Figure 5-1. Fungal subunits. (*A*) Aseptate hyphae, (*B*) septate hyphae, (*C*) pseudohyphae, and (*D*) yeasts. (Reprinted with permission from Koneman EW, Roberts GD: *Practical Laboratory Mycology,* 3rd ed. Baltimore, Williams & Wilkins, 1985, pp 69 and 71.)

—generally reproduce by **budding (blastoconidia).**

—may have a capsule (e.g., *Cryptococcus*).

—of the genus *Candida* **may elongate** to develop **into pseudohyphae** (see Figure 5-1*C*). The yeast cells of ***Candida albicans*** (found on human epithelium) also germinate, forming sprout-like projections called **germ tubes** that extend to form **true hyphae.** Along with pseudohyphae, true hyphae are found in infected tissues.

3. **Dimorphic fungi**

—are capable of **converting from a yeast** or yeast-like form **to a filamentous form** and vice versa.

—are **stimulated to convert by environmental conditions** such as temperature and availability of nutrients.

—usually exist in the yeast or yeast-like form in a mammalian body and as the filamentous form in the environment (e.g., *Coccidioides* hyphae and arthroconidia in the desert sand). Remember "yeastie beasties in body heat; bold molds in the cold."

—include the major pathogens ***Blastomyces, Histoplasma, Coccidioides,*** and ***Sporothrix*** in the United States.

4. **Pseudohyphae**

—are a series of **elongated budding yeasts** that remain attached to each other and form a hyphal-like structure, but **with constrictions at the septations** (see Figure 5-1*C*).

—are characteristic of most *Candida* species.

5. **Fungal spores**

—may be formed either asexually (without nuclear fusion) or by a sexual process involving nuclear fusion and then meiosis. Most important in clinical isolates are the **asexual spores:**

a. **Conidia**—**asexual** spores formed on the outside of a specialized piece of hyphae (Figure 5-2*A*)

b. **Blastoconidia**—**buds** from a mother yeast cell (see Figure 5-2*B*)

c. **Arthroconidia**–**conidia** formed by the fragmentation (joint formation) of the hyphal strand (see Figure 5-2*C*)

II. Fungal Diseases—Overview

A. **Fungal allergies**

—are common; molds grow on any damp organic surface, and spores are constantly in the air. **Spores and volatile fungal toxins may play a role in "sick building syndrome."**

—generally occur in individuals with other allergies.

B. **Mycotoxicoses**

—may result from **ingestion of fungal-contaminated foods** (e.g., St.

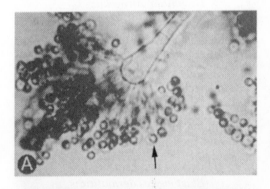
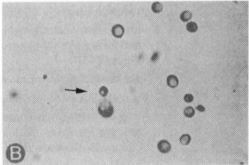
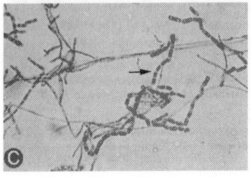

Figure 5-2. Asexual spores. (*A*) Conidia, (*B*) blasto-conidia (buds), and (*C*) arthroconidia. (Reprinted with permission from Koneman EW, Roberts GD: *Practical Laboratory Mycology,* 3rd ed. Baltimore, Williams & Wilkins, 1985, pp 71 and 73.)

Anthony's fire from ingestion of bread made with **ergot**-contaminated grain or turkey X disease caused by ingestion of poultry feed contaminated with aflatoxin, a carcinogen).

—also include **ingestion** of a **psychotropic** (e.g., *Psilocybe*) **or toxic** (e.g., *Amanita*) **mushroom.** These mushroom "poisonings" are also referred to as mycetismus.

C. Fungal infections (mycoses)

—range from **superficial to overwhelming systemic** infections that are rapidly fatal in the compromised host.

—are increasing in frequency as a result of increased use of antibiotics, corticosteroids, and cytotoxic drugs.

—are commonly classified as superficial, cutaneous, subcutaneous, and systemic infections; the systemic infections are subdivided into those caused by pathogenic fungi and those caused by opportunistic fungi (Table 5-1).

D. Diagnosis of fungal infections

1. Clinical manifestations suggestive of fungal infection

a. Pneumonia or flu-type infection that has lasted longer than or is more severe than a viral flu

b. Pneumonia resulting from exposure to dust with bird or bat

Table 5-1. Major Fungal Infections Commonly Found in the United States

Type	Disease	Causative Organism
Superficial mycoses	Tinea nigra	*Exophiala werneckii*
	Pityriasis versicolor	*Malassezia furfur*
Cutaneous mycoses	Dermatophytosis	Dermatophytes (*Microsporum, Trichophyton, Epidermophyton*)
	Candidiasis	*Candida*
Subcutaneous mycoses	Sporotrichosis	*Sporothrix schenckii*
	Chromyoblastomycosis	*Fonsecaea, Phialophora, Cladosporium*
	Eumycotic mycetoma	*Pseudallescheria boydii, Madurella*
Systemic mycoses	Pathogenic fungal infections	
	Coccidioidomycosis	*Coccidioides immitis*
	Histoplasmosis	*Histoplasma capsulatum*
	Blastomycosis	*Blastomyces dermatitidis*
	Paracoccidioidomycosis	*Paracoccidioides brasiliensis*
	Opportunistic fungal infections	
	Cryptococcal meningitis	*Cryptococcus neoformans*
	Malassezia fungemia	*Malassezia furfur*
	Aspergillosis	*Aspergillus fumigatus, Aspergillus* sp.
	Zygomycosis (phycomycosis)	*Mucor, Absidia, Rhizopus, Rhizomucor*
	Candidiasis, systemic and local	*Candida albicans, Candida* sp.

(Reprinted and modified with permission from Rippon JW: *Medical Mycology: The Pathogenic Fungi and Pathogenic Actinomycetes,* 3rd ed. Philadelphia, WB Saunders, 1988, p 3).

guano (e.g., a cave explorer) or to **desert sand** (e.g., southwestern United States)

c. **Chronic respiratory problem** with weight loss and night sweats

d. **Fever of unknown origin** that does not respond to antibacterial agents or initially responds and then worsens; mixed infections occur commonly in severely compromised patients

e. Any **infection with negative bacterial cultures** that does not respond to antibiotics and does not appear viral

f. **Signs of meningitis** in a compromised patient

2. **Microscopic examination—rapid methods**

   a. **Potassium hydroxide (KOH)** in a wet mount of skin scrapings breaks down the human cells, enhancing the visibility of the unaffected fungus.

   b. A **nigrosin or India ink** wet mount of cerebrospinal fluid (CSF) highlights the **capsule of *Cryptococcus neoformans;*** however, this method is insensitive (misses 50% of cases).

   c. A **Giemsa** or **Wright's stain** of thick blood or bone marrow smear may detect the intracellular *Histoplasma capsulatum.*

   d. **Calcofluor white stain "lights up"** fungal elements in exudates and small skin scales under a fluorescent microscope, giving them a fluorescent blue–white appearance.

3. **Histologic staining—special fungal stains for fixed tissues**

   —are necessary because fungi are not distinguished by color with hematoxylin and eosin (H and E) stain.

   a. **Gomori methenamine-silver stain** (fungi are stained dark **gray to black**)

   b. **Periodic acid-Schiff reaction** (fungi are stained **hot pink to red**)

   c. **Gridley fungus stain** (fungi are stained purplish **rose** with a yellow background)

   d. **Calcofluor white stain** (may be used on tissue sections; fungi have a **fluorescent blue–white** appearance on a dark background)

4. **Laboratory cultures for fungi**

   —must be specially ordered.

   —use special media (e.g., **Sabouraud's dextrose medium**), enriched media (e.g., **blood agar**) with antibiotics to inhibit bacterial growth, and enriched media with both **antibiotics and cycloheximide** (which inhibits many saprophytic fungi).

   a. **Identification of yeast cultures**

      —traditionally has been based on **morphologic characteristics** (presence of capsule, formation of germ tubes in serum, and morphology on cornmeal agar) and **biochemical tests** (urease, nitrate reduction, and carbohydrate assimilations and fermentations).

      —can also be accomplished with DNA probes, which are available for *Cryptococcus.*

   b. **Identification of filamentous fungal cultures**

      —is based on morphologic criteria or uses an immunologic method called **exoantigen testing,** in which antigens extracted from the culture to be identified are immunodiffused against known antisera.

—can also be accomplished with DNA probes, but only some are available.

5. **Serologic testing**

—is used **to identify patient antibodies** specific to the fungi.

—generally requires acute and convalescent sera.

—is complicated by **some cross-reactivity** among pathogenic fungi.

6. **Fungal antigen detection**

—uses known antibodies to identify circulating fungal antigens in a patient's serum, CSF, or urine.

E. **Treatment with antifungal drugs**

1. **Amphotericin B**

—is a **polyene** antifungal agent administered **intravenously** (IV).

—**binds to membranes with ergosterol** causing cell membrane damage.

—is the drug of choice in most life-threatening fungal infections.

2. **5-Fluorocytosine (5-FC, flucytosine)**

—is an **antimetabolite** that is administered **orally.**

—is used primarily in combination **with amphotericin B in the treatment of cryptococcal meningitis.** Some fungal infections develop a resistance to the drug.

3. **Miconazole**

—**inhibits ergosterol synthesis,** as do all imidazoles.

—is an **imidazole** requiring **IV** administration and exhibiting greater toxicity than ketoconazole.

—is used **topically** for mucocutaneous infections.

4. **Ketoconazole**

—is an **orally** administered **imidazole.**

—is useful in non–life-threatening systemic fungal infections, in chronic mucocutaneous candidiasis, and in many other cutaneous infections. It is ineffective against *Aspergillus*.

5. **Fluconazole**

—is a **systemic triazole** antifungal drug.

—is used in systemic **candidal infections** (e.g., **candidemias**), for coccidioidomycoses [including coccidioidal meningitis in acquired immunodeficiency syndrome (AIDS) patients], and as maintenance therapy after cryptococcal meningitis.

6. **Itraconazole**

—is an imidazole drug that is administered orally.

—may be used for treatment of non–life-threatening *Aspergillus* infection, moderate or severe histoplasmosis or blastomycosis, or sporotrichosis.

7. **Potassium iodide (KI)**

—is given **orally in milk** in the treatment of subcutaneous sporotrichosis, but it has no direct antifungal effect.

8. **Griseofulvin**

—is an **inhibitor of microtubules;** it is administered orally and localizes in the stratum corneum epidermidis.

—is effective against **dermatophytes** but may worsen yeast infections.

9. **Nystatin**

—is a **polyene** drug that is not absorbed from the gastrointestinal tract. It is used topically, intravaginally, or orally to treat **yeast infections** or reduce yeast growth in the gastrointestinal tract of compromised patients.

10. **Tolnaftate, miconazole, clotrimazole, econazole, ciclopirox, olamine, naftifine, haloprogin,** and **terbinafine**

—are antifungals used in the treatment of dermatophytic infections.

III. Superficial Mycoses

—affect the outermost layer of **skin** and **hair.**

—generally do not induce a cellular response to the infection.

—have primarily cosmetic symptoms.

—include pityriasis (tinea) versicolor, tinea nigra, and white or black piedra.

A. Pityriasis (tinea) versicolor

—is a fungal infection of the **stratum corneum epidermidis** that manifests as **hypopigmented or hyperpigmented skin patches, usually on the trunk of the body.** The color of the patch varies with pigmentation of skin, exposure to sun, and severity of disease.

—is **caused by *Malassezia furfur,*** which is found in skin scales as **short, curved, septate hyphae and yeast-like cells** ("spaghetti and meatballs" appearance).

—is diagnosed by KOH mount of skin scales; under a Wood's lamp, it fluoresces yellow.

B. Tinea nigra

—is a superficial infection of the stratum corneum epidermidis on the palmar surfaces causing benign, flat, dark, melanoma-like lesions.

—is caused by a dematiaceous fungus that produces melanin, which colors the skin.

C. Piedra

—is a fungal infection of the **hair shaft** that produces hair breakage.

IV. Cutaneous Mycoses

—may be a **dermatophytosis** caused by any of the dermatophytes, a homogeneous group of filamentous fungi with three genera, ***Epidermophyton, Microsporum,*** and *Trichophyton,* or may be a **yeast infection** caused by some of the yeasts, primarily *Candida* (Table 5-2).

—**may give rise (during successful treatment) to a hypersensitive state known as the dermatophytid (or "id") reaction, which is a result of circulating fungal antigens.**

—may involve the **skin, hair,** or **nails.**

—are classified by the area of the body involved.

—may be acquired from animals (**zoophilic**), in which case the lesions are **quite inflammatory.** Two common zoophilic species are *Microsporum canis* and *Trichophyton rubrum.*

—may be acquired from humans (**anthropophilic**), in which case there is less inflammation. Two common anthropophilic species are *Epidermophyton floccosum* and *Microsporum audouinii.*

—may fluoresce under a Wood's lamp when the infecting agent is *Microsporum.*

—are diagnosed primarily by microscopic examination of skin, hair, or nail material mounted in 10% KOH.

A. **Tinea capitis (ringworm of the scalp skin and hair)**

—is diagnosed by Wood's lamp examination (most species of *Microsporum* fluoresce) and microscopic examination of a KOH mount of skin and plucked hairs.

1. **Anthropophilic tinea capitis** (spread by head gear such as hats and combs)

—occurs in prepubescent **children** and is **epidemic.**

—is caused by *M audouinii.*

—is usually **noninflammatory** and produces **gray patches** of hair.

2. **Zoophilic tinea capitis (nonepidemic)**

—is usually transmitted by **pets** and occasionally by **farm animals,** which also need to be treated.

—is most commonly caused by *M canis* or by *Trichophyton mentagrophytes.*

—is more **inflammatory** and occurs with kerion in *T mentagrophytes* infections.

—may result in temporary alopecia, kerion, keloid, and inflammation.

3. **Black-dot tinea capitis**

Table 5-2. Tissues Infected by Dermatophytes and *Candida*

Group	Genus	Tissue Infected			Fluoresces
		Hair	Skin	Nails	
Dermatophytes	*Trichophyton*	yes	yes	yes	. . .
	Epidermophyton	. . .	yes	yes	. . .
	Microsporum	yes	yes	. . .	yes
Yeasts	*Candida*	. . .	yes	yes	. . .

—occurs in **adults** and is a **chronic infection** characterized by **hair breakage,** followed by filling of follicles with dark conidia.

—is caused by *Trichophyton tonsurans.*

4. **Favus (tinea favosa)**

—occurs in both **children and adults.**

—is caused by *Trichophyton schoenleinii.*

—is a **highly contagious and severe form of tinea capitis with scutula formation and permanent hair loss** caused by scarring. Prophylaxis of all close contacts is needed.

B. **Tinea barbae**

—is an acute or chronic **folliculitis** of the beard, neck, or face.

—is most commonly caused by *Trichophyton verrucosum* (the most common causative agent in dairy farmers, acquired from cows), *T mentagrophytes,* and *T rubrum.*

—results in **pustular or dry, scaly lesions.**

—may be superinfected with bacteria.

C. **Tinea corporis**

—is a dermatophytic infection of the **glabrous skin.** (Where the infection is limited to inside skinfolds, it is usually a **yeast infection** rather than a dermatophytic infection.)

—is most commonly caused by *T rubrum, T mentagrophytes,* or *M canis.*

—is characterized by **annular lesions** with an active border that may be pustular or vesicular.

D. **Tinea cruris**

—is an acute or chronic fungal infection of the **groin,** commonly called jock itch.

—is often accompanied by athlete's foot, which also must be treated.

—is caused by *E floccosum, T rubrum, T mentagrophytes,* or yeasts like *Candida.*

E. **Tinea pedis**

—is an acute to chronic fungal infection of the **feet,** commonly called athlete's foot.

—is most commonly caused by *T rubrum, T mentagrophytes,* or *E floccosum.*

—may be superinfected with bacteria, which may require antibiotic treatment before tinea pedis is treated.

1. **Chronic intertriginous tinea pedis** (usually white macerated tissue between the **toes)**

2. **Chronic dry, scaly tinea pedis** (hyperkeratotic scales on the **heels, soles, or sides of the feet)**

3. **Vesicular tinea pedis** (vesicles and vesiculopustules)

V. Subcutaneous Mycoses

—are mycoses that generally begin with **traumatic implantation** of normally saprobic fungi that remain localized in the cutaneous and subcutaneous tissues. In some cases, there is limited, slow spread via the lymphatics.

—are uncommon in the United States. Sporotrichosis, mycetoma (eumycotic and actinomycotic), and chromomycosis have been reported.

A. Sporotrichosis

—is caused by *Sporothrix schenckii,* which is a dimorphic fungus that grows at 37°C as a cigar-shaped, budding yeast and at 25°C as a sporulating hyphae. *S schenckii* is found in or **on plant materials such as roses, plum trees, sphagnum moss,** and mine timbers and is **traumatically introduced** into subcutaneous tissues.

—is a **subcutaneous, nodular, fungal disease** that is **generally not painful** and **may spread via the lymphatics** (lymphocutaneous sporotrichosis).

—classically presents with a **chain of lesions on the extremities;** lower lesions are often ulcerating and follow the lymph nodes along a limb.

—is known as the "**rose gardener's disease.**"

—is diagnosed by culture; histologic findings are generally negative.

—is treated with itraconazole or **KI drops** given orally in milk.

B. Eumycotic mycetoma

—is a subcutaneous fungal disease characterized by **swelling, sinus tract formation** (if not treated), and presence of "**sulfur" granules** (microcolonies) in the exudate.

—is caused by *Pseudallescheria boydii* and *Madurella,* which are **filamentous true fungi** found in soil or on vegetation; entry is by traumatic implantation.

—usually occurs in rural, third-world agricultural workers in the tropics.

C. Chromoblastomycosis

—is one of a **group of infections** caused by dematiaceous fungi and seen in tissues as dark, yeast-like bodies.

—begins with **traumatic implantation** of the spores, usually on a **limb or shoulder;** this is often seen in farm workers in the tropics.

—has **colored lesions** that start out scaly and become **raised, cauliflower-like lesions.**

VI. Fungal Pneumonias and Systemic Mycoses

—are caused by inhaled **pathogenic fungi,** which may cause disease in healthy individuals and often disseminate in compromised hosts.

—in the United States are caused by the **dimorphic fungal pathogens** *Histoplasma, Coccidioides,* and *Blastomyces,* which have specific environmental associations, produce airborne spores, and are endemic to specific geographic regions.

—occur primarily in people who are exposed to large amounts of **airborne dust or sand** containing the fungus.

—occur in three disease forms: **acute self-limited pulmonary** (asymptomatic to severe), **chronic** (pulmonary or disseminated), and **disseminated.** Dissemination may occur during the primary infection or may arise years later when the person has T-cell immunosuppression. These reactivations result from viable organisms being released from granulomas.

A. Histoplasmosis

—is a granulomatous **fungal infection caused by *H capsulatum.***

—must be differentiated from influenza and other pneumonias.

—infections are most often **(95%) inapparent, subclinical, or self-resolving pneumonia,** depending on the health, lung structure, and immune system of the host and on the dose of the inoculum.

1. *Histoplasma capsulatum*

—is a small, **dimorphic** fungus that is a **facultative intracellular yeast,** localizing **in humans** in phagocytic cells, including circulating monocytes.

—does not have a capsule.

—is found as the **filamentous form** in **soil enriched with bat or bird guano.**

—can be isolated from most areas of the world; the **major endemic regions are in the drainage areas of the Ohio, Missouri, and Mississippi rivers and the St. Lawrence Seaway.**

2. Laboratory diagnosis

a. Microscopic examination for **small intracellular yeasts** in thick blood, bone marrow smear, buffy coat, or liver biopsy, all stained with Wright's or Giemsa stain, or in a KOH mount of sputum

b. Culture of sputum or bronchial washings and **blood** for dimorphic fungus

(1) At **25°C** in the laboratory or in nature, *H capsulatum* is found as **hyphae** with round, **tuberculate macroconidia** and small, tear-shaped microconidia.

(2) Inside human cells or at **37°C** on enriched medium, *H capsulatum* is a **small, nondescript, budding yeast.**

c. Serologic testing, including complement fixation, immunodiffusion, and radioimmunoassay

d. Skin testing

—detects exposure to the antigen but **does not prove** active disease.

—if negative in a patient with known active histoplasmosis, is a poor prognostic sign.

—can boost antibody levels if performed before serology testing.

3. Forms of histoplasmosis

a. Acute histoplasmosis

—is known as the "**fungus flu.**"

—ranges from an **asymptomatic to a severe** flu-like but self-resolving **pulmonary disease** with a transient, hematogenous spread of *Histoplasma* in macrophages.

—shows a highly variable x-ray pattern with hilar lymphadenopathy; calcification is extremely common on healing, especially in young persons. Characteristically, **both lungs** are involved.

—is treated in healthy persons with bed rest and good nutrition.

  b. **Disseminated histoplasmosis (chronic to fulminant)**

  (1) **Symptoms** include

  —**mucous membrane lesions or focus of infection other than the lungs.** (Pulmonary symptoms are not always present.)

  —**prominent hepatosplenomegaly.**

  —decreases in white blood cells, hemoglobin, and platelets.

  —disseminated intravascular coagulation.

  —weight loss.

  —Addison's disease (in approximately 50% of fulminant cases).

  (2) **Predisposition to disseminated histoplasmosis**

  —occurs in individuals with underlying **immune cell defects** (e.g., patients with AIDS, T-cell deficits, or lymphoma).

  —occurs in children younger than 1 year of age who appear to have a **defect in dendritic cell function.**

B. **Blastomycosis (North American)**

—is a **pulmonary, disseminated, or cutaneous** fungal disease that is **caused by the dimorphic fungus *Blastomyces dermatitidis.***

—type of infection depends on the patient's underlying state of health.

  1. *Blastomyces dermatitidis*

  —is a **thermally dimorphic fungus.**

  —is found in the **tissues** as a **large,** mainly free **yeast with a double refractile wall** and **broad-based buds.**

  —is most likely **inhaled** as **conidia** and transformed into the yeast form in the lung.

  —is **endemic mainly to areas around the St. Lawrence, Mississippi, and Ohio rivers and to the southeastern United States (excluding Florida).**

  —has been environmentally associated with **rotting wood, including beaver dams.**

  2. **Laboratory diagnosis of blastomycosis**

  a. **Radiology**—infiltrative pattern, nodular pattern, and single lesion resembling a neoplasm are most common. Generally there is no calcification.

  b. **Direct microscopic examination**—pus, skin scrapings, or sputum is examined after KOH digestion for the **double-walled, large yeasts with broad-based buds** characteristic of *Blastomyces.*

  c. **Culture for dimorphic fungi**—is performed in the laboratory at or below 30°C to grow the filamentous form. Conversion to yeasts at 37°C, morphology, and DNA probes are used to identify the culture.

    d. Pathology—*B dermatitidis* may be extracellular or may be found in giant cells; suppurative reaction is most common.

    e. Serologic testing—is performed by complement fixation and immunodiffusion, although cross-reactions are still a problem; radioimmunoassay is more sensitive.

3. Forms of blastomycosis

    a. Acute pulmonary blastomycosis

        —may resolve without treatment; however, **itraconazole** is often used.

    b. Chronic pulmonary blastomycosis

        —usually has suppurative or granulomatous **lesions** in the upper lobe.

        —is often misdiagnosed as carcinoma.

        —most often occurs with an **infiltrative pattern** without cavitation or calcification.

    c. Disseminated blastomycosis

        —generally occurs in individuals with a low stimulation index to the antigen and a negative skin test.

        —is caused by **organisms** carried by macrophages to remote sites, most commonly skin and bones.

        —is often diagnosed by the demonstration of broad-based, budding **yeasts** in KOH mounts of scrapings of skin lesion edges.

C. Coccidioidomycosis

  —is a subclinical, acute or chronic pulmonary, or disseminated fungal **infection caused by *Coccidioides immitis*.**

  —is commonly known as "**valley fever.**"

1. *Coccidioides immitis*

    —is a **thermally dimorphic** fungus.

    —is found **in the human body as large spherules within which endospores develop;** spherules break and release **endospores,** which enlarge to form new spherules.

    —is found in **sand** as **arthroconidia,** which are inhaled.

    —is highly endemic in the San Joaquin Valley and the Lower Sonoran Desert of the **southwestern United States.**

2. Laboratory diagnosis of coccidioidomycosis

    a. Direct examination—is made of scrapings of any lesions, specimens of sputum, or bronchial washings.

    b. Culture—is only done by reference laboratories.

    c. Serologic testing

        (1) Tube precipitin test measures **IgM.**

        (2) Complement fixation test measures **IgG.**

        (3) Latex particle **agglutination and immunodiffusion tests** are used as screening tools in endemic areas and can detect 93% of cases.

      d. Skin test—becomes **positive** early in the infection; anergy is a poor prognostic sign.

  3. **Forms of coccidioidomycosis**

      a. Acute self-limiting coccidioidomycosis is **similar to acute histoplasmosis** except that erythema nodosum or multiforme is more likely to be present.

      b. Chronic coccidioidomycosis does not self-resolve.

      c. Disseminated coccidioidomycosis is similar to disseminated histoplasmosis with dissemination to the meninges and mucous membranes occurring in many AIDS patients in the endemic region. Pregnant women who acquire *Coccidioides* in the third trimester, African Americans, and certain other races have an increased risk of dissemination.

VII. Opportunistic Mycoses (Table 5-3)

—range from annoying or painful **mucous membrane or cutaneous infections** in mildly compromised patients **to serious disseminated infections** in severely compromised patients.

—are caused by endogenous or ubiquitous organisms of low inherent virulence that cause infection in debilitated, compromised patients.

—are caused most commonly by *Candida, Cryptococcus, Geotrichum, Aspergillus, Rhizopus, Mucor,* and *Absidia.*

—may be caused by any fungus if a patient is immunocompromised.

—are increasing as the number of compromised patients increases.

—may be life threatening in compromised patients, but are rarely serious in well-nourished, drug-free, healthy persons.

  A. Candidiases

    —are acute to chronic fungal infections involving the mouth, vagina, skin, nails, bronchi or lung, alimentary tract, blood stream, urinary tract, and, less commonly, the heart or meninges.

    —**are caused by *C. albicans*** or other species of *Candida.*

    —are predisposed by extremes of age, wasting and nutritional diseases, excessive moisture, pregnancy, diabetes, long-term antibiotic and steroid use, indwelling catheters, immunosuppression, and AIDS.

    —are generally treated with imidazoles, polyenes, or both.

    1. ***Candida albicans***

      —is seen as yeasts on body surfaces.

      —is part of the **normal flora of the skin, mucous membranes, and gastrointestinal tract,** along with other *Candida* species. Normal colonization must be distinguished from infection, when *Candida* invades the tissues forming pseudohyphae and true hyphae.

      —is seen in infected tissues as **pseudohyphae, true hyphae,** blastoconidia, and yeast cells.

    2. **Laboratory diagnosis of candidiases**

      a. KOH mount of skin or nail scrapings or exudate

      b. Demonstration of the **presence of pseudohyphae or true hyphae** in the tissues

Table 5-3. Symptoms and Conditions Associated With Opportunistic Mycoses

Symptoms	Common Underlying Condition	Fungal Disease
Vaginitis (erythema and pain)	Antibiotic use; pregnancy	*Candida* vaginitis
Facial swelling; lethargy; red exudate from eyes and nares	Diabetes, leukemia	Rhinocerebral mucormycosis
Fever without pulmonary symptoms	Indwelling catheter; lipid supplements	Fungemia (*Candida* or *Malassezia*)
Fever; pain on urination	Urinary catheter	Urinary candidiasis
Difficulty in swallowing	AIDS	Esophageal candidiasis
Meningeal symptoms	AIDS	Cryptococcal meningitis, *Histoplasma* or coccidioidal meningitis, *Candida* cerebritis
	Severe neutropenia	*Aspergillus* central nervous system infection
	Hodgkin's disease; diabetes	Cryptococcal meningitis (chronic)
Pulmonary symptoms	Immunocompromised patient, particularly if neutropenic	Invasive *Aspergillosis*
	AIDS	*Pneumocystis* pneumonia Histoplasmosis, coccidioidomycosis
	Alcoholism (urban)	Sporotrichosis (pulmonary)
Hemoptysis	Previous lung damage, especially cavities	Aspergilloma
Endocarditis	Intravenous drug abuse	*Candida* or *Aspergillus* endocarditis
Enteritis (often with anal pruritus)	Antibiotic use	*Candida* enteritis (irritable bowel syndrome)
Whitish covering in mouth	Premature infants, children on antibiotics	*Candida* thrush
Corners of mouth sore	Elderly suffering from malnourishment	Perlèche
Sore gums	Dentures	Denture stomatitis or allergy to antifungal used in treatment of denture stomatitis
Skin lesions; endophthalmitis	Indwelling catheter	Candidemia

    c. **Cultures** of normally sterile parts of the body (such as CSF), with cultures **identified by germ tube** ("sprouts" formed from the yeast cells) **formation** and morphologic and chemical tests

    d. **Serologic testing** demonstrating high levels of *Candida* precipitins or antigens

    e. **Chromatographic methods** to detect fungal products

  3. Forms of candidiases

    a. **Oral thrush**

      —is a yeast infection of the oral **mucocutaneous membranes.**

      —manifests as **white curd-like patches** in the oral cavity.

—occurs in premature infants, older infants being treated with antibiotics, immunosuppressed patients on long-term antibiotics, and AIDS patients.

b. Vulvovaginitis or vaginal thrush

—is a **yeast infection** of the vagina that tends to recur.

—manifests with a **thick yellow-white discharge,** a burning sensation, curd-like patches on the vaginal mucosa, and inflammation of the peritoneum.

—is predisposed by diabetes, antibiotic therapy, oral contraceptive use, and pregnancy.

c. Cutaneous candidiasis

—involves the **nails, skin folds (visible as creamy growth), or groin.**

—may be eczematoid or vesicular and pustular.

—is predisposed by **moist conditions.**

d. Alimentary tract disease

—is usually an extension of oral thrush and may include **esophagitis** and, ultimately, the **entire gastrointestinal tract.**

—is found in patients with AIDS or other **immunosuppressive disorders,** particularly those patients on long-term antibiotic therapy.

—is reduced in highly susceptible populations by fungal prophylaxis.

e. Candidemias or blood-borne infections

—occur most commonly in patients with **indwelling catheters** or gastrointestinal tract overgrowth; these infections are manifested by fever, macronodular skin lesions, and endophthalmitis.

f. Endocarditis

—occurs in patients who have manipulated or damaged valves or in IV drug abusers.

g. Bronchopulmonary infection

—occurs in patients with chronic lung disease; it is usually manifested by persistent cough.

h. Cerebromeningeal infection

—may occur in compromised patients.

i. Chronic mucocutaneous candidiasis

—is a chronic, often disfiguring infection of the **epithelial surfaces** of the body.

—is diagnosed microscopically and by the lack of cell-mediated immunity (anergy) to *Candida* antigens.

B. *Malassezia furfur* septicemia

—is a **blood-borne infection** caused by the lipophilic skin organism *M. furfur.*

—occurs in patients (primarily neonates) who are on **IV lipid emulsions.**

—is diagnosed by culturing blood on fungal medium that is either lightly overlaid with sterile olive oil or has lipids incorporated into the medium.

—may resolve by halting the lipid supplements.

C. Cryptococcal meningitis

—is the most common clinical form of cryptococcal infection. (Cryptococcal pneumonia is generally only seen in pigeon breeders who are assumed to be exposed to high levels of *C neoformans*).

—is caused by *C neoformans*.

1. *Cryptococcus neoformans*

 —is a **yeast** that possesses an **antigenic polysaccharide capsule.**

 —may be isolated from fruit, milk, vegetation, soil, and **pigeon feces.**

 —is considered to be an **opportunist** in the presence of underlying disease in patients with Hodgkin's disease, leukemias, or leukocyte enzyme deficiency diseases.

2. **Clinical presentation—cryptococcal meningitis or meningoencephalitis**

 —presents most commonly with a headache of increasing severity, usually with fever, followed by typical signs of meningitis.

 —is the most common meningitis occurring in AIDS patients.

 —also occurs in diabetic patients and patients with Hodgkin's disease.

3. **Laboratory diagnosis**

 a. **Detection of cryptococcal capsular material in the CSF** by the cryptococcal antigen **latex-particle agglutination test**

 b. Demonstration of **encapsulated yeast in CSF sediment** on a wet mount in nigrosin or **India ink** (However, this technique misses approximately 50% of the culturally proven cases of cryptococcal meningitis.)

 c. Confirmation by isolation of *C neoformans* in culture of CSF

D. Aspergilloses

—are a variety of **infections** and **allergic** diseases that are caused by *Aspergillus fumigatus* and a variety of other species of *Aspergillus.*

1. *Aspergillus fumigatus*

 —is a ubiquitous filamentous fungus (one of our major recyclers) whose **airborne spores (conidia)** are constantly in the air.

 —is recognized both in tissue and in culture by its characteristic septate hyphae with **dichotomous branching and an acute branching angle.**

 —is an **opportunistic** organism.

2. **Forms of aspergilloses**

 a. **Allergic bronchopulmonary aspergillosis**

 —is an **allergic disease** in which the organism colonizes the mucous plugs formed in the lungs but does not invade lung tissues.

 —is diagnosed by the finding of high titers of IgE antibodies to *Aspergillus.*

 b. **Aspergilloma**

 —is a roughly spherical growth of *Aspergillus* in preexisting lung cavities; growth does not invade the lung tissues.

—presents clinically as **recurrent hemoptysis.**

—is diagnosed by radiologic methods; an "air sign" shift will be seen with a change in the position of the patient.

c. Invasive aspergillosis

—occurs most commonly during severe **neutropenia** in leukemia and transplant patients.

—most commonly occurs as fever of unknown origin in patients with fewer than 500 neutrophils/mm^3 and pneumonia. It may begin as sinusitis; from either the sinuses or the lungs, it disseminates to any part of the body, most frequently the brain.

—is diagnosed by microscopy and culture of lung biopsy material.

—is treated aggressively with amphotericin B or itraconazole, but it still has a high fatality rate unless neutrophil numbers become elevated.

E. Zygomycoses

—are also known as **phycomycoses or mucormycoses.**

—are infections most commonly caused by the genera *Rhizopus, Absidia, Mucor,* and *Rhizomucor,* which belong to the phylum Zygomycota (**the nonseptate fungi**).

1. Zygomycota

—have **nonseptate** hyphae.

—**grow rapidly.**

—**have a predilection for invading blood vessels and the brain.**

2. Rhinocerebral infection

—is the most common form of zygomycosis; it occurs in patients with **acidotic diabetes.**

—presents with **facial swelling** and **blood-tinged exudate in the turbinate bones and eyes, mental lethargy, and fixated pupils.**

—must be diagnosed rapidly, usually by a KOH mount of necrotic tissue or exudates from the eye, ear, or nose.

—is **rarely treated successfully;** treatment consists of **control of diabetes, surgical débridement,** and aggressive treatment with **amphotericin B.**

F. Pneumocystis pneumonitis and pneumonia

—are infections caused by *Pneumocystis carinii.*

1. *Pneumocystis carinii*

—**is considered a fungus, based on molecular biologic techniques such as ribotyping and DNA homology.**

—is an **obligate parasite of humans (cannot be grown in vitro) but is extracellular,** growing on the surfactant layer over the alveolar epithelium.

—colonizes most humans early in life, without apparent disease.

—causes severe disease only in malnourished infants, immunosuppressed patients, and AIDS patients with low $CD4^+$ cell counts.

—is seen in the alveolar spaces as both small trophozoites and larger cysts. Cysts are seen in methenamine silver or calcofluor stains to contain 4–8 intracystic bodies (called nuclei or sporozoites).

2. **Forms of disease**

   a. **Interstitial plasma cell pneumonitis**

   —occurs in malnourished infants, transplant patients, patients on antineoplastic chemotherapy, and patients on corticosteroid therapy.

   —is characterized on radiographs by a patchy, diffuse appearance, sometimes referred to as a ground-glass appearance.

   —is diagnosed as for *Pneumocystis carinii* pneumonia.

   b. ***Pneumocystis carinii* pneumonia**

   —was the major cause of death in AIDS patients and is currently responsible for approximately 30% of deaths in AIDS patients.

   —causes morbidity and mortality when $CD4^+$ counts decrease to less than $200/mm^3$ unless prevented with prophylaxis.

   —lacks plasma cells in the alveolar spaces of AIDS patients.

   —has a PO_2 decline that is out of proportion to radiologic appearance.

   —is characterized on radiographs as having a ground-glass appearance.

   —is diagnosed by microscopy of biopsy specimen or alveolar fluids (Giemsa, specific fluorescent antibody, toluidine blue, methenamine silver, or calcofluor stains). Presence of serum antibodies is not a useful indicator of infection because almost all healthy and immunocompromised individuals have antibodies to *Pneumocystis*.

   —is treated prophylactically with trimethoprim-sulfamethoxazole or trimethoprim and dapsone.

VIII. Review Chart

—Table 5-4 summarizes superficial, cutaneous, mucocutaneous, subcutaneous, and allergic fungal diseases in a format useful for solving case-history questions on the USMLE.

—Table 5-5 summarizes systemic infections in immunocompetent patients.

Table 5-4. Symptoms and Clues to Diagnosis of Fungal Diseases in Generally Healthy Patients With Superficial, Cutaneous, Mucocutaneous, Subcutaneous, or Allergic Fungal Diseases*

Presenting Symptoms	Possible Disease	Clues†	Most Common Fungal Agent
Hyperpigmented or hypopigmented skin macules with little inflammation, generally on trunk of body	Pityriasis versicolor	KOH: yeast-like cells and short, curved, septate hyphae	*Malassezia furfur*
Cutaneous lesions with various degrees of inflammation	Tineas	KOH: hyphae and arthroconidia	Dermatophytes: *Epidermophyton, Trichophyton, Microsporum*
	Candidiasis of skin	KOH: pseudohyphae and yeasts	*Candida albicans* and related species
Mucocutaneous lesion (vaginitis, diaper rash)	Candidiasis	KOH: pseudohyphae and yeast	*Candida albicans* and related species
Subcutaneous lesions following lymph nodes or solitary nodule	Sporotrichosis	KOH: cigar-shaped yeast in tissue Hyphae and conidia at 25°C	*Sporothrix schenckii* (most likely in the United States)
Colorful subcutaneous lesions, often pedunculated	Chromoblastomycosis	KOH: dark, yeast-like cells with planar septations (sclerotic bodies) in giant cells	*Fonsecaea pedrosoi* and related forms
Subcutaneous swelling with sinus tracts and granules in exudate	Mycotic mycetoma	Granules that are microcolonies of fungus	*Pseudallescheria boydii*
Allergic reactions	Allergic bronchopulmonary aspergillosis	High IgE levels against *Aspergillus*	*Aspergillus* sp.

*See Table 5-3 for causes for infections in immunocompromised patients.
†Examination of skin scrapings or other tissue mounted in and cleared with potassium hydroxide (KOH) and examined microscopically.

Table 5-5. Symptoms and Clues to Diagnosis of Fungal Diseases in Generally Healthy Patients With Systemic Symptoms

Presenting Symptoms	Possible Disease	Clues	Most Common Fungal Agent
Acute pulmonary disease (cough, fever, night sweats)	Histoplasmosis	Exposure to soil/dust contaminated with bird (especially chicken and starling) or bat feces	*Histoplasma capsulatum*
		Environmental form or 25°C culture: hyphae with micro-conidia and large tuberculate macroconidia	
		Endemic region: Ohio, Mississippi, Missouri riverbeds	
		Tissue: small, intracellular yeast	
	Blastomycosis	Exposure to rotting wood	*Blastomyces dermatitidis*
		Environmental form or 25°C culture: hyphae with micro-conidia	
		Endemic region: as for *Histoplasma* plus southeastern seaboard of the U.S.	
		Tissue: large, budding yeast with double refractile wall	
	Coccidioidomycosis	Exposure to desert sand with arthroconidia	*Coccidioides immitis*
		Environmental form: hyphae with arthroconidia	
		Endemic region: deserts of the southwestern U.S.	
		Tissue form: spherules with endospores	
Chronic pulmonary disease (cough, fever, night sweats, weight loss, protracted)	Histoplasmosis; blastomycosis; coccidioidomycosis	Same as for acute pulmonary disease; sedimentation rate elevated	Same as above
Disseminated disease (extrapulmonary sites such as skin, mucous membrane lesions, brain)	Histoplasmosis; blastomycosis; coccidioidomycosis	Same as for acute pulmonary disease; once diagnosed, anergy (negative skin test)	Same as above

Review Test

1. A florist presents with a subcutaneous lesion on the hand, which she thinks resulted from a jab wound she received while she was making a sphagnum moss-wire frame for a floral wreath. The lesion has not healed despite use of antibacterial cream and has begun to spread up her arm with the lymph node raised and red and beginning to look like it might ulcerate, like the original lesion. The lymph node above is also beginning to redden and is slightly raised. What is most likely to be an appropriate treatment for this infection?

(A) Oral itraconazole or potassium iodide
(B) Miconazole cream
(C) Cortisone cream
(D) Oral griseofulvin
(E) Penicillin

2. What would you expect to see in the above patient's tissue biopsy?

(A) Lots of hyphae
(B) Long, branching hyphae with acute angles
(C) Yeasts with broad-based buds
(D) Cigar-shaped yeasts
(E) Yeast with multiple buds (mariner's wheel)

3. A patient presents with paranasal swelling and bloody exudate from both his eyes and nares, and he is nearly comatose. What is the most likely compromising condition underlying this infection caused by *Rhizopus, Mucor,* or *Absidia* (phylum Zygomycota, class Phycomycetes)?

(A) AIDS
(B) Diabetes (with patient in ketoacidosis)
(C) Neutropenia
(D) B-cell defects
(E) Chronic sinusitis

4. What type of fungal skin lesions would show only hyphae and possible arthroconidia in a biopsy?

(A) Blastomycosis (disseminated)
(B) Chronic mucocutaneous candidiasis
(C) Coccidioidomycosis
(D) Dermatophytosis (e.g., tinea pedis)
(E) Pityriasis versicolor

5. A severely neutropenic patient presents with pneumonia. Bronchial alveolar fluid shows dichotomously branching (generally with acute angles), septate hyphae. What is the most likely causative agent?

(A) *Aspergillus*
(B) *Cryptococcus*
(C) *Candida*
(D) *Malassezia*
(E) *Rhizopus*

6. What is a mass of fungal filaments called?

(A) Pseudohypha
(B) Hypha
(C) Mycelium
(D) Septum
(E) Yeast

7. A premature infant on intravenous nutrients and high-lipid fluids has developed a septicemia that cultures out on blood agar only when overlaid with sterile olive oil. What is the most likely causative agent?

(A) *Aspergillus*
(B) *Candida*
(C) *Cryptococcus*
(D) *Malassezia*
(E) *Sporothrix*

8. A filamentous fungus subunit is a

(A) coenocyte.
(B) hypha.
(C) mycelium.
(D) septum.
(E) yeast.

9. Which of the following oral antifungal agents inhibits microtubule formation and may be used to treat dermatophytic infections?

(A) Amphotericin B
(B) Griseofulvin
(C) Ketoconazole
(D) Miconazole
(E) Nystatin

10. A 15-year-old dirt biker visiting southern California has pneumonia caused by an organism whose environmental form consists of hyphae that break up into arthroconidia, which become airborne. What is the agent?

(A) *Aspergillus fumigatus*
(B) *Blastomyces dermatitidis*
(C) *Coccidioides immitis*
(D) *Histoplasma capsulatum*
(E) *Sporothrix schenckii*

11. Which of the following inhibits ergosterol synthesis, is important in treating *Candida* fungemias, and is used orally to suppress relapses of cryptococcal meningitis in AIDS patients?

(A) Amphotericin B
(B) Fluconazole
(C) Griseofulvin
(D) Miconazole
(E) Nystatin

12. A patient has splotchy hypopigmentation on the chest and back with only slight itchiness. What is most likely to be seen on a potassium hydroxide (KOH) mount of the skin scraping?

(A) Yeasts, pseudohyphae, and true hyphae
(B) Filaments with lots of arthroconidia
(C) Clusters of round fungal cells with short, curved, septate hyphae
(D) Darkly pigmented, round cells with sharp interior septations
(E) Cigar-shaped yeasts

13. A patient has a dry, scaly, erythematous penis. Skin scales stained with calcofluor white show fluorescent blue-white yeasts and a few pseudohyphae. What is the causative agent of this dermatophytic look-alike?

(A) *Candida*
(B) *Trichosporon*
(C) *Trichophyton*
(D) *Malassezia*
(E) *Microsporum*

14. A recent immigrant from rural Brazil presents with a swollen face and extremely poor dental hygiene, including loss of an adult tooth, which appears to be the focus of the current infection. There are two open ulcers on the outside of the swollen cheek. Small yellow "grains" are seen in one of the ulcers. Gram stain shows purple-staining fine filaments. What is the most likely disease?

(A) Actinomycotic mycetoma
(B) Chromomycosis
(C) Eumycotic mycetoma
(D) Sporotrichosis
(E) Paracoccidioidomycosis

15. A patient who is a recent immigrant from a tropical, remote, rural area with no medical care is now working with a group of migrant crop harvesters. He has a large, raised, colored, cauliflower-like ankle lesion. Darkly pigmented, yeast-like sclerotic bodies are seen in the tissue biopsy. Which of the following is the most likely diagnosis?

(A) Actinomycotic mycetoma
(B) Chromoblastomycosis
(C) Eumycotic mycetoma
(D) Sporotrichosis
(E) Tinea nigra

16. A premature baby, now 4 days old, has developed a white coating on her buccal mucosa extending onto her lips. It appears to be painful. What is the most likely causative agent?

(A) *Actinomyces*
(B) *Aspergillus*
(C) *Candida*
(D) *Fusobacterium*
(E) *Microsporum*

17. Which of the following stains allows differentiation of fungus from human tissue by staining the fungus a pink-red color?

(A) Calcofluor white stain
(B) Gomori methenamine-silver stain
(C) Periodic acid-Schiff stain
(D) Hematoxylin and eosin stain

18. A normally healthy 8-year-old boy from Florida is visiting friends on a farm in Iowa during the month of July. He presents July 28 with a fever, cough, and lower respiratory symptoms (no upper respiratory tract symptoms). He has been ill for 4 days. His chest sounds are consistent with pneumonia, so a chest radiograph is obtained. The radiograph shows small, patchy infiltrates with hilar adenopathy. His blood smear shows small, nondescript yeast forms inside monocytic cells. What is the most likely causative agent?

(A) *Aspergillus fumigatus*
(B) *Blastomyces dermatitidis*
(C) *Coccidioides immitis*
(D) *Histoplasma capsulatum*
(E) *Pneumocystis carinii*

19. Which of the following is a polyene antifungal agent used for many life-threatening fungal infections?

(A) Amphotericin B
(B) Griseofulvin
(C) Itraconazole
(D) Miconazole
(E) Nystatin

20. A logger undergoing chemotherapy for cancer has developed pneumonia and skin lesions. Biopsy of the skin lesions demonstrates the presence of large yeasts with thick cell walls and broad-based buds. What is the most likely causative agent?

(A) *Aspergillus fumigatus*
(B) *Blastomyces dermatitidis*
(C) *Coccidioides immitis*
(D) *Histoplasma capsulatum*
(E) *Sporothrix schenckii*

21. What is the scientific name for a fungal cross-wall?

(A) Coenocyte
(B) Hypha
(C) Mycelium
(D) Septum
(E) Yeast

22. An uncooperative human immunodeficiency virus (HIV)-positive patient has been complaining of a stiff neck and a severe headache. The headache was initially lessened by analgesics, but the analgesics are no longer effective. His current CD4$^+$ count is 180/mm^3. He is not on any prophylactic drugs. What is the most likely causative agent?

(A) *Aspergillus*
(B) *Cryptococcus*
(C) *Candida*
(D) *Malassezia*
(E) *Sporothrix*

23. What characteristically sets fungal cells apart from human cells?

(A) 80S ribosomes
(B) Presence of an endoplasmic reticulum
(C) Ergosterol as the major membrane sterol
(D) Enzymes that allow them to use carbon dioxide as their sole carbon source
(E) Presence of chloroplasts

Answers and Explanations

1–A. This is a classic case of lymphocutaneous sporotrichosis in which a gardener or florist is infected via a puncture wound. The drug of choice is either itraconazole or potassium iodide (administered orally in milk). Topical antifungals are not effective, and the cortisone cream would probably enhance the spread of the disease. Griseofulvin localizes in the keratinized tissues and would not halt the subcutaneous spread of this infection. Penicillin would have no effect because *Sporothrix* is not a bacterium.

2–D. *Sporothrix schenckii* is dimorphic; the tissue form is cigar-shaped yeasts.

3–B. Zygomycota are aseptate fungi that cause serious infections, primarily in ketoacidotic diabetic patients and cancer patients. Fungal infections common in AIDS patients include *Candida* infections (ranging from oral thrush early to fungemias later), cryptococcal meningitis, and disseminated histoplasmosis and coccidioidomycoses. Severely neutropenic patients are most likely to have invasive *Aspergillus* infections.

4–D. Of the choices listed, only the dermatophytes would show hyphae and arthroconidia and cause cutaneous lesions. Blastomycosis (caused by *Blastomyces*) would show big, broad-based, budding yeasts. Candidiasis would show yeasts, pseudohyphae, and true hyphae. Coccidioidomycosis would show spherules of various sizes with round endospores visible in the large, "mature" spherules. Pityriasis versicolor would have clusters of yeasts with short, septate, curved hyphae ("spaghetti and meatballs" appearance).

5–A. *Aspergillus* spores are commonly airborne. Invasive infections with *Aspergillus* are controlled by phagocytic cells. In severe neutropenia, risk of infection is high.

6–C. A mycelium is a mass of hyphae (fungal filaments).

7–D. *Malassezia furfur* is a lipophilic fungus that is found on skin. It causes fungemia, primarily in premature infants on high-lipid intravenous supplements.

8–B. The fungal subunit, called a hypha, is a filamentous structure with or without cell walls.

9–B. Griseofulvin, which localizes in the keratinized tissues, inhibits the growth of dermatophytes by inhibiting microtubule assembly.

10–C. *Coccidioides immitis* is found in desert sand, primarily as arthroconidia and hyphae.

11–B. Fluconazole is an imidazole; all imidazoles inhibit ergosterol synthesis. Fluconazole has become the mainstay in the treatment of serious candidal infections, and it is used to prevent relapse of fungal central nervous system infections in compromised patients. Miconazole, also an imidazole, is available in topical or intravenous preparations and has been largely replaced by the oral fluconazole.

12–C. *Malassezia furfur* is seen in tissues as clusters of round fungal cells with short, curved, septate hyphae ("spaghetti and meatballs") and is the causative agent of pityriasis or tinea versicolor; *M furfur* overgrowth causes pigmentation disturbances.

13–A. *Candida* may cause skin infections that resemble some dermatophytic infections. The patient described in the question has *Candida* balanitis. In tinea cruris, the penis is not usually involved.

14–A. The disease syndrome is lumpy jaw, which is a form of mycetoma. The presenting signs seen in this patient suggest actinomycotic mycetoma, a bacterial infection caused by *Actinomyces*. (Students: you needed a nonfungal question.) Yeasts will also stain gram-positive. Remember that *Actinomyces* is a gram-positive anaerobe that is not acid-fast.

15–B. The finding of dematiaceous (dark), yeast-like forms with sharp planar division lines and the clinical presentation are both characteristic of chromoblastomycosis. Tinea nigra would show dematiaceous hyphae.

16–C. The disease described is thrush, and it is caused by *Candida*.

17–C. Calcofluor white stain, Gomori methenamine-silver stain, and periodic acid-Schiff stain are all differential stains, but only the periodic acid-Schiff stain turns fungi a pink-red color. The hematoxylin and eosin stain turns fungi a pink-red color also, but does not differentiate between the fungi and human tissue.

18–D. *Histoplasma* and *Blastomyces* are both endemic in Iowa, but only *Histoplasma* fits the description of a facultative intracellular parasite circulating in the reticuloendothelial system.

19–A. Amphotericin B, a polyene, is the most effective treatment for many life-threatening fungal infections. Nystatin, also a polyene, is used topically or orally, but is not absorbed.

20–B. *Blastomyces* has a double refractile wall and buds with a broad base of attachment to the mother cell. The environmental association appears to be rotting wood.

21–D. The cross-wall of a hypha is called a septum or septation.

22–B. *Cryptococcus,* an encapsulated yeast, is the major causative agent of meningitis in patients with AIDS.

23–C. Ergosterol is the major fungus membrane sterol, and its presence is important in chemotherapy of fungal infections. For example, amphotericin B binds to ergosterol, producing pores that leak out cellular contents, killing the fungus. Imidazole drugs inhibit the synthesis of ergosterol. Both fungi and humans have 80S ribosomes and endoplasmic reticulum. Fungi are heterotrophic rather than autotrophic and thus cannot use carbon dioxide as their carbon source; instead, fungi break down organic carbon compounds. Fungi are also not photosynthetic.

6

Parasitology

I. Characteristics of Parasites and Their Hosts

A. Parasites

—are classified as **ectoparasites** if they live on the skin or hair (e.g., lice) or as **endoparasites** if they live in the host.

—may be **obligate (entirely dependent on the host)** or **facultative** (free living or associated with the host).

—rival malnutrition as the major cause of morbidity and mortality worldwide.

B. Hosts

—may be one of three types:

1. **Definitive,** in which the adult parasite reaches sexual maturity
2. **Intermediate,** in which the larval or intermediate parasite stages develop
3. A **reservoir,** which is essential to parasite survival and a focus for spread to other hosts (e.g., swine for *Trichinella* organisms)

C. Vectors

—are living transmitters of disease.

—may be one of two types:

1. **Mechanical,** or nonessential to the life cycle of the parasite
2. **Biological,** serving as the site of some developmental events in the life cycle of the parasite

II. Protozoan Parasites

A. General characteristics–protozoan parasites

—are single-celled animals.

—may cause infections.

—generally have two distinctive forms:

1. **Trophozoite,** the actively motile form
2. **Cyst,** the resting stage (the stage most often transmitted from host to host)

B. **Classification**

1. **Amebas** move by **pseudopods.**
2. **Flagellates** move by the action of **flagella.**
3. **Ciliates** move by the action of **cilia.**
4. **Apicomplexa** (also called sporozoa or coccidia) are intracellular protozoans with complex life cycles involving more than one host and an apical complex that allows them to be taken up by host cells.

C. **Important intestinal and urogenital protozoans** (Table 6-1)

—include *Entamoeba histolytica, Giardia lamblia, Cryptosporidium* species, *Balantidium coli,* and *Trichomonas vaginalis.*

1. *Cryptosporidium* is gaining importance in the United States because of its increased frequency in patients with acquired immunodeficiency syndrome (AIDS), in whom it can cause severe diarrhea. Furthermore, because of its resistance to chlorination, there have been major outbreaks of *Cryptosporidium* infection in immunocompetent people exposed to high-level contamination in swimming pools or drinking water.
2. *E histolytica,* a pathogen, must be differentiated from *Entamoeba coli,* a nonpathogenic commensal. *E histolytica* has a nucleus that looks like a wagon wheel with a sharp central dot (karyosome), fine radiating "spokes" of nucleoplasm, and a fine peripheral rim of nucleoplasm. *E histolytica* ingests both white blood cells and red blood cells, which may be seen inside the cytoplasm as dark dots. (Thus fecal polymorphonuclear counts may not be as elevated as would be expected from this highly invasive organism.)

D. **Important tissue or blood protozoans**

—include *Plasmodium, Toxoplasma, Pneumocystis, Babesia, Trypanosoma,* and *Leishmania.*

1. **Plasmodia**

—have **two distinct hosts.**

a. A **vertebrate** (human or cattle) is the intermediate host where the asexual phase of the parasite's life cycle (schizogony) takes place in the liver and red blood cells.

b. The *Anopheles* mosquito is the definitive host and is the site of the sexual phase of the parasite's life cycle (sporogony).

—**are transmitted to humans by the bite of an infected *Anopheles* mosquito.** The injected sporozoites infect only liver parenchymal cells. Merozoites released from those liver cells infect only red blood cells. Details of the life cycle are seen in Figure 6-1.

—cause disease by a wide variety of mechanisms:

Table 6-1. Intestinal and Urogenital Protozoan Parasites and Associated Diseases

Species	Morphology	Associated Diseases	Mode/Form of Transmission	Diagnosis	Treatment
Entamoeba histolytica		Amebiasis (dysentery; extra intestinal abscesses common)	Fecal–oral by water, fresh fruits, and vegetables; via cysts	Trophozoites Cysts in stool; serologic testing Pathologic appearance (inverted flask-shaped lesions)	Metronidazole followed by iodoquinol
Giardia lamblia		Giardiasis (diarrhea with malabsorption)	Fecal (e.g., human, beaver, muskrat) by water, food, oral–anal intercourse, day care; via cysts	Trophozoites Cysts in stool	Quinacrine hydrochloride or metronidazole
Cryptosporidium species		Cryptosporidiosis (transient diarrhea in healthy persons; severe diarrhea in immunocompromised persons)	Undercooked meat; via cysts	Acid-fast oocysts in stool Biopsy: dots (cysts) in intestinal glands	Under study
Balantidium coli		Dysentery; colitis; diarrhea to severe dysentery	Contaminated food or water; via cysts	Trophozoites Cysts in feces	Tetracycline
Trichomonas vaginalis		Trichomoniasis (asymptomatic or vaginal discharge associated with burning or itching, or, in males, urethral discharge)	Sexual contact; via trophozoites	Motile trophozoites and excessive neutrophils in methylene blue wet mount	Metronidazole

Illustrations are not to scale.

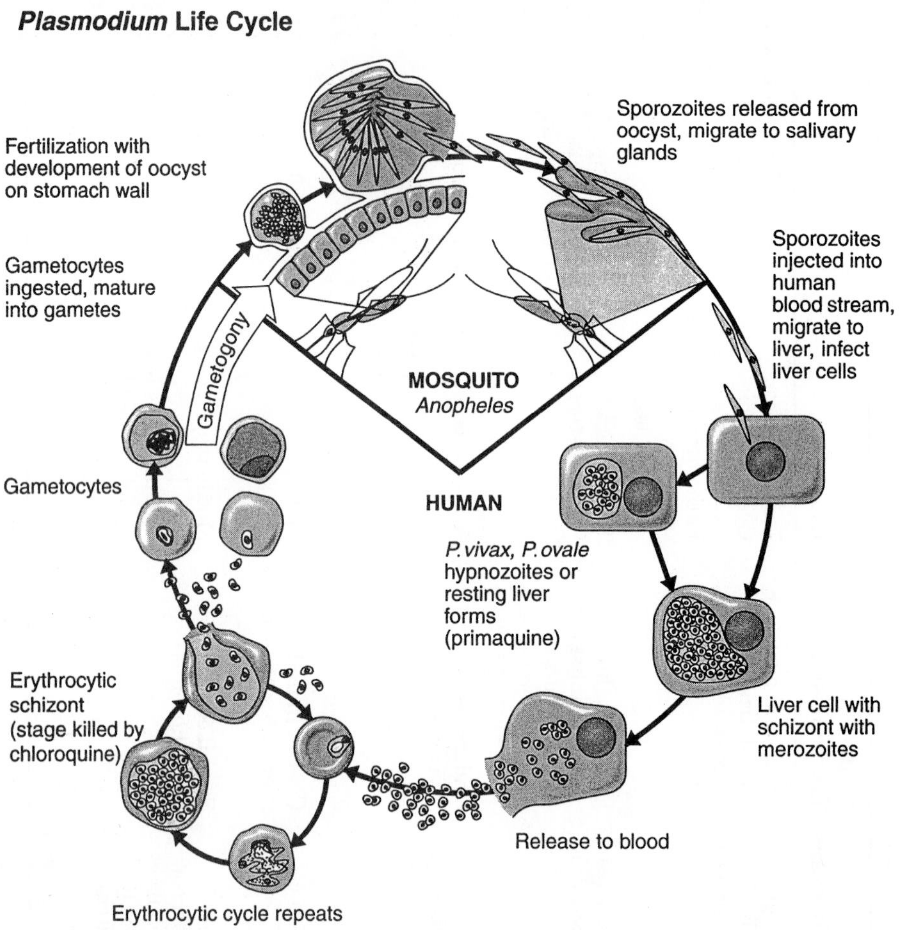

Plasmodium Life Cycle

Figure 6-1. The general life cycle of the *Plasmodium* species that cause malaria. (Reprinted with permission from Hawley L: *High-Yield Microbiology and Infectious Diseases.* Philadelphia, Lippincott Williams & Wilkins, 2000, p 133.)

  a. Paroxysms (chills, fever, and rigors) from release of toxic hemoglobin metabolites

  b. Anemia from loss of red blood cells

  c. Cerebral malaria (*Plasmodium falciparum*) from adherence of infected erythrocytes in cerebral venules and effects of metabolic byproducts in the central nervous system

  —species differences are presented in Table 6-2.

2. *Toxoplasma gondii*

  —can cause severe disease in immunosuppressed patients, such as those with AIDS, and can cause mononucleosis-like symptoms in healthy adults.

  —can cross the placenta (generally in women with no or low antibody levels) and cause **congenital infections characterized by intracerebral calcifications, chorioretinitis, hydrocephaly or microcephaly, and convulsions.**

Table 6-2. Plasmodial Organisms and Associated Diseases

Species*	Associated Diseases	Diagnosis	Treatment
Plasmodium vivax	Tertian malaria	Oval-shaped host cells with Schüffner's granules and ragged cell walls, seen on thick and thin blood examination	Chloroquine phosphate then primaquine
Plasmodium malariae	Quartan malaria†	Bar and band forms; rosette schizonts	Chloroquine
Plasmodium falciparum	Malignant tertian malaria‡	Multiple ring forms and crescents (gametocytes); schizonts rare in peripheral blood	Chloroquine-resistant strains with quinine sulfate with doxycycline

*Plasmodium ovale (rare) causes benign tertian (ovale) malaria. Transmission, diagnosis, and treatment are similar to those for *P vivax*. Both *P ovale* and *P vivax* form hypnozoites (or sleeping forms) in the liver that may not progress to merozoite production until months later (and like other liver forms are not sensitive to chloroquine).
†Recurrence of *P malariae* symptoms, called *recrudescence*, may result from a persistent low level of parasites in the *red* blood *cells.*
‡*P falciparium*-infected red blood cells adhere to the endothelium of peripheral capillaries, resulting in "sludging." Severe anemia results from multiple infections of both immature and mature red blood cells. The severe disease that results constitutes a medical emergency.

    —is acquired primarily from the **ingestion of undercooked or raw meat**.

    —may be acquired from **cat feces,** although a wide variety of animals carry *Toxoplasma*. Pregnant women should not change litter boxes, or they should wear gloves and change the box daily because the infectious form takes more than 24 hours to develop in the soil (Figure 6-2).

3. *Babesia microti*

    —is a malaria-like parasite that primarily causes disease in cattle.

    —may cause anemia with malaria-like symptoms in humans (babesiosis).

    —is transmitted by the ***Ixodes*** tick, so **coinfections with *Borrelia burgdorferi* occur.**

    —is diagnosed by the presence of multiple ring-like forms in the red blood cells.

4. *Trypanosoma* and *Leishmania* species

    —are **hemoflagellates.**

    —infect blood and tissues.

    —have life cycles involving several forms.

    a. Trypomastigotes are free-living, elongated, flagellated forms with an undulating membrane. They are seen extracellularly in blood in *Trypanosoma* infections.

    b. Amastigotes are "oval" cells that do not have a flagellum or an undulating membrane. They are seen in infected tissue (e.g., heart tissue infected with *Trypanosoma cruzi*) or macrophages (*Leishmania*).

    —cause several diseases.

Toxoplasma gondii Life Cycle

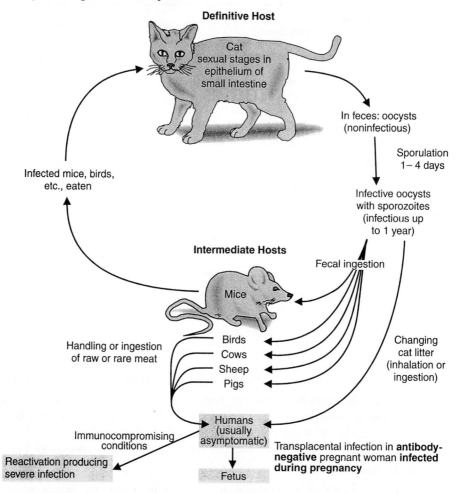

Figure 6-2. The life cycle of *Toxoplasma gondii*. Infection during pregnancy can cause toxoplasmosis in the baby. (Reprinted with permission from Hawley L: *High-Yield Microbiology and Infectious Diseases*. Philadelphia, Lippincott Williams & Wilkins, 2000, p 135.)

a. ***Leishmania donovani*** complex causes **visceral leishmaniasis.** ("Complex" means that the taxonomy is not straightforward and that it is a group of closely related leishmaniae.) *Leishmania braziliensis* causes mucocutaneous leishmaniasis. **Sandflies** are the vectors for both *L donovani* and *L braziliensis*.

b. ***T cruzi*** causes **Chagas' disease,** which is generally an acute disease in babies or young children that may infect the brain. In adults, the initial infection is likely to be more mild with a high rate of chronic disease leading to flabby heart tissue and heart failure later in life. Romaña's sign (unilateral eyelid swelling) is an early sign of Chagas' disease. The vector is variously called *Triatoma* (genus name), reduviid bugs (after the family), cone-nose bugs (for "head" shape), and kissing bugs (for propensity to bite around the mouth or eyes). The bug deposits the trypanosome in feces and the host scratches to implant in bite wound.

    c. ***Trypanosoma brucei gambiense*** and ***Trypanosoma brucei rhodesiense*** (subspecies of *Trypanosoma brucei*) both cause **African sleeping sickness.** They are transmitted by **tsetse flies.** The extreme **antigenic variation** of *T. brucei* is responsible for the decline to death in some untreated cases.

    d. Details are given in Table 6-3.

  5. Free-living amebas

    —include *Naegleria* and *Acanthamoeba.*

    a. ***Naegleria fowleri***

      —causes **primary amebic meningoencephalitis (PAM),** which is most commonly acquired by active children.

      —is most commonly acquired while **diving** and **swimming during hot weather** in brackish or fresh water and, rarely, in swimming pools.

      —generally presents with **fever, severe headache, confusion,** and **odor auras.** Coma and death follow in a few days.

      —is seen in the purulent cerebrospinal fluid as "slug-like" amebas.

    b. ***Acanthamoeba***

      —causes keratitis.

      —is acquired from contaminated homemade contact saline.

      —is characterized by **severe ocular pain** not usually seen in herpetic keratitis.

      —may cause a chronic central nervous system infection called **granulomatous amebic encephalitis (GAE),** generally **in debilitated or immunocompromised patients.** Altered mental status is the most common presentation of GAE.

      —infections do not appear to be associated with swimming. The ameba causing GAE may come from some other infected site in the body.

III. Trematodes

  A. General characteristics–trematodes

    —are called **flukes.**

    —are generally flat and fleshy.

    —are **hermaphroditic,** except for *Schistosoma,* which has separate males and females.

    —have complicated life cycles occurring in two or more hosts.

    —have **operculated** eggs (except for *Schistosoma*); these eggs:

    1. Contaminate water, perpetuating the life cycle.

    2. Are used to diagnose infections.

    3. Produce a swimming ciliated larval form, called a **miracidium,** when they hatch.

Table 6-3. Hemoflagellates and Associated Diseases

Species	Associated Diseases	Reservoir Host	Mode of Transmission	Diagnosis	Treatment
Trypanosoma cruzi	Chagas' disease (American trypanosomiasis)	Cat, dog, armadillo, opossum	Passage of trypomastigote in feces at site of reduviid bug bite	Blood films; blood or lymph node culture; serologic testing	Nifurtimox
Trypanosoma brucei gambiense; Trypanosoma brucei rhodesiense	African sleeping sickness (African trypanosomiasis)	Gambia: mostly humans; Rhodesia: wild animals	Contamination of bite site by trypomastigote in saliva of tsetse fly	Blood films; lymph node aspiration; cerebrospinal fluid; serologic testing	Suramin (acute therapy); melarsoprol (chronic therapy)
Leishmania donovani	Visceral leishmaniasis (kala-azar, Dumdum fever)	Urban areas: humans; rural areas: rodents and wild animals	Sandfly* bite	Aspiration or culture of bone marrow, liver, or spleen; serologic testing	Stibogluconate sodium
Leishmania tropica; Leishmania mexicana; Leishmania peruviana	Dermal leishmaniasis	(Same as *L donovani*)	(Same as *L donovani*)	Scrapings or biopsies of lesion or skin test	Stibogluconate sodium
Leishmania braziliensis	Mucocutaneous leishmaniasis	(Same as *L donovani*)	(Same as *L donovani*)	(Same as *L donovani*)	Stibogluconate sodium

Phlebotomus sandfly genus carries Old World *Leishmania; Lutzomyia* sandfly genus carries New World *Leishmania* in South and Central America (*L mexicana, L braziliensis,* and *L donovani* in the Americas).

B. Intermediate hosts

—are **snails or other mollusks.**

—are sometimes two in number.

C. Clinical manifestations (Table 6-4)

—vary greatly, from no symptoms for a light intestinal infection with *Fasciolopsis buski* to systemic symptoms with anemia and hepatomegaly with *Fasciola hepatica.*

D. Therapy

—is with **praziquantel** for serious trematode disease.

—is with calamine, trimeprazine, and sometimes sedatives for swimmer's itch.

IV. Cestodes

A. General characteristics–cestodes

—are commonly called **tapeworms.**

—have three basic portions:

1. Head, or scolex

2. Neck, which produces the segments, or proglottids

3. Proglottids, which mature as they move away from the scolex (collectively, the neck and proglottids are termed the **strobila**)

—are **hermaphroditic,** with both male and female reproductive organs developing in each proglottid and mature eggs developing in the most distal proglottids.

—adhere to the mucosa via the **scolex,** a knobby structure with suckers or a sucking groove for attachment to the small intestine.

—**lack a gastrointestinal tract;** instead, they absorb nutrients from the host's gastrointestinal tract.

—cause infections that can be diagnosed by demonstration of eggs or proglottids in the feces.

—typically have complex life cycles involving:

1. Extraintestinal **larval** forms in **intermediate hosts**

2. Adult **tapeworms** in **definitive hosts**

B. Clinical manifestations

1. When humans are the definitive host, the presence of the **adult tapeworm in the small intestine** is generally **without symptoms,** but it may affect nutrition. Human adult tapeworms include *Taenia saginata* (beef), *Taenia solium* (pork), *Diphyllobothrium latum* (cool lake region

Table 6-4. Trematodes (Flukes)

Organism	Associated Diseases	Reservoir Host*	Mode of Transmission	Progression in Humans
Schistosoma japonicum; Schistosoma mansoni	Intestinal schistosomiasis	Cats, dogs, cattle, pigs (*S japonicum*); primates, marsupials, rodents (*S mansoni*)	Contact with contaminated water	Cercaria enter skin, then circulation; mature into adults in intrahepatic portal blood[†]
Schistosoma haematobium	Vesicular schistosomiasis	Primates	Contact with contaminated water	See *S japonicum*[‡]
Nonhuman schistosomes	Swimmer's itch	Birds	Contact with contaminated water	Penetration of skin, causing dermatitis without further development; itching is most intense at 2–3 days
Clonorchis (Opisthorchis) sinensis (Chinese liver fluke)	Clonorchiasis	Cats, dogs, humans	Ingestion of contaminated raw fish	Cysts germinate in duodenum, exit through wall into liver, and proceed to bile ducts, where they mature; eggs enter feces in bile
Fasciola hepatica (sheep liver fluke)	Fascioliasis	Sheep, cattle, humans	Ingestion of contaminated aquatic plants (watercress)	Cysts germinate in duodenum, exit through wall into liver, and proceed to bile ducts, where they mature; eggs enter feces in bile
Fasciolopsis buski (giant intestinal fluke)	Fasciolopsiasis	Pigs, dogs, rabbits, humans	Ingestion of contaminated aquatic plants (water chestnuts)	Cysts germinate in duodenum; adults attach to mucosa of small intestine, where eggs are produced
Paragonimus westermani (lung fluke)	Paragonimiasis	Humans, pigs, felines, canines	Ingestion of contaminated raw crabs, crayfish	Excyst in stomach, migrate to lung; eggs in sputum or feces

*Snails or clams are the intermediate hosts for all flukes. The second intermediate host for *Clonorchis* is freshwater fish; for *Paragonimus*, freshwater crabs or crayfish.

[†]Adult forms mate in mesenteric veins.

[‡]Adult forms mate in bladder veins.

fish), *Hymenolepis nana* (humans and rodents), and *Dipylidium caninum* (dogs and cats).

2. When humans serve as the intermediate host, more serious disease results. Symptoms depend on the **migration of the larval forms.**

   a. **Cysticercosis** is caused by the larvae of ***T solium.*** The eggs are ingested from contaminated water or food and hatch in the gastrointestinal tract. Larvae migrate into the blood and then the tissues. Cysticerci in the eye and brain have the most serious consequences; calcifications occur when cysticerci die.

   b. **Sparganosis (*D latum*)** is acquired by drinking pond water contaminated with crustaceans containing early larval forms of *D latum.* Because humans are dead-end hosts, only the subcutaneous or eye lesions develop.

   c. **Unilocular hydatid cyst disease** occurs when eggs of ***Echinococcus granulosus*** are ingested. Oncospheres escape the intestine and enter the blood, liver, and lungs, where cysts containing brood capsules develop. This disease is most common in sheep-raising areas.

   d. **Alveolar hydatid cyst disease (*Echinococcus multilocularis*)** is transmitted via ingestion or inhalation of contaminated cat, wolf, or dog feces. Progression usually resembles that for diseases caused by *E granulosus.*

3. Table 6-5 presents additional details on cestodes.

V. Nematodes

A. General characteristics–nematodes

—are called **roundworms.**

—have round, unsegmented bodies covered by a tough cuticle.

—are transmitted in several ways:

1. **Ingestion of eggs** (*Enterobius, Ascaris, Trichuris,* and *Toxocara*)

2. **Direct invasion** of skin by larval forms (*Necator, Ancylostoma,* and *Strongyloides*)

3. **Ingestion of larvae** (*Trichinella*)

4. **Larvae transmission via insect bite** (*Wuchereria, Loa, Mansonella, Onchocerca,* and *Dracunculus*)

B. Clinical manifestations–nematodes

—cause a wide variety of diseases, including ascariasis, pinworm infection (enterobiasis), whipworm infection (trichuriasis), hookworm infection, trichinosis, strongyloidiasis (threadworm infection), filariasis, and river blindness (onchocerciasis).

—are transmitted as eggs (Table 6-6).

—are transmitted as larval forms (Table 6-7).

Table 6-5. Important Cestodes (Tapeworms)*

Organism	Common Intermediate Host	Disease When Human is Intermediate Host	Common Definitive Host	Disease When Human is Definitive Host
Taenia saginata (beef tapeworm)	Cattle	Extremely rare	Humans	**Intestinal tapeworm:** generally vague abdominal pain
Taenia solium (pork tapeworm)	Pigs	**Cysticercosis: ingested eggs** (from human fecal contamination of food or water) hatch and larvae migrate out of intestines; commonly diagnosed when the cysticercus larvae develop in the CNS, causing **neurocysticercosis;** in tissues, cysticercus larvae look like opalescent white kidney beans	Humans	**Intestinal tapeworm:** generally vague abdominal pain
Diphyllobothrium latum (fish tapeworm)†	Microscopic crustaceans; fish	**Sparganosis:** human **drinks water** with copepods (tiny crustaceans) **carrying early larval forms;** also acquired from ingesting raw tadpoles or using raw snake or frog meat as wound dressing; symptoms develop when larvae localize in tissues and grow, eliciting a strong inflammatory response; most painful are eye and CNS lesions	Humans	**Intestinal tapeworm:** vitamin B_{12} anemia results if *D latum* attaches in the proximal portion of the jejunum in genetically predisposed individuals
Echinococcus granulosus	Herbivores (mainly sheep)	**Hydatid cyst disease:** space-filling lesion (up to large grapefruit size); slow growing; damage by compression, unless cyst ruptures, then anaphylaxis and dissemination	Carnivores (humans not definitive host)	None
Echinococcus multilocularis	Rodents	**Alveolar hydatid cysts:** most commonly in the liver (called "alveolar" because of multilobar shape, not location)	Carnivores (humans not definitive host)	None

*Treatment for all tapeworm infections is praziquantel, with the exception of the hydatid cyst diseases, which require albendazole and careful drainage or surgery.
†Adult tapeworms attach to the small intestine and absorb food from the human intestine.

Table 6-6. Nematodes Transmitted by Eggs

Species	Associated Diseases/Symptoms	Mode of Transmission	Diagnosis	Treatment
Enterobius vermicularis (pinworm)*	Enterobiasis (perianal itching)	Ingestion of eggs from dust or autoinfection	Microscopic detection of eggs from perianal area	Pyrantel pamoate given to entire family; damp mop dusting
Trichuris trichiura (whipworm)	Trichuriasis (generally asymptomatic; severe: abdominal pain, bloody diarrhea, appendicitis, rectal prolapse)	Ingestion of eggs (e.g., use of human feces as vegetable fertilizer, contaminated food and water)	Microscopic detection of barrel-shaped eggs with bipolar plugs	Mebendazole
Ascaris lumbricoides†	Ascariasis [pneumonitis (larvae in lungs); asymptomatic to heavy bowel infections; anesthetics, fever, drugs may induce adult worms to migrate to places such as the bile ducts or pancreas. Intestinal blockage may occur in children with heavy worm burden.]	Ingestion of eggs (e.g., use of human feces as vegetable fertilizer, contaminated food and water)	Bile-stained knobby eggs or 6–12 inch long roundworms seen on radiograph or cholangiogram; serologic test shows some cross-reaction with *Trichuris*	Supportive therapy during pneumonitis; surgery for ectopic migrations; mebendazole
Toxocara canis; Toxocara catis‡	Toxocariasis (visceral larva migrans); generally asymptomatic because humans are dead-end hosts)	Ingestion of eggs [e.g., handling puppy or eating dirt (pica)]	Clinical findings; serologic testing	Diethylcarbamazine or thiabendazole§

*Most common helminth in the United States. Worm is 2–5 mm long.
†Most common helminth worldwide. Adult worms are 20–35 cm long.
‡Affects approximately 80% of puppies; high transmission rate to children in household.
§Disease usually is self-limiting; therefore, treatment may not be needed.

Table 6-7. Nematodes Transmitted by Larvae

Species	Associated Diseases/Symptoms	Mode of Transmission	Progression in Humans	Diagnosis	Treatment
Nector americanus (New World hookworm); *Ancylostoma duodenale* (Old World hookworm)	Hookworm infection (ground itch, diarrhea, vomiting, abdominal pain, iron deficiency anemia)	Filariform larvae in soil penetrate intact **skin** of bare feet* (shoes reduce transmission)	Larvae travel from skin to circulation to lungs, then ascend to epiglottis, and are swallowed; adult worms attach and mature in small intestine	Non-bile-staining segmented eggs in stool†; possible occult blood in stools	Mebendazole and treat anemia
Ancylostoma braziliense; Ancylostoma caninum	Cutaneous larva migrans	Filariform larvae penetrate intact **skin** (beaches with free-roaming dogs; cat feces in sandboxes)	Larvae migrate from skin to subcutaneous tissues; they do not mature but "creep" in subcutaneous tissues	Usually a presumptive diagnosis from clinical symptoms; no reliable test exists	Thiabendazole
Strongyloides stercoralis	Strongyloidiasis (skin pruritis, mild pneumonitis; asymptomatic to severe diarrhea with malapsorption)	Filariform larvae penetrate intact **skin** of bare feet; free-living cycle occurs outside host	Larvae migrate from skin to blood to lung to small intestine as do *Necator* and *Ancylostoma*; **auto-infection** also occurs	Larvae in stool; serologic testing	Thiabendazole
Trichinella spiralis	Trichinosis (asympto-matic to gastritis, then fever, muscle aches and eosino-philia)	Consumption of encysted larvae in **undercooked meat** (bear, pork, horse meat)	Larvae leave meat in small intestine and mature into adult worms, which migrate into blood stream and muscle tissue	Splinter hemorrhages beneath nails; muscle biopsy; marked eosinophilia; serologic testing	Steroids for severe symptoms and mebendazole

Organism	Disease	Transmission	Life cycle	Diagnosis	Treatment
Wuchereria bancrofti; Brugia malayi	Filariasis (asymptomatic to elephantiasis)	Infective larvae enter in **mosquito** bite	Larvae migrate to lymphatics and mature; adult worms live in lymph nodes, producing elephantiasis	Blood films, clinical findings	Diethylcarbamazine
Loa loa (African eye worm)	Filariasis (subcutaneous migration, Calabar swellings)	Infective larvae in *Chrysops* (mango fly) bite	Adult *Loa loa* migrate through subcutaneous tissue, often crossing conjunctiva	Calabar swelling; worms in eye; eosinophilia; blood films	Diethylcarbamazine and surgical removal
Onchocerca volvulus	River blindness (subcutaneous nodules, dermatitis, wrinkled skin, eye infections)	Larvae-infected black fly bite	Adult worms develop in subcutaneous nodules, migrate to skin and other tissues	Microfilariae seen on skin examination	Surgical removal of subcutaneous nodules and ivermectin
Dracunculus medinensis (guinea worm)	Dracunculosis (subcutaneous nodules with systemic symptoms: nausea, vomiting, or diarrhea; asthma)	Consumption of water contaminated with *Cyclops* organisms containing larvae or direct contact as in step wells	Ingested larvae exit the small intestine and develop into adults; females migrate to surface, causing ulcers, and release motile larvae	Clinical symptoms or flood ulcer to induce worm release	Slow worm removal; metronidazole

*Rhabditiform stage initially released is noninfective and feeds on bacteria and detritus in soil.
†The two species cannot (and need not) be distinguished by eggs.

Review Test

1. A biology graduate student who recently visited a tropical region of Africa presents with new visual impairment and the sensation that something is moving in her eye. She tells you that she is concerned because she had been warned about eye disease transmitted by black flies. When in Africa, she was in a river area, and despite her best efforts she received a lot of black fly bites. She also has some subcutaneous nodules. If her infection was acquired by black fly bite, what is the most likely causative agent?

(A) Ancylostoma braziliense
(B) Dracunculus medinensis
(C) Loa loa
(D) Onchocerca volvulus
(E) Wuchereria bancrofti

2. A surgical patient who imports food from Mexico, and so spends several months each year in rural Mexico, returns several days after her mastectomy with signs of acute appendicitis. When her appendix is removed it is found to contain a light-colored, 20.5-cm long roundworm and bile-stained, knobby eggs consistent with Ascaris. How did she acquire this infection?

(A) Ingestion of water containing filariform larvae
(B) Skin penetration by filariform larvae
(C) Skin penetration by rhabditiform larvae
(D) Ingestion of food contaminated with the eggs
(E) Inhalation of dust carrying the cysts

3. A patient whose major source of protein is smoked and cooked fish develops what appears to be pernicious anemia. What parasite is noted for causing a look-alike vitamin B_{12} anemia in certain genetically predisposed infected individuals?

(A) Echinococcus granulosus
(B) Diphyllobothrium latum
(C) Hymenolepis nana
(D) Dipylidium caninum
(E) Taenia solium

4. Which of the following protozoans is free living and acquisition does not generally indicate fecal contamination?

(A) Acanthamoeba
(B) Dientamoeba fragilis
(C) Entamoeba histolytica
(D) Entamoeba coli
(E) Giardia

5. What is the most likely reason for a chloroquine-treated case of Plasmodium vivax relapsing?

(A) P vivax has a significant level of chloroquine resistance.
(B) P vivax has a persistent erythrocytic stage.
(C) P vivax has a persistent exoerythrocytic stage (hypnozoite).
(D) Chloroquine is not one of the drugs of choice.

6. How is Leishmania donovani transmitted?

(A) Anopheles mosquito bite
(B) Black fly bite
(C) Culex mosquito bite
(D) Sandfly bite
(E) Skin penetration by trauma

7. How is Schistosoma haematobium transmitted?

(A) Ingestion of raw or undercooked snail, frog, or snake
(B) Invasion of filariform larvae from soil
(C) Handling aquatic birds
(D) Standing or swimming in contaminated water
(E) Tsetse fly bite

8. An untreated human immunodeficiency virus (HIV)-positive patient (CD4$^+$ count = 180 cells/mm^3) from southern California has developed progressively severe headache and mental confusion, along with ataxia and retinochoroiditis. Focal lesions are present on a computed tomography scan of his brain. No mucocutaneous lesions are found. He has been living under a bridge for the last 2 years. His level of immunoglobulin G to the infectious agent is high. What is the most likely explanation for how this current infection started?

(A) Earlier exposure to pigeons
(B) Earlier exposure to desert sand
(C) Reactivation of bradyzoites in cysts from an earlier infection
(D) Recent exposure to cat feces
(E) Recent exposure to bats

9. Which of the following is the tapeworm acquired from eating undercooked pork?

(A) *Dipylidium* spp
(B) *Echinococcus granulosus*
(C) *Taenia saginata*
(D) *Taenia solium*
(E) *Trichinella spiralis*

10. What roundworm is most likely to be transmitted by ingestion of food or water contaminated with feces?

(A) *Ascaris lumbricoides*
(B) *Enterobius vermicularis*
(C) *Necator americanus*
(D) *Taenia saginata*
(E) *Toxocara canis*

11. What roundworm is transmitted by filariform larvae that are found in the soil and penetrate the skin?

(A) *Dracunculus medinensis*
(B) *Enterobius vermicularis*
(C) *Strongyloides stercoralis*
(D) *Taenia saginata*
(E) *Toxocara canis*

12. How is *Clonorchis sinensis* (Chinese liver fluke) most likely transmitted to humans?

(A) Fish ingestion
(B) Mosquito bite
(C) Swimming or water contact
(D) Water chestnut ingestion
(E) Watercress ingestion

13. A rural subsistence farmer from Brazil died of heart failure. His autopsy showed a greatly enlarged heart. What was the most likely vector for the most likely infectious agent that may have been responsible for his death?

(A) *Ixodes* tick
(B) Mosquito
(C) Reduviid bug
(D) Sandfly
(E) Tsetse fly

14. A patient who recently returned from camping in Canada presents with malabsorption diarrhea. How does the most likely agent cause the diarrhea?

(A) Coinfection with bacteria
(B) Enterotoxin production
(C) Suction disk attachment
(D) Tissue invasion leading to an inflammatory response and prostaglandin production

15. Which of the following protozoans is transmitted primarily by the motile trophozoite form?

(A) *Balantidium coli*
(B) *Entamoeba histolytica*
(C) *Giardia lamblia*
(D) *Taenia solium*
(E) *Trichomonas vaginalis*

Answers and Explanations

1–D. *Onchocerca volvulus* causes river blindness and is transmitted by the bite of a black fly. The patient may be able to detect movement in the eye.

2–D. Fertilized *Ascaris* eggs released in feces may contaminate food or water, which is then consumed. *Ascaris* does not attach to the intestine but maintains its position by mobility. The worm may become hypermotile (e.g., during febrile periods, anesthetic use, or antibiotic use) and may migrate into the appendix or bile duct.

3–B. *Diphyllobothrium* is the tapeworm associated with fish found in cool lake regions.

4–A. *Acanthamoeba* is a free-living organism with a sturdy cyst stage that is found in dust. A common way of acquiring *Acanthamoeba* infections in the United States is through homemade saline solutions for soft contact lenses.

5–C. Both *Plasmodium ovale* and *Plasmodium vivax* may form liver hypnozoites, which are very slow to develop into schizonts with merozoites and proceed onto the chloroquine-sensitive erythrocytic stages. (It's not *over* with *P ovale* or *P vivax* unless you also treat with primaquine phosphate, which kills the liver stages.)

6–D. All leishmaniae are transmitted by sandflies.

7–D. All schistosomes are transmitted by skin penetration from standing or swimming in contaminated water. Remember that snails are intermediate hosts.

8–C. The most likely disease in this case is encephalitis with focal lesions. Because of the mention of high levels of immunoglobulin G, the current infection is likely a reactivation of an earlier infection; therefore, recent exposures (choices D and E) can be eliminated. Exposure to pigeons suggests cryptococcosis, which is often a reactivational infection. However, in cryptococcosis antibody levels are rarely monitored, and there is no mention of India ink stain or capsular polysaccharide in the cerebrospinal fluid, which are the major diagnostic methods. In addition, based on the patient's symptoms, the infection is more likely to be encephalitis rather than meningitis or meningoencephalitis; also, retinochoroiditis is usually not present in cryptococcosis. The retinochoroiditis and lack of mucocutaneous lesions makes infection with *Coccidioides* less likely. Reactivation of toxoplasmosis is most likely.

9–D. If you answered *Trichinella spiralis,* you fell for a typical testing "bait and switch." *T spiralis* is the pork roundworm and *Taenia solium* is the pork tapeworm. *Dipylidium caninum* is the common tapeworm of both cats and dogs. It may be transmitted by ingestion of fleas harboring cysticercoid larvae. Transmission to humans usually occurs when crushed fleas harboring the disease are transmitted from a pet when it licks a child's mouth.

10–A. *Ascaris lumbricoides* is transmitted via the fecal-oral route. *Enterobius* is most likely transmitted via contaminated hands, clothing, or bedding. *Necator* enters by skin penetration. *Taenia* is not a roundworm. *Toxocara* is most commonly acquired from eating fecally contaminated dirt or soil.

11–C. *Strongyloides stercoralis* is a type of hookworm (also a roundworm). The filariform larvae of *S stercoralis* are picked up when walking barefoot or sitting on the ground. *Dracunculus medinensis* (the guinea worm) is picked up by drinking water with copepods containing the larvae. Filtration of all drinking water through clean sari silk or T-shirt material is reducing the incidence of new cases dramatically and may allow its eradication. (For those who are infected with *D medinensis,* adults in subcutaneous nodules are slowly removed by rolling them out on a pencil.) *Toxocara canis* and Toxocara cati are acquired most commonly by pica, the ingestion of inert material; in this case, dirt or sand with animal feces. *Taenia saginata* is a flatworm. *Enterobius* (pinworm) eggs are ingested.

12–A. Raw, undercooked, smoked, or pickled fresh-water fish are the most common route of transmission of *Clonorchis sinensis.*

13–C. The case of the Brazilian farmer is a classic description of heart failure from chronic Chagas' disease, which is caused by *Trypanosoma cruzi*. *T cruzi* is transmitted by reduviid bugs (cone-nose bugs or kissing bugs) that defecate as they bite. Scratching the bite spreads the trypanosome into the bite site, initiating the infection.

14–C. In this case, *Giardia lamblia* is the causative agent. *G lamblia* is carried by muskrats and beavers, which is why it can be picked up in pristine northern lakes, such as those found in Canada. Attachment of numerous *Giardia* via their ventral sucking disks in the duodenal-jejunal area leads to maladsorption diarrhea and temporary lactose intolerance.

15–E. Protozoans transmitted by the fecal-oral route are transmitted in the cyst form, which survives stomach acid. Only the sexually transmitted *Trichomonas vaginalis* is transmitted in the motile form. *Taenia solium* is not a protozoan, but a flatworm.

7
Immunology

I. Overview

A. Immunity

—is defined as an "enhanced state" of responsiveness to a specific substance, induced by prior contact with that substance.

1. Natural immunity

—is present from birth and is **nonspecific.**

—consists of various barriers to external insults; for example, skin, mucous membranes, macrophages, monocytes, neutrophils, eosinophils, and the contents of these cells.

2. Acquired immunity

—is expressed after exposure to a given substance and is **specific.**

—involves specific receptors on lymphocytes and the participation of macrophages for its expression.

—consists of:

a. Humoral immunity, mediated by antibodies
b. Cell-mediated immunity, mediated by lymphocytes

B. Immune system

—consists of the cellular and molecular components derived from the central and peripheral lymphoid organs.

1. Central lymphoid organs

—consist of the bone marrow and thymus.

—are the location of maturation of lymphoid cells.

2. Peripheral lymphoid organs

—consist of the spleen, lymph nodes and lymphatic channels, tonsils, adenoids, Peyer's patches, and appendix.

—are the location of reactivity of lymphoid cells.

3. Cells of the immune system

—include the white blood cells (approximately 8000/mm³ of blood), which are composed of:

a. Granulocytes—50%–80% of white blood cells

b. Lymphocytes—20%–45% of white blood cells

c. Monocytes and macrophages—3%–8% of white blood cells

4. Molecules of the immune system

a. Antibodies (immunoglobulins) are protein products of certain lymphocytes with a precise specificity for a particular antigen.

b. Lymphokines are secreted lymphocyte products that play a role in the activation of the immune response.

C. Development of the immune system

—involves the maturation of pluripotential stem cells in the bone marrow or thymus into B cells and T cells, respectively.

—includes the generation of specific receptors on the cell surface of B cells and T cells.

1. Pluripotential stem-cell sources

a. Embryonic yolk sac

b. Fetal liver

c. Adult bone marrow

2. B cells

—mature in the bursa (hence the name "B" cells) of Fabricius in birds and in the fetal liver and adult bone marrow in humans (bursal equivalents).

—are involved in the generation of humoral immunity.

—have specific receptors (**immunoglobulins**) on their surface for antigen recognition.

—mature into antibody-producing plasma cells.

—are sessile and located predominantly in the germinal centers of the lymph nodes and spleen.

3. T cells

—mature in the thymus.

—are involved in "helping" B cells become antibody-producing plasma cells.

—have specific receptors (T-cell receptors) on their surface for antigen recognition.

—are involved in cell-mediated immunity.

—participate in suppression of the immune response.

—are the predominant (95%) lymphocytes in the circulation.

—are found in the paracortical and interfollicular areas of the lymph nodes and spleen.

D. Physiology of immunity

—involves the following series of events that culminate in B-cell or T-cell activation (or both) and response to the introduction of a foreign entity into the circulation:

1. **"Processing"** of the foreign entity by a macrophage or B cell
2. **Recognition** of this foreign entity by specific, preformed receptors on certain B cells and T cells
3. **Proliferation** of these B cells and T cells, as stimulated by soluble signals (interleukins) between macrophages, B cells, and T cells
4. **Blast transformation** and a series of mitotic divisions leading to the generation (from B cells) of **plasma cells that produce immunoglobulins** and (from T cells) of **sensitized T cells**—all capable of interacting with the original foreign stimulus

II. Antigens (Immunogens)

A. Characteristics

1. **Immunogenicity**—the capacity to stimulate production of specific, protective humoral or cellular immunity.
2. **Specific reactivity**—the capacity to be recognized by the antibodies and T cells produced.
3. **Foreignness**—the recognition of a body as nonself (foreign proteins are excellent antigens).
4. **Size**—must be at least approximately 10 kilodaltons (kd) to be recognized.
5. **Shape**—tertiary and quaternary structure determines the extent of antigenicity.

B. Definitions

1. **Epitope**
   —is the restricted portion of an antigen molecule that determines the specificity of the reaction with an antibody.
   —is the antibody-binding site on an antigen for a specific antibody.
   —generally contains four to six amino acid or sugar residues.
2. **Hapten**
   —is a small foreign molecule that is not immunogenic by itself but can bind to an antibody molecule already formed to it.
   —can be immunogenic if coupled to a sufficiently large carrier molecule.

III. Antibodies (Immunoglobulins)

A. Characteristics—antibodies

—are a heterogeneous group of proteins that contain carbohydrate.

—have sedimentation coefficients ranging from 7S to 19S.

—are found predominantly in the γ-globulin fraction of serum; some antibodies are also found in the α- and β-globulin fractions.

—consist of **polypeptide chains** linked by disulfide bonds, such that each antibody contains a minimum of two identical heavy (H) chains and two identical light (L) chains.

—have interchain disulfide bonds holding the chains together (i.e., L to H and H to H).

—have antigen-binding capacity defined by their specific H and L chains.

B. Enzymatic treatment of antibody molecules

1. Reduction of disulfide bonds

—breaks disulfide bonds between polypeptide chains.

—produces two identical H chains and two identical L chains per antibody molecule.

—destroys antigen-binding activity.

—shows that H chains have a molecular weight of approximately 50 kd.

—shows that L chains have a molecular weight of approximately 25 kd.

2. Papain treatment

—produces two identical antigen-binding fragments (Fab) per antibody molecule.

—produces one crystallizable fragment (Fc) per antibody molecule.

—shows that Fab has univalent binding capability (i.e., can bind to antigen but cannot precipitate antigen).

3. Pepsin digestion

—yields a large fragment [(Fab′)$_2$] that can precipitate antigen.

—shows that (Fab′)$_2$ fragments have bivalent binding capacity.

C. Structure of antibody molecules (Figure 7-1)

1. H chains

—are polypeptide chains of 440–550 amino acid residues in length.

—have intrachain domains of approximately 110 amino acid residues, formed by intrachain disulfide bonds.

—have an amino-terminal variable domain, followed by three to four constant domains.

—are structurally different for each of the defined classes of antibody [mu (μ), gamma (γ), alpha (α), delta (δ), and epsilon (ε)].

2. L chains

—are polypeptide chains of approximately 220 amino acid residues in length.

—have intrachain domains of approximately 110 amino acid residues, formed by intrachain disulfide bonds.

—have an amino-terminal variable domain and a carboxy-terminal constant domain.

—have two structurally distinct classes: kappa (κ) chains and lambda (λ) chains.

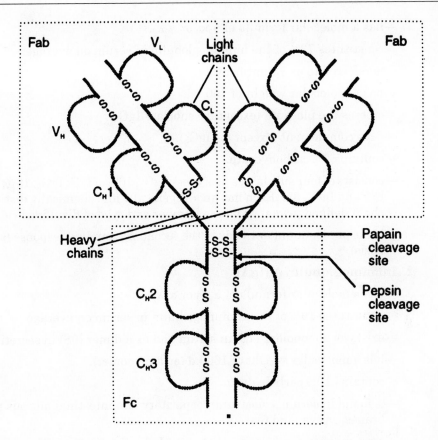

Figure 7-1. Diagrammatic representation of a typical immunoglobulin G (IgG) molecule. L = light chain; H = heavy chain; V_L = variable domain of L chain; S-S = disulfide bonds; C_L = constant domain of L chain; V_H = variable domain of H chain; C_H1, C_H2, C_H3 = constant domains of H chains; *Fab* = antigen-binding fragment; *Fc* = crystallizable fragment.

3. Variable domains

—exist in both H and L chains.

—are involved in antigen specificity of the antibody.

—contain the **hypervariable regions** (complementarity-determining regions, or CDRs), which:

a. Exist in both H- and L-chain variable domains

b. Appear approximately at amino acid positions 25–35, 50–58, and 95–108

c. Define the paratope (antigen-binding site) of the antibody, which binds to the epitope of the antigen

D. Classes (isotypes) of antibody molecules

—are found in all species and all individuals.

—are defined by the type of H chain, of which there are five: γ, μ, α, ϵ, δ.

1. Immunoglobulin G (IgG)

—has a molecular formula of $\gamma_2\kappa_2$ or $\gamma_2\lambda_2$.

—constitutes 73% of the immunoglobulin in serum on average.

—is referred to as 7S antibody.

—has a molecular weight of 150 kd.

—crosses the placenta (except for subclass IgG_4).

—fixes complement (except for IgG_4).

—contains 3% carbohydrate.

—consists of four subclasses (isotypes): IgG_1, 70% of IgG; IgG_2, 19%; IgG_3, 8%; and IgG_4, 3%. Each has an antigenically and chemically distinct H chain defined primarily by the number and type of disulfide bridges.

—is the predominant antibody in the secondary immune response (anamnesis).

2. Immunoglobulin A (IgA)

—has a molecular formula of $\alpha_2\kappa_2$ or $\alpha_2\lambda_2$.

—constitutes 19% of the immunoglobulin in serum on average.

—exists as a monomer (7S) in serum and as a dimer (9S) in secretions.

—has a molecular weight of 160 kd (as a monomer).

—contains 10% carbohydrate.

—is found in serum, colostrum, respiratory and intestinal mucous membranes, saliva, and tears.

—consists of two subclasses: IgA_1 and IgA_2; the former is the predominant form in serum, and the latter is the predominant form in secretions. IgA_2 has no covalent bonds between the L and the α_2 chains.

—may have a joining (J) polypeptide chain holding two molecules together.

—may contain a secretory (transport) piece synthesized in the local epithelium, which may help retard autodigestion.

—is an important component of mucosal immunity.

3. Immunoglobulin M (IgM)

—is a pentamer and has a molecular formula of $(\mu_2\kappa_2)_5$ or $(\mu_2\lambda_2)_5$.

—constitutes 7% of the immunoglobulin in serum on average.

—is referred to as the 19S antibody.

—is referred to as a macroglobulin.

—has a molecular weight of 900 kd.

—contains 15% carbohydrate.

—is the first immunoglobulin to appear in phylogeny (the lamprey eel has IgM).

—is the first immunoglobulin to appear in ontogeny.

—is the first immunoglobulin to appear in response to antigen stimulation.

—has a J polypeptide chain that holds the IgM pentamer together.

—has four constant domains on each H chain: $C\mu$ 1, $C\mu$ 2, $C\mu$ 3, and $C\mu$ 4.

4. Immunoglobulin D (IgD)

—has a molecular formula of $\delta_2\kappa_2$ or $\delta_2\lambda_2$.

—constitutes an average of 1% of the immunoglobulin in serum.

—has a molecular weight of 150 kd.

—contains 18% carbohydrate.

—has an unknown function in serum.

—serves as a receptor on the B-cell surface.

5. Immunoglobulin E (IgE)

—has a molecular formula of $\epsilon_2\kappa_2$ or $\epsilon_2\lambda_2$.

—constitutes less than 0.01% of serum immunoglobulin.

—has a molecular weight of 200 kd.

—contains 18% carbohydrate.

—is referred to as **reaginic** antibody.

—is involved in allergic reactions.

—has four constant domains on each H chain (three in the Fc region, as in IgM): Cϵ 1, Cϵ 2, Cϵ 3, and Cϵ 4.

—has an Fc region that binds to receptors on basophils and mast cells.

E. Allotypes of immunoglobulins

—are defined as small, regular structural differences among molecules of a particular immunoglobulin isotype.

—are genetically defined and codominantly expressed.

—may be as simple as a single amino acid substitution in the H or L chains.

—may be detected by immunologic means.

—exist in IgG molecules as Gm_1-Gm_{20}, in IgA molecules as Am_1-Am_3, and in κ chains as Km_1-Km_3.

F. Idiotype of antibody molecules

—is the antibody paratope to the antigenic epitope.

—is defined by the hypervariable regions (CDRs) of the variable domain of the L and H chains.

—involves those determinants that define the binding capability of a given antibody.

—can be defined by immunologic means.

—number in the 10^6 range.

G. Idiotypic–anti-idiotype network

—is the concept that a given antibody idiotype can evoke the generation of an anti-idiotypic antibody; this process may control the generation and level of the antibody response.

IV. Immunoglobulin Genetics

A. Exons

—are defined as minigenes or gene segments.

—encode for distinct parts of polypeptide chain.

—of immunoglobulin genes are:

1. **L exon**—leader segment
2. **V exon**—variable segment
3. **D exon**—diversity segment
4. **J exon**—joining segment
5. **C exon**—constant segment

B. Introns

—are intervening sequences between exons.

—are spliced out via mRNA transcription.

C. L-chain formation

—is genetically determined on human chromosome 2 (κ) or 22 (λ).

—involves selection, at the germline level, of 1 of 30 V genes, 1 of 5 J genes, and the C exon.

—is preceded by DNA arrangement and deletion of "unused" minigenes (exons) at the germline level and by RNA splicing to remove intervening sequences (introns) in translation for the secreted L chain.

D. H-chain formation

—is genetically determined on human chromosome 14.

—involves selection, at the germline level, of 1 of 65 V exons, 1 of 6 J exons, 1 of 27 D exons, and 1 C exon, as indicated below.

—is preceded, as in L-chain formation, by DNA rearrangement and deletion of unused minigenes and by RNA splicing to remove introns before translation into the completed H chains.

E. Isotype formation

—is defined by expression of one of the C exons on the H chain encoding for μ, δ, γ3, γ1, α1, γ2, γ4, ε, or α2, in that order, on chromosome 14.

—occurs after the determination of idiotype (i.e., the assembly of the V-D-J exons).

F. Immunoglobulin assembly

—is initiated by the formation of a functional L chain from either chromosome 2 (κ) or chromosome 22 (λ).

—has as its second major step the assembly of a specific H-chain isotype.

—has as its final stage the joining of H chains and the joining of L chains to H chains by disulfide bonding.

—ends with secretion of the completed immunoglobulin molecule.

G. Antibody diversity

—is genetically determined and independent of antigen availability.

—allows for the expression of more than 10^6 different idiotypes.

—is generated by:

1. Random joining of V and J genes in L chains
2. Random joining of V, D, and J genes in H chains
3. Random assembly of H and L chains
4. "Errors" in recombination of the V, D, and J genes
5. Somatic mutations

V. Antigen–Antibody Reactions

A. Forces holding antigen–antibody complexes together

—are identical to any protein–protein interaction.

—are not covalent.

—include the following:

1. **Ionic bonds**—attraction of oppositely charged groups (e.g., NH_3^+ and ^-OOC)
2. **Hydrogen bonds**—sharing of hydrogen by hydrophilic groups
3. **Hydrophobic interactions**—exclusion of water by such amino acids as valine, leucine, and phenylalanine
4. **Van der Waals forces**—weak magnetic field

B. Definitions

1. Affinity

—is the tendency to form a stable complex.

—applies to a specific antibody directed against a specified epitope (i.e., a single antigen–antibody reaction).

—is defined by the formula:

$$\text{Affinity} = \frac{k}{k'} = \frac{[SL]}{[S][L]}$$

where

k = association constant

k' = disassociation constant

S = binding site of antibody (paratope)

L = ligand (epitope of antigen)

[ ] = concentration

which is derived from the standard protein (enzyme) formula: S + L = SL

2. Avidity

—is the sum of the affinities.

—refers to the total antibody response to all of the epitopes associated with a given antigen.

3. Lattice theory

—states that a precipitate will form in a lattice arrangement under optimum relationships between antibody and antigen.

—states that antibody or antigen excess will diminish a lattice network and decrease the amount of precipitate.

C. Types of antigen–antibody reactions

1. Quantitative precipitin curve

—is generated by a series of reactions usually involving a constant amount of antibody titrated against increasing amounts of antigen.

—is set as follows:

a. Nine test tubes are prepared, each with 0.1 mL of antiserum to ovalbumin (i.e., anti-OA antibody).

b. Each tube receives increasing amounts of antigen (tube 1 = 0 μg OA; tube 2 = 10 μg OA; tube 3 = 20 μg OA; and so on through tube 9 = 80 μg OA).

c. Upon incubation, there is a zone of antibody excess (tubes 1–3), a zone of equivalence (tubes 4–6), and a zone of antigen excess (tubes 7–9); precipitation occurs in all zones but is greatest at equivalence.

2. Ring test

—is a precipitation reaction that takes place at the interface between two solutions, one containing antigen and one containing antibody.

3. Oudin (single diffusion)

—is a precipitation technique, usually accomplished in a test tube, in which antibody (or antigen) in a gel is allowed to react with soluble antigen (or antibody) diffusing through it from a liquid interface.

4. Ouchterlony (double diffusion) [Figure 7-2]

—is a precipitation technique in agar, usually accomplished in a Petri dish, in which antigen and antibody are allowed to diffuse against each other and permit the formation of a precipitin line between the sample wells.

—If two or more sample (antigen) wells are diffused against a single antiserum (antibody) well, the following distinctions can be made:

a. **Lines of identity**—a single precipitin line indicating uniformity and identity of the antigens in the sample wells

b. **Lines of nonidentity**—two distinct and crossing precipitin lines indicating no cross-reactivity or identity between the antigens in the two sample wells

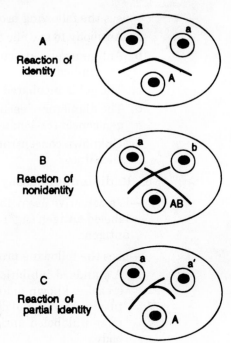

A
Reaction of
identity

B
Reaction of
nonidentity

C
Reaction of
partial identity

Figure 7-2. Ouchterlony double diffusion reactions showing (*A*) reaction of identity, (*B*) reaction of nonidentity, and (*C*) reaction of partial identity. *A* = antiserum to antigen a; *B* = antiserum to antigen b; *a* = antigen a; *b* = antigen b; *a′* = antigen with some antigenic determinants similar to those of a.

    c. Lines of partial identity—a spur formation, indicating that some of the antigenic determinants (epitopes) are shared between the antigens in the two sample wells

5. Immunoelectrophoresis (IEP)

    —is an antigen–antibody reaction technique developed to resolve and identify highly complex mixtures of antigens.

    a. Antigen is placed in a well in agar on a glass slide and subjected to **electrophoresis,** using an electric current, to separate the serum proteins at a given pH (usually pH 8.4) into their constituent parts (albumin, α_1, α_2, β_1, β_2, and γ-globulin fractions) according to their electrical charge.

    b. The separated proteins react with their specific antibody diffusing from an antiserum trough, and form a series of arcs of precipitate.

6. Rocket IEP

    —is a rapid method for estimating antigen concentration.

    —uses the following procedure:

    a. Sample wells are punched at one end of a gel plate in which antibody to a specific antigen has been dissolved.

    b. Samples are applied and electrophoresed.

    c. Rocket-like precipitate lines form. The length of the lines depends on the initial antigen sample concentration; a reference line is determined.

    d. Unknown concentration is determined by the length of the arc relative to the standard reference line.

7. Radial immunodiffusion

    —is a method for estimating antigen concentration.

—uses the following procedure:

a. Antibody to specific antigen is diffused in an agar gel or slab.

b. Antigen wells are cut, and samples of various known concentrations are applied.

c. The gel is incubated and precipitin rings are developed.

d. The diameter of each precipitin ring is proportional to the initial antigen concentration; a reference line is determined.

e. Unknown concentration is determined by comparison with the reference line.

8. **Radioimmunoassay (RIA)**

—is a sensitive assay for **antigen** that usually uses a known amount of labeled antigen (Ag*) and a known amount of specific antibody for that antigen.

—uses the following procedure:

a. A standard inhibition ("quench") curve is generated by reacting increasing known amounts of unlabeled antigen with the constant antibody amount and determining the ratio of bound Ag* to free Ag*; the more unlabeled antigen present, the less Ag* will be bound to antibody.

b. Unknown concentration is determined by interpolation of the standard inhibition curve.

9. **Radioimmunosorbent test (RIST)**

—is an RIA for **total IgE.**

—uses the following procedure:

a. A solid phase surface (e.g., dextran beads) is coupled with anti-IgE antibody.

b. A known concentration of labeled IgE (IgE*) is reacted with the bound antibody along with increasing known concentrations of unlabeled IgE to produce a standard inhibition curve.

c. An unknown serum sample is tested, and its IgE concentration is determined by interpolation of the standard inhibition curve.

10. **Radioallergosorbent test (RAST)**

—is an RIA to determine **specific IgE concentration.**

—uses the following procedure:

a. Solid phase beads are coupled with specific antigen.

b. Known amounts of specific IgE are reacted with the solid phase–antigen complex.

c. Labeled anti-IgE (anti-IgE*) is reacted with the solid phase–antigen complex.

d. Anti-IgE* is added, and the concentration of specific IgE is determined from the standard curve.

11. **Enzyme-linked immunosorbent assay (ELISA)**

—is the same test as RIA (RIST and RAST) except that an enzyme is attached to an antibody instead of a radioactive label, and different immunoglobulins are detected (not just IgE).

—involves measurement of a color change, which results from addition of substrate that is specific for the enzyme; the intensity of the color is proportional to the amount of antigen detected in the sample.

VI. Immunocompetent Cells in the Immune Response

—include macrophages, monocytes, and other antigen-presenting cells (APCs) as well as T cells and B cells.

A. Antigen-presenting cells

—include macrophages and monocytes and their derivatives, including microglial cells, Kupffer's cells, and Langerhans' cells of the skin.

—are characterized by dendritic extensions and by the ability to phagocytose, internalize, and process antigen.

—possess Ia antigens, Fc receptors, and C3b receptors.

—produce interleukin (IL)-1.

B. T cells

—are thymus-dependent lymphocytes.

—develop in the thymus.

—have a unique antigen receptor of a specific idiotype [T-cell receptor (TCR)].

—develop a series of thymus-induced differentiation markers labeled as cluster of differentiation (CD) antigens.

—have Fc receptors on some subsets and C3b receptors.

1. TCR (Figure 7-3)

—is the antigen-specific (idiotype) receptor on T cells.

—consists of a heterodimer—usually a 43-kd α chain and a 49-kd β chain, each having two external domains, a transmembrane segment, and a cytoplasmic extension. Most T cells (95%) possess the αβ TCR.

—may exist as a γδ heterodimer in a small subset of T cells (5% of total). The γδ TCR is not usually associated with either CD4 or CD8 and may have tumor or microbial antigen specificity.

—α chain is encoded on chromosome 14; β chain is encoded on chromosome 7.

—is encoded by a DNA rearrangement of V, D, and J exons for the V region, and a C gene for the C region.

—is associated with CD3.

2. CD markers

—arise on T cells during maturation in the thymus.

—appear on T cells in the following sequence: CD2 (formerly known as T11), CD3 (T3), CD4 (T4), and CD8 (T8).

a. CD2

—is the earliest T-cell marker.

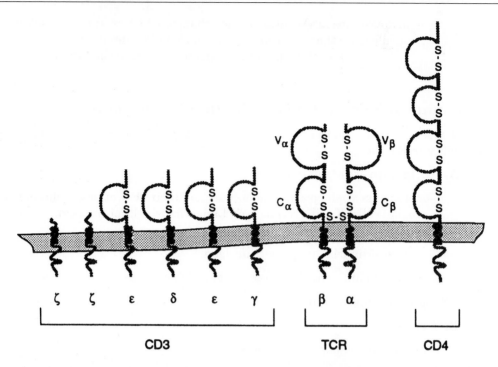

Figure 7-3. The T-cell receptor (TCR) complex consists of the TCR, CD3, and either CD4 or CD8 markers. The TCR is a heterodimer consisting of an alpha (α) and beta (β) chain, each of which has variable (V_α, V_β) and constant (C_α, C_β) domains. The TCR is associated with the CD3 molecule, which consists of three sets of dimers: gamma-epsilon (γ-ϵ), delta-epsilon (δ-ϵ), and two zeta (ζ) chains. CD3 transduces the external signal from the TCR to the cell cytoplasm. CD4 appears on helper T cells and binds to the class II histocompatibility antigens on antigen-presenting cells. CD8 is an analogous molecule that appears on cytotoxic T cells and binds the class I histocompatibility antigens found on all nucleated cells.

    —is the sheep red blood cell (SRBC) receptor.

    —is an adhesion molecule with a natural ligand of lymphocyte function associated antigen (LFA)-3 (CD58); the interaction allows T cells to bind to many other cells.

    —is present on virtually every peripheral T cell.

    —is a 50-kd polypeptide.

b. CD3

    —is intimately associated with TCR.

    —is composed of six molecules [consisting of a γ, δ, two ϵ, and two zeta (ζ) polypeptide chains], essentially transmembrane and cytoplasmic, that transduce signals from TCR.

    —exists as three sets of dimers: γ-ϵ, δ-ϵ, and ζ-ζ.

c. CD4

    —is present mainly on helper T (T_H) cells.

    —is involved in interaction with class II human leukocyte antigens (HLAs).

    —has a molecular weight of 62 kd.

d. CD8

    —is present mainly on cytotoxic T (T_C) cells.

—recognizes class I HLAs.

—has a molecular weight of 76 kd.

3. Ontogeny of T cells

—occurs as stem cells flow through the thymic cortex, into the medulla, and then out into the general circulation.

—begins in the thymic cortex with the appearance of CD2, followed by the appearance of CD3 (with TCR), then with concomitant expression of CD4 and CD8.

—in the thymic medulla consists of a loss of marker to produce two populations of cells—one $CD2^+$, $CD3^+$, TCR^+, $CD4^+$ (65%) and the other $CD2^+$, $CD3^+$, TCR^+, $CD8^+$ (35%)—that are then released into the peripheral circulation.

—is the time when both positive selection and negative selection occur.

a. Positive selection of thymocytes

—occurs in the cortical region of the thymus during the maturation process and involves the interaction of immature thymocytes with cortical epithelial cells, which bear major histocompatibility complex (MHC) molecules.

—selects those cells whose TCR binds with self-MHC molecules on the epithelial cells. The thymocytes that do not bind with self-MHC molecules die by apoptosis.

—results in cells that are self-MHC restricted.

b. Negative selection of thymocytes

—occurs in the medulla of the thymus and involves immature thymocytes that have survived positive selection.

—involves interaction of these thymocytes with dendritic cells and macrophages that bear self-MHC molecules and self-antigens. Thymocytes that have receptors for self-antigen in the presence of self-MHC molecules will die by apoptosis.

—results in thymocytes that are both self-MHC restricted and self-tolerant.

4. Other important T-cell markers

a. CD28

—is present on all $CD4^+$ cells and 50% of $CD8^+$ cells.

—is the natural ligand for B7.1 or B7.2 on APCs.

—acts as a costimulatory molecule for T cells.

—increases T-cell proliferation in addition to TCR activities.

b. CTLA-4 (CD152)

—is present on activated T cells.

—has considerable sequence homology with CD28.

—is the natural ligand for B7.1 or B7.2 on APCs.

—acts in an inhibitory manner on T cells, possibly causing apoptosis of activated cells.

c. LFA-1

—is an adhesion molecule.

—is also known as CD11a/CD18.

—has intercellular adhesion molecule-1 (ICAM-1; CD54) as its ligand, which is present on APCs and other cells.

d. CD40L

—appears on activated T_H cells.

—is the natural ligand for CD40 on B cells.

—allows B cells to switch isotype.

—Congenital immunodeficiency results in hyper-IgM syndrome, with no IgG, IgA, or IgE produced.

5. Subpopulations of T_H cells

a. T_H1 cells

—secrete IL-2, interferon (IFN)-γ, and tumor necrosis factor (TNF)-β.

—promote cell-mediated immunity by activating T_C cells and intracellular killing of pathogens by activating macrophages and other APCs.

b. T_H2 cells

—secrete IL-4, IL-5, IL-6, IL-10, and IL-13.

—promote B-cell transformation and proliferation.

—are potent chemoattractants of B cells, basophils, eosinophils, and mast cells.

—promote the humoral immune response by causing B cells to increase antibody production and to switch the antibody class.

—promote the production of IgE through IL-4 action on activated B cells.

C. B cells

—are thymus-independent lymphocytes.

—develop independent of antigen.

—arise from stem cells and mature in the bone marrow (bursa of Fabricius in birds), bursal equivalent, or both.

—have a unique surface immunoglobulin (S-Ig) receptor for antigen.

—develop a series of markers during the differentiation process.

1. S-Ig

—is the antigen-specific idiotype receptor on B cells.

—is equivalent to an antibody molecule with a transmembrane projection.

—exists in 100,000 copies per mature B cell.

—is associated with signal transduction molecules, Ig-α and Ig-β.

—undergoes capping and endocytosis after activation by antigen.

2. Ontogeny of B cells

—is the process by which a stem cell undergoes differentiation from a pre–B cell, to an immature B cell, to a mature B cell that is driven by antigen to become an activated B cell, and finally becomes a plasma cell that is capable of producing immunoglobulin.

—is initiated in the fetal liver and adult bone marrow and usually terminates in the germinal centers of the lymph nodes, in the spleen, and in the red pulp of the spleen.

3. **Sequential appearance of B-cell markers in B-cell maturation**

   a. **Hematopoietic stem cell**—CD34 marker present

   b. **Pro–B cell**—D-J gene rearrangement

   c. **Pre–B cell**—V-D-J rearrangement; cytoplasmic μ chains

   d. **Late pre–B cell**—surface μ chains and surrogate L chains; Ig-α and Ig-β transduction molecules

      —Stage at which **positive selection** of B cells occurs. Only cells that have produced a viable μ chain continue to mature.

   e. **Immature B cell**—V-J rearrangement of L chain; membrane-bound IgM subunits; C3b, Fc, Epstein-Barr virus (EBV) receptors

      —Stage at which **negative selection** of B cells occurs. Cells encountering cell-bound self-antigen on the surface of bone marrow cells die by apoptosis (deletion); cells encountering soluble antigen are inactivated (anergy).

   f. **Mature B cell**—membrane-bound IgM and IgD

   g. **Activated B cell**—presence of antigen; "capping" of S-Ig; proliferation of B cells

   h. **Plasma cell**—few S-Ig and HLA-DR molecules; no Fc, C3b, and EBV receptors; immunoglobulin secretion

   i. **Memory cells**—surface immunoglobulin expressed

4. **B-cell surface molecules** (partial list)

   a. **S-Ig**—antigen-binding components

   b. **Ig-α and Ig-β**—signal transduction molecules

   c. **CD19, CD20, and CD81**—additional transduction molecules

   d. **CD32**—Fc receptor for IgG (FcγRII)

   e. **Class II MHC**—presents processed peptide to CD4 T_H cells; binds to TCR and CD4

   f. **CD40**—binds to CD40L on T cells to induce immunoglobulin class switch

   g. **B7.1 and B7.2**—interact with CD28 on T cells; costimulatory molecules

   h. **CD5**—marker on B-1 cells, which arise earlier in ontogeny than conventional B cells (B-2 cells); B-1 cells produce low-affinity IgM against bacterial polysaccharide antigen

VII. Actions and Products of Immune System Cells

A. **Actions of immune system cells**

1. **APCs—macrophages**

   —phagocytose, process, and degrade the antigen.

   —express antigenic determinants (epitopes) of the antigen on their surface in the context of class II HLA molecules.

—produce IL-1 and possibly other monokines.

2. T$_H$ cells

—recognize antigen epitopes in the context of class II HLA molecules by TCR and CD4.

—use the CD3 molecules to transduce the antigenic signal internally.

—react with IL-1 from APCs.

—produce IL-2 and express IL-2 receptors.

—become activated when the IL-2 receptors are occupied by IL-2.

—produce a variety of lymphokines, which have a stimulatory role in B-cell growth and differentiation.

3. B cells

—recognize antigen epitopes via surface immunoglobulin receptors.

—cross-link these antigen epitopes on the B-cell surface.

—undergo capping and internalization (by pinocytosis) of these "occupied" surface receptors.

—are stimulated to blastogenesis and differentiated into plasma cells by lymphokines produced by T$_H$ cells.

B. Products of immune system cells (Table 7-1)

1. IL-1

—is produced by many different cell types, with relatively high concentrations being produced by macrophages, monocytes, Langerhans' cells of the skin, and other dendritic cells.

—was formerly known as lymphocyte-activating factor (LAF).

—augments the activity of many cell types, especially T cells.

—is an endogenous pyrogen (EP).

—induces an increase in acute phase reactants.

—is a heat-stable and pH-stable peptide with a molecular weight of 17.5 kd.

—occurs in two forms: IL-1α and IL-1β.

2. IL-2

—is produced by T cells and large granular lymphocytes (LGLs).

—was formerly known as T-cell growth factor (TCGF).

—augments proliferation of T and B cells.

—enhances activity of T cells and natural killer (NK) cells.

—is a heat-labile glycoprotein with a molecular weight of 15.5 kd.

3. IFN-γ (Table 7-2)

—is produced by activated T cells and LGLs.

—increases the expression of class II HLAs on B cells, macrophages, and other APCs.

—has antiviral properties.

Table 7-1. Cytokines and Their Actions

Cytokine	Major Cell Source	Major Immunologic Action
IL-1 (α, β)	Macrophages Endothelial cells Dendritic cells Langerhans' cells	Stimulates IL-2 receptor emergence in T cells Enhances B-cell activation Induces fever, acute phase reactants, and IL-6 Increases nonspecific resistance Inhibited by an endogenous IL-1 receptor antagonist
IL-2	T_H1 cells	T-cell growth factor Activates NK and B cells
IL-3	T cells	Stimulates hematopoiesis
IL-4	T cells	Stimulates B-cell synthesis of IgE Down-regulation of IFN-γ
IL-5	T cells	Stimulates growth and differentiation of eosinophils B-cell growth factor Enhances IgA synthesis
IL-6	Monocytes T cells Endothelial cells	Induces acute phase reactants, fever, and late B-cell differentiation
IL-7	Bone marrow	Stimulates pre–B and pre–T cells
IL-8	Monocytes Endothelial cells Lymphocytes Fibroblasts	Chemotactic factor for neutrophils and T cells
IL-9	T_H cells	T-cell mitogen
IL-10	T_H2 cells	Inhibits IFN-γ synthesis by T_H1 cells Suppresses other cytokine synthesis
IL-11	Bone marrow	Stimulates hematopoiesis Enhances acute phase protein synthesis
IL-12	Macrophages B cells	Promotes T_H1 differentiation and IFN-γ synthesis Stimulates NK cells and $CD8^+$ T cells to cytolysis Acts synergistically with IL-2
IL-13	T_H2 cells	Inhibits inflammatory cytokines (IL-1, IL-6, IL-8, IL-10, MCP)
IL-15	T cells	T-cell mitogen Enhances growth of intestinal epithelium
IL-16	$CD8^+$ T cells Eosinophils	Increases class II MHC, chemotaxis, and $CD4^+$ T-cell cytokines Decreases antigen-induced proliferation
IL-17	T cells	Increases the inflammatory response
IL-18	Activated macrophages	Increases IFN-γ production and NK cell action
TNF-α	Macrophages T cells B cells Large granular lymphocytes	Cytotoxic for tumors Causes cachexia Mediates bacterial shock
TNF-β	T cells	Cytotoxic for tumors
Transforming growth factor β	Almost all normal cell types	Inhibits proliferation of both T and B cells Reduces cytokine receptors Potent chemotactic agent for leukocytes Mediates inflammation and tissue repair

IFN = interferon; Ig = immunoglobulin; IL = interleukin; MCP = macrophage chemotactic protein; MHC = major histocompatibility complex; NK = natural killer; TNF = tumor necrosis factor.

Table 7-2. Interferons

Type	Characteristic
Alpha	At least 17 different subtypes
	Produced in B and null lymphocytes, macrophages, and epithelial cells
	Induced by viruses, bacteria, and tumor and foreign cells
	Inhibits viral replication
Beta	Only a single entity
	Produced in fibroblasts, macrophages, and epithelial cells
	Induced by viruses and bacterial products
	Inhibits viral replication
Gamma	Only a single entity
	Produced by T_H1 and NK cells
	Potent activator of macrophages
	Strong immunomodulating agent
	Inhibits IL-4 activation of mast cells and IgE synthesis

Ig = immunoglobulin; IL = interleukin; NK = natural killer; T_H = helper T cells.

    —provides regulatory control in the immune response.

    —has a heat-labile glycoprotein with a molecular weight of 17 kd.

4. IL-3

    —is produced by T cells.

    —enhances hematopoiesis.

5. IL-4

    —is produced by T cells.

    —is mitogenic for B cells.

    —promotes a switch to IgE production.

    —stimulates mast cells.

6. IL-5

    —is produced by T cells.

    —stimulates B-cell differentiation and maturation.

    —enhances IL-2 receptor expression.

    —enhances IgA synthesis.

7. IL-6

    —is produced by B cells, T cells, monocytes, and fibroblasts.

    —induces acute phase reactants.

    —induces B-cell differentiation.

VIII. Initiators of the Immune Response

A. T-dependent antigens

    —are the predominant type of initiator of the immune response.

    —necessarily need the presence of an APC and the activation of T_H cells and their concomitant lymphokines to activate and differentiate B cells to become plasma cells and secrete antibody.

B. T-independent antigens

—do not need T_H cell activity, T-cell activation, or the production of lymphokines.

—are polymeric in nature.

—produce a primary (IgM) immune response; they produce neither memory cells nor an anamnestic, secondary (IgG) immune response.

—include endotoxin, lipopolysaccharide, polysaccharide capsules, dextran, polyvinylpyrrolidone, polymerized flagellin, and EBV.

C. T-cell mitogens

—are polyclonal activators of T cells.

—stimulate general T-cell activation by cross-linking specific sugars on the cell surface.

—include concanavalin A (Con A) and phytohemagglutinin (PHA).

D. B-cell mitogens

—are polyclonal activators of B cells.

—include all of the T-independent antigens.

IX. Immunology of Acquired Immunodeficiency Syndrome (AIDS)

A. Acquired immunodeficiency syndrome

—is caused by human immunodeficiency virus 1 (HIV-1).

—is characterized by the loss of T_H (CD4$^+$) cells, specifically the T_H1 subset.

—results in an increase in opportunistic infections [e.g., *Pneumocystis carinii* (fungal infection), *Mycobacterium tuberculosis*], neoplasms (e.g., Kaposi's sarcoma, tumor of blood vessel tissue of skin and internal organs), skin disorders, and neurologic disease.

B. History

—The current epidemic has been ongoing since 1981, probably originating in central Africa and moving to the United States and Europe via the Caribbean Islands.

—The causative agent was identified as lymphadenopathy-associated virus (LAV) in 1983 by Luc Montagnier of the Pasteur Institute; in 1984, the human T lymphotropic virus-III (HTLV-III) was identified by Robert Gallo of the National Institutes of Health.

—The virus is now referred to as HIV-1 (the prevalent form in the United States, Europe, the Caribbean, and South America) and HIV-2 (a less virulent form prevalent in Africa and Asia).

—Testing for anti–HIV-1 antibody has been available since 1985, a crucial step in ensuring the safety of the blood banking industry.

—In 1987, the book, *And the Band Played On,* presented the early attempts to identify and control this epidemic.

—In 1988, azidothymidine (**AZT, zidovudine**), a reverse transcriptase inhibitor, was approved as a treatment for AIDS.

—In 1992, dideoxyinosine didanosine (**ddI**) and dideoxycytidine (**ddC**) were approved as treatments for patients with AIDS.

—In 1996, drug cocktails, which included **protease inhibitors** (saquinavir, ritonavir), were being used with some effectiveness. These agents prevent the production of HIV proteins. (See the December, 1996 issue of *Time* magazine, Man of the Year story.)

—Since 1998, parenterally administered vaccines (gp120 and gp41) are being tested.

C. Human immunodeficiency virus

—is a member of the lentivirus family of retroviruses.

—has an external membrane derived from the host cell.

—has glycoproteins on and in the membrane (gp120 and gp41) that are encoded by the *env* gene.

—has a protein core (p17 matrix, p24 capsid, and p7 nucleocapsid) encoded by *gag* genes.

—has two copies of the viral RNA genome and the reverse transcriptase, ribonuclease, and protease encoded by the *pol* gene within the core.

D. Transmission of human immunodeficiency virus

—is most effective via whole infected cells:

1. **Sexual contact** [e.g., blood, semen; risk increases with large number of partners, "rough" sex, and other sexually transmitted diseases (i.e., gonorrhea, herpesvirus type 2)]

2. **Drug users,** via shared needles

3. **Blood** and blood products (hemophiliacs at risk)

4. **Perinatally,** from mother to infant (transmission rate is 25%; AZT is now usually administered to pregnant HIV patients)

E. Prevalence of acquired immunodeficiency syndrome

—was estimated at approximately 860,000 cases in the United States as of January, 1998; these cases were distributed as follows:

1. Homosexual and bisexual men: 52%

2. Intravenous drug users: 24%

3. Homosexual and bisexual persons and intravenous drug users: 7%

4. Persons with hemophilia and coagulation disorders: 1%

5. Heterosexual persons: 7%

6. Persons who received a blood transfusion: 1%

7. Undetermined: 7%

F. Incidence of acquired immunodeficiency syndrome

—is estimated by the World Health Organization; the number of adults and children living with HIV or AIDS as of January, 1998 is as follows:

1. North America: 860,000
2. Caribbean Islands: 310,000
3. Latin America (Central and South America): 1.3 million
4. Western Europe: 530,000
5. Eastern Europe and Central Asia: 150,000
6. East Asia and Pacific Islands: 440,000
7. South and Southeast Asia: 6.0 million
8. Australia and New Zealand: 12,000
9. North Africa and Middle East: 210,000
10. Sub-Sahara Africa: 20.8 million

G. Acquired immunodeficiency syndrome testing techniques

1. ELISA

—is the primary test to detect HIV-1 infection.

—detects the presence of anti-HIV antibodies (anti-gp120 and anti-p24) in the circulation.

—is a test by which purified native or recombinant virion proteins (e.g., HIV-1) are immobilized on plastic beads or multiwell trays and bind to antibodies in test serum specific to those proteins; an enzyme-linked anti-antibody added to the well is then read colorimetrically.

—is both highly sensitive (> 99%) and highly specific (> 99%).

2. Western blot

—is the **confirming** test for HIV infection.

—detects the presence of antibodies to the various protein components of HIV (e.g., anti-p18, anti-p24, anti-gp41).

—consists of four steps:

a. Electrophoresis of HIV proteins on cellulose acetate
b. Reacting putative serum antibodies of patients with the bound HIV proteins
c. Reacting conjugated (enzyme or radiolabeled) anti-antibody with the serum antibodies and the HIV proteins
d. Reading color change or radioactivity for positive result

H. Effect of human immunodeficiency virus infection on the immune system

1. HIV-1 destroys $CD4^+$ (T_H) cells, which are pivotal in the immune response.

2. The receptor for HIV is the CD4 molecule, probably via gp120 and gp41.

   —More recent findings (1996) indicate that HIV needs a coreceptor for entry into target cells (via the V3 loop of gp120).

    a. HIV that has an affinity for macrophages predominates during the early part of an HIV infection. The coreceptor (in addition to CD4) on the macrophage is CCR-5 (a 7tM molecule).

    b. HIV that has an affinity for T cells has as its coreceptor (in addition to CD4) the molecule CXCR4 (fusin). This type of HIV predominates in the late stages of AIDS development.

  3. The HIV envelope proteins may mimic parts of class II HLAs, leading to binding of HIV to CD4 and loss of the immune response.

  4. Macrophages and some brain cells may have low levels of CD4 on the surface, allowing for tropism by HIV and multiplication of HIV in these cells but not destruction of the carrier cells. This would allow HIV to be hidden from the immune system for an indefinite period.

I. **Sequential events in human immunodeficiency virus infection**

  1. After binding to CD4$^+$, the virus is engulfed and uncoated.

  2. RNA is transcribed to DNA by reverse transcriptase (*pol* gene product) and is inserted into human chromosomal DNA by endonuclease (*pol* product) as the provirion.

  3. The provirus is the latent stage.

    —More recent findings (1996) indicate that there may not actually be a "latent period" in HIV infection.

    a. It is now believed that within days or weeks after primary HIV infection, the virus is found in huge numbers throughout the circulation and all lymphoid tissue.

    b. As many as 10^9 lymphocytes are killed daily, especially "naive" CD4 cells. The dead cells are replaced daily until the body can no longer sustain this insult.

    c. Antibody levels to HIV epitopes are phenomenal and free virus in serum is kept in check, but virus in cells continues to multiply and be released.

    d. Long-term survivors of HIV infection appear to have a greater T_H1 response, producing IL-2 and IFN, leading to heightened cell-mediated immunity to HIV. Also, CD8 cells appear to produce cytokines, which have CCR-5 and CXCR4 as receptors and, thus, effectively block HIV entry.

    e. A small group has been shown to be resistant to HIV infection because of an inherited deficiency of the CCR-5 chemokine coreceptor.

  4. Activation of the cell causes DNA $\rightarrow$ RNA $\rightarrow$ mRNA transcription $\rightarrow$ protein synthesis $\rightarrow$ virus $\rightarrow$ virus budding with destruction of the CD4$^+$ cell and release of the HIV virus.

  5. Death of the cell may be due to formation of **syncytia** by the infected cell gp120 interaction with CD4 of the noninfected cell.

  6. The number of CD4$^+$ cells is approximately 1200/mm^3 of blood. HIV infection gradually decreases this number over time. When the number of CD4$^+$ cells falls below 200/mm^3 of blood, clinical AIDS ensues.

J. **Treatment modalities for human immunodeficiency virus infection and acquired immunodeficiency syndrome**

1. **AZT** is the drug treatment of choice. It probably prevents the virus from replicating, interferes with reverse transcriptase, or acts as a false building block in viral DNA assembly.

2. The drugs **ddI, ddC,** and **3TC** have similar modes of action and may be used in concert with AZT.

3. Protease inhibitors, which prevent the virus assembly of its surface protein coat subunits, has had marked effectiveness in many cases, especially when administered in combination with drugs that inhibit reverse transcriptase (AZT, ddC, ddI).

4. **Parenteral injection of gp120 and gp41 proteins** to enhance the immune response of HIV-infected persons and as a potential vaccine have thus far had only limited success, which is most likely due to the extensive mutability of the virus envelope.

X. Histocompatibility Antigens

A. Major histocompatibility complex (MHC) [Figure 7-4]

—is located on the short (p) arm of human chromosome 6.

—encodes for the major histocompatibility antigens, known in humans as **human leukocyte antigens (HLA).**

—encodes for the class I antigens by the genes HLA-A, HLA-B, and HLA-C.

—encodes for the class II antigens, defined by the genes in the D (immune response) region, HLA-DR, HLA-DP, and HLA-DQ.

—encodes for the class III antigens, which include various complement components such as C2, C4, factor B, and the C3b receptor.

1. Class I MHC molecules (see Figure 7-4)

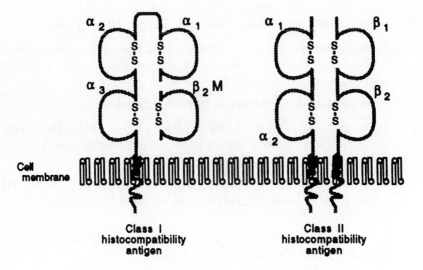

Figure 7-4. Class I and class II histocompatibility antigens α_1, α_2, α_3 are the three external domains of a class I histocompatibility antigen. $\beta_2M = \beta_2$ microglobulin; α_1 and α_2 = external domains of class II histocompatibility antigen; β_1 and β_2 = external domains of class II histocompatibility antigen.

—are encoded by HLA-A, HLA-B, and HLA-C genes.

—are expressed on every nucleated cell in the body.

—are associated noncovalently with a 12-kd polypeptide, β_2-microglobulin, which is encoded on chromosome 15.

—consist of a 44-kd polypeptide chain containing transmembrane and cytoplasmic components.

—have three external domains analogous to immunoglobulin domains (β_2-microglobulin defines the fourth domain).

—are involved in recognition (restriction) by T_C cells, which bear appropriate receptors for the class I molecules (CD8).

—are associated with the presentation of antigen on virus-infected or transformed cells.

2. **Class II MHC molecules** (see Figure 7-4)

—are encoded by genes in the HLA-D region: HLA-DR, HLA-DQ, and HLA-DP.

—are expressed mainly on B cells, macrophages, activated T cells, and other APCs.

—consist of an α-chain (29 kd) and β-chain (34 kd) heterodimer, with cytoplasmic and transmembrane components.

—possess two external domains on each of the polypeptide chains.

—allow interaction (restriction) between APCs and T cells via CD4.

—are associated with the presentation of antigen on APCs.

B. **Immunologic role of the histocompatibility antigens**

—Antigens are recognized by the appropriate TCR only in the context of the histocompatibility antigens.

—Exogenous antigens (e.g., bacteria), which would undergo processing by an APC, would be expressed on the surface of the APC in the context of a class II MHC molecule and be recognized by $CD4^+$ T_H cells.

—Endogenous antigens (e.g., virally transformed cell proteins) would be expressed on the surface of any cell in the context of a class I MHC molecule and be recognized by a $CD8^+$ T_C cell.

C. **Histocompatibility antigens in transplantation**

—Because the MHC gene products, both class I and class II, are cell-surface proteins and very antigenic, it is important that tissues be typed before transplantation.

—The histocompatibility antigens are very polymorphic. In the HLA class I, there are at least 167 specificities encoded by HLA-A, 149 by HLA-B, and 39 by HLA-C.

—In the class II HLA, there are at least 180 specificities encoded for HLA-DR, 50 for HLA-DQ, and 8 for HLA-DP.

D. **Human leukocyte antigens and disease association**

—Certain diseases have a propensity for persons with a particular HLA.

—Relative risk quantifies the chance of an individual with the specific HLA to acquire a specific disease compared with an individual who does not have that HLA.

—Examples are included in Table 7-3.

XI. Tumor Immunology

A. Tumor cells

—are cells that have been transformed by virus or by chemical or physical means.

—are usually not well differentiated.

—lack contact inhibition and usually proliferate uncontrollably.

—have tumor-associated antigen (TAA) expression on their surface.

1. Viral tumors

—are caused by RNA and DNA oncogenic viruses.

—share TAA epitopes with cells transformed by the same or similar viruses and may have cross-reactivity.

2. Chemically induced tumors

—are caused by a variety of chemical carcinogens (e.g., coal tar and 3-methylcholanthrene).

—share virtually no TAA epitopes and have no cross-reactivity.

3. Physically induced tumors

—are caused by physical "insult" such as contact with ultraviolet light, radiographs, or γ-radiation.

—behave akin to chemically induced tumors (i.e., no cross-reactivity).

4. Oncofetal antigens

—are antigenic epitopes that are found in normal fetal development and on some transformed (tumor) cells.

—are not usually present on normal adult cells.

a. Carcinoembryonic antigen (CEA)

Table 7-3. Human Leukocyte Antigens (HLA) and Disease Association

Disease	HLA	Risk*
Ankylosing spondylitis	B27	87
Dermatitis herpetiformis	DR3	56
Reiter's syndrome	B27	40
Insulin-dependent diabetes	DR3/DR4	33
Psoriasis vulgaris	C6	13
Goodpasture's syndrome	DR2	13
Sjögren's syndrome	DR3	6
Behçet's disease	B5	4

*Times more likely to acquire the disease than a person who does not have the specific HLA

—is normally found in the intestine, liver, and pancreas in months 2 to 6 of gestation.

—appears in 90% of pancreatic cancers, 70% of colon cancers, 35% of breast cancers, and 5% of normal persons.

—increases during pregnancy and in recurrence of the relevant tumor.

b. α-Fetoprotein (AFP)

—is the normal α-globulin of embryonic and fetal serum.

—appears in hepatomas, cirrhosis, and hepatitis.

B. Immune mechanisms in tumor-cell destruction

—include both the humoral and the cell-mediated mechanisms elicited by TAAs.

1. Humoral immunity to tumor cells

—starts with antibody binding to tumor cells and can lead to killing of tumor cells by:

a. Attachment of antibody to Fc receptors on macrophages and neutrophils, followed by phagocytosis

b. Attachment of antibody to Fc receptors on null (killer) cells, followed by lysis by antibody-dependent cell-mediated cytotoxicity (ADCC)

c. Activation of the complete complement sequence, causing tumor lysis

d. Activation of the complement sequence to produce C3b on the tumor-cell surface, which reacts with C3b receptors on macrophages and neutrophils to enhance phagocytosis

2. Cell-mediated immunity to tumor cells

—leads to killing of tumor cells by:

a. Production of lymphokines by T_H cells, thereby mobilizing and activating macrophages against tumor cells; these lymphokines include macrophage-activating factor (MAF), macrophage migration inhibition factor (MIF), and macrophage chemotactic factor (MCF)

b. Production of monokines by activated macrophages (e.g., TNF)

c. Activation of $CD8^+$ T_C cells that recognize TAA on virally transformed cells in association with class I histocompatibility antigens

d. Killing of tumor cells—spontaneously and without previous sensitization—by NK cells

XII. Blood Group Immunology

A. ABO system

—is defined by the presence of alloantigens A and B on the surface of red blood cells.

—is characterized by natural isohemagglutinins (predominantly IgM) in the circulation.

—is determined genetically by the A, B, and O alleles, where A and B are dominant over O.

1. Type (phenotype) A

—has A alloantigen on red blood cells.

—has anti-B isohemagglutinin in serum.

—can be genotype AA (homozygous) or AO (heterozygous).

2. **Type B**

—has B alloantigen on red blood cells.

—has anti-A isohemagglutinin in serum.

—can be genotype BB or BO.

3. **Type AB**

—has both A and B alloantigens on red blood cells.

—has no isohemagglutinins.

—is genotype AB.

4. **Type O**

—has neither A nor B alloantigens on red blood cells.

—has both anti-A and anti-B isohemagglutinins.

—is genotype OO; the O allele does not code for any product.

—has H antigen fully expressed.

B. Rh antigens

—are determined by a complex of genes, DCE/dce; the D antigen is the most important medically.

—have codominant expression.

—are called "positive" if the D gene is expressed and "negative" if D is not expressed.

—Incompatibility can lead to hemolytic disease of the newborn, which can be prevented if the Rh-negative mother is inoculated with anti-Rh antibody within 72 hours after delivery of an Rh-positive infant.

XIII. The Complement System

A. Complement-mediated cell cytotoxicity

—causes lysis of a target cell.

—may be initiated by antibody fixation to a cell-surface antigen.

—may be caused by antigen–antibody complex formation.

—occurs by activation of either:

1. **Classic complement cascade**—mediated by IgG, IgG2, IgG3, or IgM antibody

2. **Alternative pathway**—initiated by certain antigens (i.e., lipopolysaccharide, endotoxin, zymosan) or antigen–antibody complexes

B. Complement components

—is a collective term for a group of heterogeneous proteins involved in a sequential activation, culminating in target cell lysis.

—are not immunoglobulins.

—are present in normal serum.

—do not increase as a result of antigen stimulation.

—are manufactured early in ontogeny (first trimester).

—are made in macrophages and liver (except C1, which is made and assembled in gastrointestinal epithelium).

—are heat labile.

—are defined by number (C1, C2, C3) and letter (factor B, factor D) designations.

C. **Classic activation pathway** (Figure 7-5)

1. A singlet of IgM or a doublet of IgG1, IgG2, or IgG3, very closely spaced on the cell surface, binds C1 by the C1q region via a receptor in the Fc region (Cμ4 or Cγ3).

2. C1 consists of subunits of C1q, C1r, and C1s bound by Ca^{2+} and is activated from a proesterase to an esterase, cleaving both C4 and C2 sequentially.

3. C4 is cleaved into C4b and C4a, with C4b attaching at the site of antibody fixation and C4a going off in the fluid phase; C4a may act as an anaphylatoxin.

4. C2 is cleaved into C2a and C2b, with C2a attaching to C4b via Mg^{2+}; C2b is released in the fluid phase and acts as a kinin.

5. Antibody-C1–C4bC2a complex is C3 convertase.

6. C3 is cleaved into C3a and C3b; C3b has receptors on many cell surfaces, including neutrophils and macrophages; C3a is anaphylatoxin I and attaches preferentially to C3a receptors on mast cells and causes histamine release.

7. C5 is analogous to C3 and is cleaved into C5b and C5a; C5b causes activation of C6 and C7; C5a is anaphylatoxin II, has receptors on mast cells for histamine release, and is chemotactic for neutrophils and macrophages.

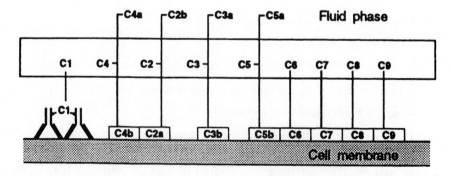

Figure 7-5. Diagrammatic presentation of the classic pathway of complement activation. C1 attaches to a doublet of immunoglobulin G (IgG) on the cell surface. C4 is cleaved to C4a (goes to fluid phase) and C4b. C2 is cleaved to C2a, which attaches to C4b to yield C3 convertase and C2b (fluid phase). C3 is cleaved to yield C3a (fluid phase) and C3b on the cell surface. C5 is cleaved to yield C5a (fluid phase) and C5b on the surface. C6, C7, C8, and C9 are then placed on the cell surface in equimolar concentrations and probably form a circular channel to allow fluid influx.

8. C6 and C7 are activated by C5b and exist as an activated entity C5b67, which is chemotactic for neutrophils and macrophages.

9. C8 and C9 cause permeability changes and allow water influx, resulting in cell swelling and lysis.

D. Control mechanisms of complement activation

1. Instability of components

—includes the short half-lives of C2a and C5b.

2. Inhibitors

—include C1 inhibitor (C1-INH), which stops continued activation of C1; congenital lack of C1-INH is called hereditary angioedema.

3. Inactivators

—include:

a. **C3b inactivator**—an enzyme that destroys C3b activity

b. **C6 inactivator**—destroys C6 activity

c. **Anaphylatoxin inactivator**—cleaves C-terminal arginine from C3a and C5a

E. Alternative activation pathway

—is caused by the presence of zymosan, endotoxin, or complexes of aggregated human immunoglobulins, including $F(ab')_2$ fragments.

—bypasses the need for specific antibody and early components C1, C4, and C2.

1. Low levels of C3b are present in serum under normal circumstances.

2. In the presence of factor D, factor B can be cleaved into Bb and Ba; Bb assembles with C3b.

3. Properdin (P) stabilizes C3bBb on the surface of zymosan or endotoxin and allows this entity (P.C3b.Bb) to cleave another molecule of C3 to continue the cascade.

XIV. Hypersensitivity Reactions

—are categorized according to the **Gell and Coombs classification.**

A. Type I hypersensitivity—anaphylaxis

—occurs in atopic persons.

—occurs in response to environmental antigens (e.g., allergens) or administered antigens (e.g., penicillin).

—is mediated by IgE (reaginic) antibody bound to the surface of mast cells or basophils.

—may be localized or systemic.

1. IgE in immediate hypersensitivity

—is produced in response to environmental antigens.

—binds by the Fc portion of IgE to mast cells or basophils.

—causes release of vasoactive and chemotactic factors from mast cells upon cross-linking of antigen on the surface.

—can be measured in toto by use of **RIST.**

—can also be measured for specific idiotypes by **RAST.**

2. **Products released by mast cells upon stimulation of surface IgE**
   a. **Vasoactive mediators**
      (1) **Histamine**—causes smooth muscle contraction in bronchioles and small blood vessels and increased permeability of capillaries; molecular weight is 111 daltons.
      (2) **Platelet-activating factor (PAF)**—activates platelets.
      (3) **Slow-reacting substance of anaphylaxis (SRS-A)**—consists of metabolite of arachidonic acid and includes the leukotrienes LTC4, LTD4, and LTE4.
      (4) **Prostaglandins and thromboxanes**—products of cyclooxygenase metabolism or arachidonic acid; cause erythema and vasopermeability. These metabolites are potent inducers of smooth muscle contractility, bronchoconstriction, and increased vascular permeability.
   b. **Chemotactic factors**
      (1) **Eosinophil chemotactic factor of anaphylaxis (ECF-A)**—causes influx of eosinophils; molecular weight is 2 kd.
      (2) **Neutrophil chemotactic factor**—has a high molecular weight (660 kd); is chemotactic for neutrophils.

3. **Treatment of allergic reactions**
   a. Eliminate or avoid the allergen.
   b. Tie up IgE molecules with haptens of allergens or with monovalent antigens.
   c. Inject patient with solubilized allergen to cause production of IgG, which competes with IgE for allergen (**hypersensitization**).
   d. Administer **cromolyn sodium;** stabilize the mast-cell membrane and decrease the amount of histamine released.
   e. Increase cyclic adenosine monophosphate (AMP) levels, which stabilizes the mast-cell membrane and decreases the amount of vasoactive and chemotactic molecules released; this may be done by an increase of adenyl cyclase activity (stimulation of β-receptors, isoproterenol) or by a decrease in phosphodiesterase activity (methylxanthines—aminophylline, theophylline).

B. **Type II hypersensitivity—cytotoxic reactions**

—involve the production of antibody to specific cell-surface epitopes, which cause destruction of the cell.

1. **Antibody to cell-surface antigen**

   —can cause reduction in cell-surface charges.

   —can cause opsonic adherence via the Fc region of antibody to neutrophils, macrophages, and K cells (the cells responsible for ADCC); enhances cell phagocytosis and promotes cell death.

   —can activate complement to cause cell lysis.

2. Examples of type II hypersensitivity reactions

a. **Transfusion reactions**—ABO incompatibility involving IgM antibodies against A or B alloantigens

b. **Rh incompatibility**—IgG antibodies against the D antigen on fetal red blood cells

c. **Hemolytic anemia**—antibody to red blood cell epitopes

d. **Goodpasture's syndrome**—antibody to glomerular and bronchial basement membrane

e. **Myasthenia gravis**—antibody to muscle acetylcholine receptors

C. Type III hypersensitivity—immune complex reactions

—involve soluble antigen that becomes bound antigen–antibody complexes, which, especially in antigen excess, can cause a series of events that lead to pathologic expression, edema, neutrophil infiltrate, and lesions in blood vessels and kidney glomeruli.

1. Consequences of antigen–antibody complex formation

a. Platelet aggregation, leading to formation of microthrombi and release of vasoactive amines

b. Activation of complement and release of anaphylatoxins (causing histamine release) and chemotactic factors (for neutrophils)

c. Clotting factor XII activation, leading to fibrin, plasmin, and kinin formation

2. Examples of type III hypersensitivity reactions

a. **Arthus reaction**—immunization of rabbits with horse serum (classic prototype of type III reaction)

b. **Farmer's lung**—antibody to inhaled aspergillus mold

c. **Cheesemaker's lung**—antibody to fungi

d. **Pigeon fancier's disease**—antibody to pigeon dander

e. **Serum sickness**—antibody to "foreign" immunoglobulin injection

f. **Rheumatoid arthritis**—rheumatoid factor (IgM) against the Fc portion of self-IgG

D. Type IV hypersensitivity—delayed-type hypersensitivity

—is differentiated from immediate-type hypersensitivity reactions (types I, II, and III).

—is an example of cell-mediated immunity; types I, II, and III are mediated by antibody and are examples of humoral immunity.

1. Sequence of events in a type IV reaction

a. An appropriate antigen (tuberculin, purified protein derivative of *Mycobacterium tuberculosis,* tumor cell, transplanted cell, virally transformed cell) is processed by macrophages; epitopes of antigen are expressed on the macrophage surface via class II HLAs; macrophages produce IL-1.

b. T_H cells react to antigen epitope and class II antigens via TCR and CD4, respectively.

c. T_H cells are also stimulated by IL-1 from macrophages.

d. T_H cells produce IL-2, and IL-2 receptors become fully activated and release lymphokines, having an effect on T cells and macrophages.

2. Lymphokines

—that affect macrophages include MCF, MIF, and MAF.

—that affect CD8$^+$ cells include IL-2, which activates them to become fully cytotoxic.

—that are produced by CD4$^+$ and CD8$^+$ cells include **TNF,** osteoclast-activating factor (**OAF**), and histamine-releasing factor (**HRF**).

3. CD8$^+$ cytotoxic cells

—react to viral and tumor antigens and class I HLAs via TCR and CD8 molecules, respectively.

—are further stimulated by IL-2 from T_H cells.

—produce IL-2 themselves.

—produce IFN-γ.

XV. Developmental Immunologic Disorders

—are of major concern when considering the immunodeficiency diseases of neonates and children and the depressed immune response of elderly persons.

—are diagnosed using information concerning the patient's history of multiple infections, which can be verified with quantitative immunoglobulin tests, T- and B-cell ratios, and humoral and cell-mediated responses to common antigens.

A. Transient hypogammaglobulinemia of infancy

—reflects a normal condition resulting from temporal requirements for full development of the infant's immune system.

—occurs in the normal neonate who is born with an adult level of placentally transferred IgG and who possesses antibodies associated with the maternal immune experience; however, the rate of synthesis of secretable immunoglobulin by newborn infants is low and does not reach adequate levels for a number of months.

—is a transient period of physiologic hypogammaglobulinemia, generally from the third to the fifth month, beginning with the disappearance of maternally transferred IgG ($t_{1/2}$ = 22–28 days) and the onset of significant synthesis of IgG by the infant.

—results in increased susceptibility to some microorganisms.

B. Congenital agammaglobulinemia (Bruton's agammaglobulinemia)

—is a sex-linked (male) disorder characterized by recurrent pyogenic infections and digestive tract disorders beginning at 5–6 months of age.

—is diagnosed by the absence of tonsils, germinal centers, and B cells, and by serum immunoglobulin levels of less than 10%.

—defect may lie in the transition from pre–B to B cells, because the pre–B cells are normal.

—patients have an apparently normal thymus and cell-mediated immunity.

—can be treated by passive transfer of adult serum immunoglobulins to protect the patient.

C. Common variable hypogammaglobulinemia

—can be acquired at any age by either sex.

—patients generally have B cells but do not secrete immunoglobulin.

—patients have depressed serum immunoglobulin to less than 250 mg/dL of IgG and less than 50 mg/dL of IgA and IgM (normal IgG = 800–1400; IgM = 60–200; IgA = 100–300 mg/dL).

—patients are seen with increased susceptibility to pyogenic infections and autoimmune diseases.

—has multiple causes and diverse treatments.

D. Dysgammaglobulinemia

—patients are seen with a selective immunoglobulin class (one or more, but not all) deficiency.

—commonly results in depressed IgA levels (< 5 mg/dL; 1 in 600–800 individuals), leading to:

1. Loss of mucosal surface protection

2. Patients with normal numbers of IgA cells; however, these cells fail to differentiate into plasma cells

3. Increased autoimmunity

E. Congenital thymic aplasia (DiGeorge syndrome)

—is characterized by an absence of T cells, hypocalcemia, and tetany; it is not hereditary.

—is caused by an intrauterine insult to the third and fourth pharyngeal pouches, resulting in lack of development of the thymus and the parathyroid between the fifth and sixth weeks of human gestation.

—results in a depressed cell-mediated immunity that permits disease caused by opportunistic organisms (e.g., *Candida, Pneumocystis,* viral infections).

—patients can die from vaccination with live vaccines (e.g., measles, smallpox).

—patients have apparently normal germinal centers, plasma cells, and serum immunoglobulin.

—treatment with transplantation of fetal thymus is experimental and may be complicated by a graft-versus-host reaction.

F. Chronic mucocutaneous candidiasis

—is a highly specific T-cell disorder characterized by an absence of immunity to *Candida*.

—patients have apparently normal T-cell absolute numbers and other T-cell functions.

—can include endocrine dysfunctions (hypothyroidism) in about half of these patients.

G. Wiskott-Aldrich syndrome

—is a sex-linked (male) disease, with patients presenting with a triad of thrombocytopenia, eczema, and recurrent infections.

—is characterized by a depressed cell-mediated immunity and serum IgM but normal IgG and IgA levels.

—patients respond poorly to polysaccharide antigens.

—can include increased lymphoreticular malignancies or lymphomas.

—may have as its primary defect an absence of specific glycoprotein receptors on both T cells and platelets.

—patients can receive bone marrow transplantation as an experimental treatment.

H. Severe combined immunodeficiency disease (SCID)

—is characterized by a genetic defect in stem cells, resulting in absence of the thymus and T and B cells.

—involves, in half of the patients, a loss in the enzyme adenosine deaminase, resulting in accumulation of toxic deoxyadenosine triphosphate (dATP), which inhibits ribonucleotide reductase and prevents DNA synthesis. A mutation in the δ chain of the Il-z receptor gene has been found in other patients.

—results in extreme susceptibility to infections and a very short life span.

I. Chronic granulomatous disease

—is characterized by a genetic defect in the nicotinamide adenine dinucleotide phosphate (NADPH) oxidase system.

—results in defective neutrophil bactericidal activity because of depressed superoxide dismutase and decreased hydrogen peroxide levels.

—is diagnosed in the laboratory based on failure of neutrophils and macrophages to reduce a nitroblue tetrazolium (NBT) dye.

—may be treated with IFN-γ with some success.

J. Senescence of the immune response

—is manifest in the elderly by depressed humoral and cellular immune responses.

—is highly variable with chronologic age.

—is characterized primarily by a loss in some T-cell functions.

—includes an increase in occurrence of autoimmune disease.

XVI. Autoimmune Disorders

—are disorders in immune regulation resulting in antibody or cell-mediated immunity against the host's own tissues.

—may or may not result in injury to the host.

—are disorders in which persons are normally unresponsive to self-antigens due to tolerance; however, B-cell clones do exist in persons with idiotypes reacting with self-antigens.

A. Explanatory theories

1. Microbial antigens cross-reacting with host tissues induce an immune response against self

—is not a true autoimmunity because the stimulus is of exogenous origin.

—Examples include:

a. Streptococcal antigens cross-react with sarcolemmal heart muscle and kidney.

b. Anti-DNA antibodies reacting with cells in patients with systemic lupus erythematosus (SLE) may be induced by microbial DNA.

c. Deposition of viral antigens on host–cell membranes may involve an immune reaction against the host cell.

2. Host antigens previously sequestered from fetal tolerance-inducing mechanism are released and become immunogenic

—such as for some antigens in thyroid and heart tissue that emerge after tissue damage by microbes or surgery.

3. Alteration of host molecules, exposing new antigenic determinants unavailable at the time of induction of fetal tolerance

—For example, rheumatoid factor (in patients with rheumatoid arthritis) is mainly an IgM antibody against the Fc fragment of slightly altered IgG.

4. Attachment of foreign hapten to self-molecule, forming a hapten-carrier complex

—For example, when certain drugs (e.g., quinidine and sulfathiazole) attach to platelets, the antibody to the drug reacts with the drug on the platelet membrane and activates complement; then the platelet lyses.

5. Depletion of suppressor cells

—may result in autoantibodies if the normally occurring suppression by suppressor T cells of B-cell clones with idiotype specificity for self-antigens is lost or diminished.

B. Systemic autoimmune disorders

1. SLE

—is an episodic, multisystem disease usually in young women, with vasculitis as a major lesion.

—is characterized by multiple autoreactive antibodies, the most dominant of which is antinuclear antibody (ANA). Cross-reactive ANA may be induced by microbial infection.

—may include nephritis resulting from continuous insult by antigen–antibody complexes in antigen excess and complement activation at the level of the glomeruli.

—can be confused with rheumatoid arthritis, because 30% of SLE patients exhibit serum rheumatoid factor.

2. Rheumatoid arthritis

—is a chronic, systemic inflammatory disease mainly of the joints.

—is characterized by the appearance in serum and synovial fluids of rheumatoid factors (antibodies against immunoglobulin) and complement activation; resulting chemotactic factors attract inflammatory cells into joints, which damage tissues via release of pharmacologically active mediators.

—Rheumatoid factor formation may be a response by synovial lymphocytes against microbial antigens.

—may involve a genetic predisposition (HLA-D4 and HLA-DR4) for this condition.

3. Sjögren's syndrome

—is a chronic inflammatory disease, primarily of postmenopausal women, characterized by autoantibodies against salivary duct antigens.

—patients may complain of dryness of the mouth, trachea, bronchi, eyes, nose, vagina, and skin.

—may occur secondary to rheumatoid arthritis and SLE.

—is of unknown etiology.

4. Polyarteritis nodosa

—is one of a number of similar human vasculitides that can be reproduced experimentally by antigen–antibody complexes.

—often involves complexes of hepatitis B antigen with its specific antibody that are found deposited in vessel walls (30%–40% of patients).

C. Organ-specific autoimmune disorders

1. Blood disorders

a. **Autoantibodies reacting with blood cells** results in anemia; leukopenia and thrombocytopenia can occur (e.g., SLE).

b. **Malignant transformation of a single plasma cell clone (multiple myeloma)** results in the appearance of an excess of IgG or other immunoglobulin classes (termed paraproteins); such patients may also secrete Bence Jones proteins (monoclonal light chains) in their urine.

2. Central nervous system (CNS) disorders

a. **Allergic encephalitis**

—is a demyelinating disease that can occur after an infection or immunization.

—is characterized immunologically by a perivascular, mononuclear cell infiltrate in the white matter of the CNS.

—can be mimicked experimentally by immunization of animals with homologous extracts of brain or a nonapeptide from the basic protein of myelin.

—Experimental disease can be transferred with sensitized lymphocytes, thereby complicating cell-mediated immunity in the demyelination process.

b. **Multiple sclerosis**

—is a chronic, relapsing disease characterized immunologically by mononuclear cell infiltration and demyelinating lesions (plaques) in the white matter of the CNS.

—patients generally have increased IgG in the cerebrospinal fluid, containing elevated titers to measles and other viruses.

—is characterized by a decrease in suppressor T-cell function, which indicates an immunoregulatory disorder.

c. Myasthenia gravis

—is characterized by a defect in neuromuscular transmission, resulting in muscle weakness and fatigue.

—is associated with the presence of an antiacetylcholine receptor antibody, causing loss of the receptor.

—patients often have thymic hyperplasia or thymoma with increased numbers of B lymphocytes.

3. Endocrine disorders

a. Chronic thyroiditis

—is characterized by autoantibodies and cell-mediated immunity to thyroglobulin or thyroid microsomes.

—lesions can be reproduced experimentally by infection of autoantigen with an adjuvant.

—generally is a self-limiting disease of females with a probable genetic basis.

—may involve tissue damage occurring via ADCC.

b. Graves' disease (hyperthyroidism)

—is characterized by autoantibodies to the thyroid-stimulating hormone (TSH) receptor and infiltration of the thyroid gland with T cells and B cells.

—antibodies may compete with TSH for receptor site and mimic TSH activity.

c. Diabetes mellitus

—is characterized in insulin-dependent (juvenile onset, or type I) diabetes by the destruction of insulin-producing cells through either humoral or cell-mediated anti-islet cell immunity; there is no evidence for autoimmune pathogenesis in non–insulin-dependent (maturity onset, or type II) diabetes.

4. Gastrointestinal tract disorders

a. Pernicious anemia

—is characterized by autoantibodies to the gastric parietal cell and intrinsic factor.

—results in inability to absorb vitamin B_{12}.

b. Ulcerative colitis

—is characterized by chronic inflammatory lesions confined to the rectum and colon and by infiltration of monocytes, lymphocytes, and plasma cells.

—patients' lymphocytes show cytotoxicity against colonic epithelial cells in culture.

—patients have antibodies that are cross-reactive with *Escherichia coli,* but the disease is of unknown etiology.

    c. Crohn's disease

      —is an inflammatory, granulomatous disease usually occurring in the submucosal area of the terminal ileum.

      —is a chronic progressive disease often suspected, but not established, as being of microbial etiology.

    d. Chronic active hepatitis

      —is characterized by infiltration of the liver by T cells, B cells, and monocytes.

      —may be a disease of faulty immunoregulation.

Review Test

1. To which of the following classes of immunoglobulins (Ig) do the allergy-mediating antibodies belong?

(A) IgA
(B) IgG
(C) IgM
(D) IgD
(E) IgE ✓

2. What type of hypersensitivity reaction is responsible for hives, urticaria, and allergies?

(A) Type I (anaphylactic) hypersensitivity reaction
(B) Type II (cytotoxic) hypersensitivity reaction
(C) Type III (immune complex) hypersensitivity reaction
(D) Type IV (delayed) hypersensitivity reaction
(E) None of the above

3. Which of the following immunoglobulin (Ig) classes is the first to be produced in an immune response to a given antigen?

(A) IgA
(B) IgG
(C) IgM
(D) IgD
(E) IgE

4. Which of the following is a receptor for the gp120 envelope protein of the human immunodeficiency virus (HIV)?

(A) CD2
(B) CD3
(C) CD4
(D) CD8
(E) CD25

5. Which of the following substances enhances the switch from immunoglobulin G (IgG) to immunoglobulin E (IgE) production?

(A) Interleukin (IL)-1
(B) IL-2
(C) IL-3
(D) IL-4
(E) IL-5

6. In most normal persons, what percentage of the total serum immunoglobulin (Ig) is IgG?

(A) 10%
(B) 25%
(C) 50%
(D) 60%
(E) Over 70%

7. Which one of the following is the principal immunoglobulin (Ig) in exocrine secretions?

(A) IgA
(B) IgG
(C) IgM
(D) IgD
(E) IgE

8. What type of hypersensitivity reaction is responsible for farmer's lung?

(A) Type I (anaphylactic) hypersensitivity reaction
(B) Type II (cytotoxic) hypersensitivity reaction
(C) Type III (immune complex) hypersensitivity reaction
(D) Type IV (delayed) hypersensitivity reaction
(E) None of the above

9. Which of the following is a five-polypeptide transmembrane chain complex?

(A) CD2
(B) CD3
(C) CD4
(D) CD8
(E) CD25

10. Which of the following statements about immunoglobulin M (IgM) is true?

(A) It is the reaginic antibody.
(B) It is important in the first few days of the primary immune response.
(C) It increases in serum concentration after IgG has reached its peak serum concentration.
(D) It is the smallest of the immunoglobulin molecules.
(E) It is involved in allergic reactions.

11. Which of the following fragments are seen when immunoglobulin G (IgG) is split by papain?

(A) Two monovalent fragments with antibody activity [antigen-binding fragments (Fab)]
(B) Two fragments devoid of antibody activity
(C) Fab fragments that contain the variable (V) section of the heavy chain but not the light chain
(D) Fab fragments that contain the variable (V) section of the light chain but not the heavy chain
(E) Two crystallizable fragments (Fc) and one Fab fragment

12. Which of the following substances is produced by macrophages and macrophage-like cells?

(A) Interleukin (IL)-1
(B) IL-2
(C) IL-3
(D) IL-4
(E) Tumor necrosis factor (TNF)-β

13. Which of the following findings is seen in neonatally thymectomized mice?

(A) Increased numbers of blood lymphocytes
(B) Depleted T-cell areas in lymph nodes and the spleen
(C) Increased ability to reject allografts
(D) Large amounts of antibody produced in response to many antigens
(E) Large amounts of antibody of the immunoglobulin G (IgG) class

14. What is the approximate molecular weight of immunoglobulin G (IgG)?

(A) 10 kilodaltons (kd)
(B) 15 kd
(C) 150 kd
(D) 200 kd
(E) 900 kd

15. Which of the following is a receptor for lymphocyte function associated antigen (LFA)-3?

(A) CD2
(B) CD3
(C) CD4
(D) CD8
(E) CD25

16. Which of the following components determines the class-specific antigenicity of immunoglobulins?

(A) J chain
(B) T chain
(C) Light chain
(D) Heavy chain
(E) Secretory component

17. What type of hypersensitivity reaction is responsible for Addison's disease?

(A) Type I (anaphylactic) hypersensitivity reaction
(B) Type II (cytotoxic) hypersensitivity reaction
(C) Type III (immune complex) hypersensitivity reaction
(D) Type IV (delayed) hypersensitivity reaction
(E) None of the above

18. The classic complement cascade consists of a series of sequential events that eventually culminates in cell lysis. Which of the following complement components causes the cleavage of C3 into C3a and C3b?

(A) C5b
(B) C5a
(C) C1qrs
(D) C4b2a
(E) C2b

19. Which of the following substances is a potent stimulator of hematopoiesis?

(A) Interleukin (IL)-1
(B) IL-2
(C) IL-3
(D) IL-4
(E) IL-5

20. Which of the following statements about systemic lupus erythematosus (SLE) is true?

(A) Vasculitis is a basic lesion.
(B) A linear deposition of immunoglobulin on the glomerular basement membrane occurs with nephritis.
(C) Thyroid receptor antibody is present.
(D) Rheumatoid factor is rarely present.

21. What type of hypersensitivity reaction is responsible for myasthenia gravis?

(A) Type I (anaphylactic) hypersensitivity reaction
(B) Type II (cytotoxic) hypersensitivity reaction
(C) Type III (immune complex) hypersensitivity reaction
(D) Type IV (delayed) hypersensitivity reaction
(E) None of the above

22. Which of the following is the structure responsible for T-cell rosettes in the presence of sheep red blood cells?

(A) CD2
(B) CD3
(C) CD4
(D) CD8
(E) CD25

23. Which one of the following statements best describes the rheumatoid factor?

(A) It is the antigen initiating the rheumatoid inflammatory process.
(B) It is an antibody against cellular DNA.
(C) It consists primarily of DNA.
(D) It is an antibody against immunoglobulin.

24. Which of the following substances is an endogenous pyrogen?

(A) Interleukin (IL)-1
(B) IL-2
(C) IL-3
(D) IL-4
(E) IL-5

25. Susceptibility to the yeast *Candida* can occur in

(A) congenital agammaglobulinemia.
(B) congenital thymic aplasia (DiGeorge syndrome).
(C) common variable hypogammaglobulinemia.
(D) systemic lupus erythematosus (SLE).

26. Which one of the following factors characterizes the immune deficiency in chronic granulomatous disease?

(A) Reduced levels of the fifth component of complement (C5)
(B) Inability of polymorphonuclear leukocytes to ingest bacteria
(C) Dysgammaglobulinemia
(D) Inability of polymorphonuclear leukocytes to kill ingested bacteria

27. What type of hypersensitivity reaction is responsible for the reaction to purified protein derivative of *Mycobacterium tuberculosis*?

(A) Type I (anaphylactic) hypersensitivity reaction
(B) Type II (cytotoxic) hypersensitivity reaction
(C) Type III (immune complex) hypersensitivity reaction
(D) Type IV (delayed) hypersensitivity reaction
(E) None of the above

28. Which of the following autoimmune diseases occurs in 1 in 800 persons and is associated with decreased immunoglobulin A (IgA) levels?

(A) Congenital agammaglobulinemia
(B) Wiskott-Aldrich syndrome
(C) Dysgammaglobulinemia
(D) Graves' disease
(E) Chronic mucocutaneous candidiasis

29. Which of the following is the receptor for interleukin (IL)-2?

(A) CD2
(B) CD3
(C) CD4
(D) CD8
(E) CD25

30. Which of the following autoimmune diseases is characterized by demyelinating lesions, increased immunoglobulin G (IgG) in the cerebrospinal fluid, and chronic, relapsing occurrences?

(A) Ulcerative colitis
(B) Multiple sclerosis
(C) Chronic granulomatous disease
(D) Systemic lupus erythematosus (SLE)
(E) Congenital thymic aplasia

31. Which finding is associated with severe combined immunodeficiency disease (SCID)?

(A) Presence of the thymus but absence of the bursal equivalent
(B) Deficiency in the nicotinamide adenine dinucleotide phosphate (NADPH) oxidase system
(C) Deficiency in adenosine deaminase, resulting in a loss of this enzyme activity
(D) A transient low level of humoral immunity in neonates

32. What type of hypersensitivity reaction is responsible for serum sickness?

(A) Type I (anaphylactic) hypersensitivity reaction
(B) Type II (cytotoxic) hypersensitivity reaction
(C) Type III (immune complex) hypersensitivity reaction
(D) Type IV (delayed) hypersensitivity reaction
(E) None of the above

33. Which of the following substances increases expression of class II histocompatibility antigens on the surface of antigen-presenting cells (APCs)?

(A) Interleukin (IL)-4
(B) IL-5
(C) IL-6
(D) Interferon (IFN)-γ
(E) Tumor necrosis factor (TNF)-β

34. Which immunological finding is associated with aging?

(A) Interleukin-2 (IL-2) levels diminish
(B) Antibody production increases
(C) Cellular immune response increases
(D) Thymus tissue increases

35. Which of the following reactions requires complement?

(A) Immunoglobulin G (IgG)-mediated anaphylaxis
(B) Killing the cytotoxic T lymphocytes
(C) Development of glomerulonephritis caused by antigen–antibody complexes
(D) Antibody-dependent cell-mediated cytotoxicity

36. Which of the following autoimmune diseases is associated with chronic inflammatory lesions confined to the rectum and colon?

(A) Ulcerative colitis
(B) Myasthenia gravis
(C) Wiskott-Aldrich syndrome
(D) Systemic lupus erythematosus (SLE)
(E) Graves' disease

37. The first component of complement (C1) would disassemble into its component parts as a result of

(A) conditions that have minimized its polymeric behavior.
(B) autodigestion.
(C) loss of calcium.
(D) loss of magnesium.

38. Which of the following binds to class I histocompatibility antigens?

(A) CD2
(B) CD3
(C) CD4
(D) CD8
(E) CD25

39. Which one of the following substances may be passively transferred from the mother to the fetus during the third trimester of pregnancy?

(A) Immunoglobulin G (IgG)
(B) Immunoglobulin M (IgM)
(C) Anti-Rh antibody
(D) Natural isohemagglutinins

40. Which of the following is a factor made by T cells that is cytotoxic to certain tumor cells?

(A) Interleukin (IL)-4
(B) IL-5
(C) IL-6
(D) Interferon (IFN)-γ
(E) Tumor necrosis factor (TNF)-β

41. A male heterozygous for Rh factor mates with an Rh-negative female. On the basis of genetic theory, it could be predicted that

(A) no offspring would be Rh positive.
(B) 25% of the offspring would be Rh positive.
(C) 50% of the offspring would be Rh positive.
(D) 100% of the offspring would be Rh positive.

42. What type of hypersensitivity reaction is responsible for autoimmune hemolytic anemia?

(A) Type I (anaphylactic) hypersensitivity reaction
(B) Type II (cytotoxic) hypersensitivity reaction
(C) Type III (immune complex) hypersensitivity reaction
(D) Type IV (delayed) hypersensitivity reaction
(E) None of the above

43. Which of the following autoimmune diseases is a highly specific T-cell disorder with a normal absolute number of T cells?

(A) Dysgammaglobulinemia
(B) Graves' disease
(C) Chronic mucocutaneous candidiasis
(D) Congenital thymic aplasia
(E) Multiple sclerosis

44. Which statement regarding T cells is true?

(A) They mature in the bursa of Fabricius or bursal equivalent.
(B) They are found in the germinal centers of lymph nodes and the spleen.
(C) They are progenitors of plasma cells.
(D) They are involved in humoral and cell-mediated immunity.

45. Which of the following substances is a T-cell growth factor?

(A) Interleukin (IL)-1
(B) IL-2
(C) IL-3
(D) IL-4
(E) IL-5

46. Which of the following statements about B cells is correct?

(A) They arise in the spleen.
(B) They mature in the thymus.
(C) They are predominantly recirculating lymphocytes.
(D) They are involved in cell-mediated immunity.
(E) They are progenitors of plasma cells.

47. Which of the following autoimmune diseases is characterized by the absence of tonsils, germinal centers, and B cells; serum immunoglobulin of less than 10%; and cell-mediated immunity that appears normal?

(A) Pernicious anemia
(B) Congenital agammaglobulinemia
(C) Wiskott-Aldrich syndrome
(D) Chronic granulomatous disease
(E) Severe combined immunodeficiency disease (SCID)

48. Which of the following binds to class II histocompatibility antigens?

(A) CD2
(B) CD3
(C) CD4
(D) CD8
(E) CD25

49. Which of the following immunoglobulins (Ig) protects the mucosal surfaces of the respiratory, intestinal, and genitourinary tracts from pathogenic organisms?

(A) IgA
(B) IgG
(C) IgM
(D) IgD
(E) IgE

50. Which of the following substances enhances the switch from immunoglobulin G (IgG) to immunoglobulin A (IgA) production?

(A) Interleukin (IL)-1
(B) IL-2
(C) IL-3
(D) IL-4
(E) IL-5

51. Which of the following autoimmune diseases is associated with loss of adenosine deaminase enzyme in 50% of patients, resulting in accumulation of toxic deoxyadenosine triphosphate (dATP)?

(A) Severe combined immunodeficiency disease (SCID)
(B) Pernicious anemia
(C) Multiple sclerosis
(D) Systemic lupus erythematosus (SLE)
(E) Wiskott-Aldrich syndrome

52. Which of the following immunoglobulins (Ig) is at its highest level in a normal adult?

(A) IgA
(B) IgG
(C) IgM
(D) IgD
(E) IgE

53. Which of the following autoimmune diseases is associated with defective neutrophil bactericidal activity resulting from depressed superoxide dismutase?

(A) Ulcerative colitis
(B) Multiple sclerosis
(C) Chronic granulomatous disease
(D) Congenital thymic aplasia
(E) Myasthenia gravis

54. Which of the following substances stimulates interleukin (IL)-2 receptor production on the surface of T cells?

(A) IL-1
(B) IL-2
(C) IL-3
(D) IL-4
(E) IL-5

55. Which of the following is invariably a part of the T-cell receptor complex?

(A) CD2
(B) CD3
(C) CD4
(D) CD8
(E) CD25

56. Which of the following autoimmune diseases is associated with the presence of autoantibody to the thyroid-stimulating hormone receptor?

(A) Pernicious anemia
(B) Congenital agammaglobulinemia
(C) Wiskott-Aldrich syndrome
(D) Dysgammaglobulinemia
(E) Graves' disease

57. Which of the following immunoglobulins (Ig) is at its highest level in a normal 1-day-old infant?

(A) IgA
(B) IgG
(C) IgM
(D) IgD
(E) IgE

58. Which of the following autoimmune diseases is associated with an anti–acetylcholine receptor antibody?

(A) Multiple sclerosis
(B) Congenital agammaglobulinemia
(C) Chronic mucocutaneous candidiasis
(D) Myasthenia gravis
(E) Severe combined immunodeficiency disease (SCID)

59. Which of the following immunoglobulins (Ig) is implicated in an atopic response?

(A) IgA
(B) IgG
(C) IgM
(D) IgD
(E) IgE

60. Which of the following immunoglobulins (Ig) is produced by B cells in response to antigen?

(A) IgA
(B) IgG
(C) IgM
(D) IgD
(E) IgE

61. Which of the following autoimmune diseases is associated with soluble anti–DNA-DNA complexes that result in glomerulonephritis?

(A) Systemic lupus erythematosus (SLE)
(B) Dysgammaglobulinemia
(C) Graves' disease
(D) Chronic granulomatous disease
(E) Congenital thymic aplasia

62. Which of the following autoimmune diseases is characterized by autoantibodies against intrinsic factor?

(A) Pernicious anemia
(B) Congenital agammaglobulinemia
(C) Wiskott-Aldrich syndrome
(D) Dysgammaglobulinemia
(E) Graves' disease

63. Which of the following immunoglobulins (Ig) has the longest half-life?

(A) IgA
(B) IgG
(C) IgM
(D) IgD
(E) IgE

64. Which of the following autoimmune diseases is characterized by absence of T cells, hypocalcemia, and tetany with lowered cell-mediated immunity?

(A) Ulcerative colitis
(B) Multiple sclerosis
(C) Chronic granulomatous disease
(D) Systemic lupus erythematosus (SLE)
(E) Congenital thymic aplasia

65. Which of the following autoimmune diseases is characterized by the triad of thrombocytopenia, eczema, and recurrent infections?

(A) Myasthenia gravis
(B) Severe combined immunodeficiency disease (SCID)
(C) Pernicious anemia
(D) Congenital agammaglobulinemia
(E) Wiskott-Aldrich syndrome

Answers and Explanations

1–E. Immunoglobulin E (IgE), the reagin or reaginic antibody, mediates the allergic reaction. IgE binds allergens via its antigen-binding sites and is bound to tissue mast cells by its specialized Fc region.

2–A. Hives, urticaria, and allergy are clinical expressions of a type I (anaphylactic) hypersensitivity reaction.

3–C. Immunoglobulin M (IgM) is the first antibody class produced in response to an antigen, and it is also the predominant antibody in a primary immune response.

4–C. The human immunodeficiency virus (HIV) attaches to T cells via the CD4 molecule, which is an integral part of the T helper subset and is normally the receptor for class II histocompatibility antigens. The gp120 molecule probably mimics the class II histocompatibility antigen structure.

5–D. Interleukin-4 (IL-4) is the major interleukin involved in the shift to immunoglobulin E (IgE) production and concomitant stimulation of mast cells. IL-4 is therefore important in the inception and maintenance of type I hypersensitivity reactions.

6–E. Immunoglobulin (Ig) G is the predominant immunoglobulin in serum. A normal person has approximately 73% IgG, 19% IgA, 7% IgM, 1% IgD, and 0.01% IgE. These ratios remain constant even in cases of hyperimmunization.

7–A. Secretory immunoglobulin A (IgA) is the predominant antibody in exocrine secretions (e.g., milk, saliva, tears), where it is usually found in the dimeric form, held together by a J chain, and with an attached secretory component to help stabilize it against proteolytic enzymes.

8–C. Farmer's lung, a type III hypersensitivity reaction, consists of complexes of antibody to inhaled aspergillus mold.

9–B. CD3 is a five-chain entity associated with the T-cell receptor. It consists of gamma, delta, and epsilon chains and two zeta chains. After antigen binding, CD3 is probably a transducer of the signal from the T-cell receptor to the internal milieu of the cell.

10–B. Immunoglobulin M (IgM), the first antibody to be produced after antigenic stimulation, has a very important role in the first few days of a primary immune response. The largest of the immunoglobulin molecules, it is not involved in allergic (type I hypersensitivity) reactions.

11–A. Papain splits immunoglobulin G (IgG) to produce two antigen-binding fragments or fractions (Fab) and a crystallizable fragment (Fc). Because the Fab is monovalent, antigen can be bound by the Fab but not cross-linked and precipitated. A Fab fragment contains the variable (V) region of both the heavy and light chains.

12–A. Macrophage and macrophage-like cells produce interleukin (IL)-1. (All the other interleukins listed are T-cell products.) Macrophages are also known to produce tumor necrosis factor (TNF)-β and several other monokines. Some researchers believe that IL-6 and IL-8 are produced by both T cells and macrophages.

13–B. Neonatal thymectomy severely decreases the number of functional T cells throughout the body, resulting in decreased circulating blood lymphocytes (predominantly T cells) and depleted T-cell areas in the lymph nodes and spleen. Allograft rejection would be decreased because of decreased or depleted CD8$^+$ T cells, and antibody levels would be decreased due to decreased or depleted CD4$^+$ T helper cells.

14–C. Immunoglobulin (Ig) G has a molecular weight of approximately 150 kilodaltons (kd) [150,000 molecular weight]. IgD is similar in weight. IgA weighs 160 kd; IgE weighs approximately 200 kd, and IgM weighs 900 kd.

15–A. CD2 is an adhesion molecule; its natural ligand is lymphocyte function associated antigen (LFA)-3 (CD58).

16–D. The heavy chain defines the immunoglobulin (Ig) class. Gamma (γ) chains specify IgG, mu (μ) chains specify IgM, and so on. Each of the classes can contain either a kappa (κ) or lambda (λ) set of light chains. IgA and IgM can contain a J chain. Only IgA can have a secretory component, also known as a T (transport) chain.

17–B. Addison's disease is characterized by antibody to the adrenal cells and is thus a type II (cytotoxic) hypersensitivity reaction.

18–D. The classic cascade consists of the sequential activation of C1, C4, C2, C3, C5, C6, C7, C8, and C9. The formation of C4b and C2a in the presence of Mg^{2+} allows for cleavage of the C3 moiety.

19–C. Interleukin-3 (IL-3) is the major hematopoiesis stimulator of the interleukins listed.

20–A. Vasculitis and antinuclear antibody are hallmarks of systemic lupus erythematosus (SLE), as is a "lumpy-bumpy" deposition of immune complexes on and behind the glomerular basement membrane. A linear deposition occurs only when the antigen is part of this membrane, as in Goodpasture's nephritis. Rheumatoid factors are frequently present in SLE.

21–B. Myasthenia gravis is characterized by antibody directed to muscle acetylcholine receptors and is thus a class II (cytotoxic) hypersensitivity reaction.

22–A. CD2 allows for T-cell rosettes of sheep red blood cells and allows T cells to bind to many other cells and surfaces.

23–D. Rheumatoid factor is an immunoglobulin (Ig) M molecule with a specificity for the crystallizable fragment (Fc) portion of endogenous IgG.

24–A. Interleukin-1 (IL-1), or endogenous pyrogen, is a cytokine released from antigen-presenting cells and enhances T-cell responses.

25–B. Immunity to *Candida* is predominantly cell mediated; thus, susceptibility is increased in instances of depressed T-cell function, as in congenital thymic aplasia (DiGeorge syndrome).

26–D. In chronic granulomatous disease, the inability to kill ingested microorganisms, rather than a defect in simple phagocytosis, is the dominant malfunction. There is no evidence for a loss of complement components or immunoglobulins.

27–D. The Mantoux test, which measures the reaction to purified protein derivative of *Mycobacterium tuberculosis,* demonstrates a classic example of a type IV (delayed) hypersensitivity reaction.

28–C. Dysgammaglobulinemia commonly results in depressed immunoglobulin A (IgA) levels. Patients have a normal number of IgA cells, but the cells fail to differentiate into plasma cells.

29–E. CD25 is the interleukin-2 (IL-2) receptor.

30–B. Patients with multiple sclerosis generally have increased immunoglobulin G (IgG) in the cerebrospinal fluid and demyelinating lesions in the white matter of the central nervous system. Multiple sclerosis is a chronic, relapsing disease.

31–C. Severe combined immunodeficiency disease (SCID) is a devastating terminal disease involving a lesion in the stem-cell population, such that lymphoid tissue does not form. Fifty percent of patients with SCID exhibit a loss in adenosine deaminase activity. A loss in nicotinamide adenine dinucleotide phosphate (NADPH), on the other hand, characterizes the neutrophils in chronic granulomatous disease. The normal condition of transient hypogammaglobulinemia of infancy is characterized by a temporary low rate of synthesis of secretable immunoglobulin in newborn infants from approximately 3–6 months of age.

32–C. Serum sickness occurs as a result of prophylactic treatment of a patient with foreign immune globulin injection (e.g., horse tetanus antitoxin). This can result in complexes of antibody to the horse antigen and thus an immune complex (type III hypersensitivity) reaction.

33–D. Interferon (IFN)-γ is a potent stimulator of natural killer (NK) and T-cell activity and enhances the activity of antigen-presenting cells (APCs) by up-regulating the expression of class II histocompatibility antigens on the APC surface.

34-A. Generally, interleukin-2 (IL-2) levels are diminished in the elderly. This results in decreased cellular immunity and decreased antibody production.

35–C. Complement is the key mediator of the glomerulonephritis and vasculitis induced by immune complex (type III) hypersensitivity reactions.

36–A. Ulcerative colitis is characterized by chronic inflammatory lesions confined to the rectum and colon. The disease is of unknown etiology but patients have antibodies that are cross-reactive with *Escherichia coli.*

37–C. Calcium holds the C1 components together. Chelation of Ca^{2+} leads to the dissolution of C1 into its C1q, C1r, and C1s subunits.

38–D. The CD8 molecule, found on all cytotoxic T cells, binds to the class I MHC molecules found on every nucleated cell.

39–A. Immunoglobulin (Ig) G is the only immunoglobulin that passes the placental barrier. Anti-Rh antibody of the IgG type readily crosses the placenta and causes erythroblastosis fetalis. IgM does not pass the placenta nor do the majority of natural isohemagglutinins (IgM molecules predominantly).

40–E. Tumor necrosis factor (TNF)-β is manufactured by T cells. TNF-β is a similar molecule produced by macrophages.

41–C. A heterozygous individual, by definition, would be Dd with respect to Rh. An Rh-negative female would be dd. A Dd × dd cross would allow for 50% of the offspring to be Rh positive.

42–B. Antibodies directed to red blood cell epitopes cause hemolytic anemia. This is a classic case of a type II (cytotoxic) hypersensitivity reaction.

43–C. Patients with chronic mucocutaneous candidiasis have normal T-cell absolute numbers. This disorder is characterized by an absence of immunity to *Candida.*

44–D. T cells arise from stem cells in the bone marrow, and they mature in the thymus. They are the main type of lymphocyte in the circulation, are involved in cell-mediated immunity, and have helping and regulatory functions in humoral immunity.

45–B. Interleukin-2 (IL-2) was formerly called T-cell growth factor.

46–E. B cells arise in the bone marrow and are found in the germinal centers of the lymph nodes and spleen. They are progenitors of plasma cells.

47–B. Congenital agammaglobulinemia, or Bruton's disease, is diagnosed by the absence of tonsils, germinal centers, and B cells and serum immunoglobulin of less than 10% of normal values. It is a sex-linked (male) disorder characterized by recurrent pyogenic infections and digestive tract disorders that usually begin at 5–6 months of age.

48–C. The CD4 molecule, found on all helper T cells, binds to the class II MHC molecules present on antigen-presenting cells (APCs).

49–A. Immunoglobulin A (IgA) is the antibody associated with secretions and mucosal surfaces. Typically, it is an IgA dimer composed of the IgA subclass associated with a J chain and a T piece.

50–E. The synthesis of immunoglobulin A (IgA) is enhanced by interleukin-5 (IL-5) production.

51–A. Severe combined immunodeficiency disease (SCID) is characterized by a genetic defect in stem cells, resulting in absence of the thymus and T cells and B cells. Patients are extremely susceptible to infections and have a short life span.

52–B. Immunoglobulin G (IgG) is the predominant immunoglobulin (approximately 73% of total immunoglobulin) found in the adult.

53–C. Chronic granulomatous disease is characterized by a genetic defect in the nicotinamide adenine dinucleotide phosphate (NADPH) oxidase system. It may be treated with interferon-γ.

54–A. The production of interleukin (IL)-1 by macrophages stimulates production of IL-2 by the targeted T cells as well as the production of IL-2 receptors on these T cells.

55–B. CD3 is invariably part of the T-cell receptor complex. The other constituent is CD4 or CD3.

56–E. Graves' disease (hyperthyroidism) is characterized by autoantibodies to the thyroid-stimulating hormone receptor and infiltration of the thyroid gland with T cells and B cells.

57–B. Although immunoglobulin G (IgG) is not produced to any great extent in utero, IgG is readily passed transplacentally. A 1-day-old infant has adult levels of maternally derived IgG.

58–D. Myasthenia gravis is characterized by a defect in neuromuscular transmission resulting in muscle weakness and fatigue. It causes loss of the acetylcholine receptor.

59–E. Atopic allergic responses are the realm of immunoglobulin E (IgE; reaginic) antibody.

60–C. The initial immunoglobulin (Ig) produced in reaction to an antigen is IgM. IgM is also the first immunoglobulin to be synthesized in ontogeny.

61–A. Systemic lupus erythematosus (SLE) usually occurs in young women and is an episodic, multisystem disease. It is characterized by multiple autoreactive antibodies, the most dominant being antinuclear antibody.

62–A. Pernicious anemia is characterized by autoantibodies to the gastric parietal cell and intrinsic factor. It results in inability to absorb vitamin B_{12}.

63–B. Immunoglobulin (Ig) G has the longest half-life of the immunoglobulins (21-day average). The shortest half-life is that of IgE, which is approximately 48 hours.

64–E. Congenital thymic aplasia, or DiGeorge syndrome, is characterized by the absence of T cells and by hypocalcemia and tetany. It results in depressed cell-mediated immunity, which permits disease caused by opportunistic organisms.

65–E. Wiskott-Aldrich syndrome is a sex-linked (male) disease. Patients are seen with the triad of thrombocytopenia, eczema, and recurrent infections. It is characterized by depressed cell-mediated immunity and serum immunoglobulin (Ig) M but normal IgG and IgA levels.

Comprehensive Examination

1. Which of the following cells is involved in antibody-dependent cell-mediated cytotoxicity?

(A) CD4$^+$ cell
(B) CD8$^+$ cell
(C) Mature B cell
(D) Plasma cell
(E) Natural killer (NK) cell
(F) Null (K) cell

2. Over the last 2 weeks, a heterologous kidney transplant patient has had headaches of increasing severity and mental lethargy. On physical examination, macronodular skin lesions are noted. The cerebrospinal fluid (CSF) is clear, and protein and glucose concentrations are within normal levels. Microscopic examination of CSF sediment in India ink reveals encapsulated yeasts. Which of the following tests permits rapid confirmation of the identity of the infective organism?

(A) Detection of specific antibodies in the CSF
(B) Detection of polysaccharide in the CSF
(C) Detection of lipo-oligosaccharides in the CSF
(D) Detection of cell-wall antigens in the CSF
(E) Detection of serum antibody

3. Roseola (or exanthema subitum) is caused by

(A) cytomegalovirus.
(B) human herpesvirus 6.
(C) human papillomavirus.
(D) human parvovirus B19.

4. Which of the following viruses has an arthropod vector?

(A) Respiratory syncytial virus
(B) Parvovirus
(C) Reovirus
(D) Parainfluenza virus
(E) Bunyavirus
(F) Arenavirus

5. A 16-year-old boy from a rural area presents with two highly inflammatory lesions in the bearded area of his face. Both of the rashes are itchy, highly erythematous, sore to the touch, and spreading. The most advanced lesion is clearing in the center, but the periphery continues to expand. Skin scrapings from lesion margins mounted in potassium hydroxide demonstrate the presence of true hyphae and arthroconidia. Which drug or combination is most appropriate?

(A) Amoxicillin
(B) Amoxicillin and clavulanate
(C) Amphotericin B
(D) An imidazole such as itraconazole
(E) Praziquantel

6. Pieces of plasmid or bacterial chromosomal DNA may be mistakenly packaged into the capsid (head) of a bacterial virus. Assuming that no prophage state has existed in the phage production, what is the process called when the virus with the bacterial or plasmid DNA infects another bacterium?

(A) Conjugation
(B) Lysogeny
(C) Generalized transduction
(D) Specialized transduction
(E) Transformation

7. A 6-month-old child has had watery diarrhea for 6 days. The stools have no blood and no pus. The causative agent is a double-stranded RNA virus. Which of the following is the most likely causative agent?

(A) *Bacillus cereus*
(B) *Giardia lamblia*
(C) Norwalk agent
(D) Rotavirus
(E) *Salmonella enteritidis*
(F) *Staphylococcus aureus*

8. A 3-year-old child develops acute glomeru-lonephritis following impetigo. The bacterium is a catalase-negative, gram-positive coccus that has M12 surface protein. What is the most likely causative agent?

(A) *Enterococcus faecalis*
(B) *Staphylococcus aureus*
(C) *Staphylococcus epidermidis*
(D) *Streptococcus agalactiae*
(E) *Streptococcus pneumoniae*
(F) *Streptococcus pyogenes*

9. Which of the following exotoxins has a mode of action similar to that of *Pseudomonas* exo-toxin A?

(A) Botulinus toxin
(B) Diphtheria toxin
(C) Pertussis toxin
(D) Shiga toxin
(E) Tetanus toxin

10. A patient presents with paranasal swelling, hemorrhagic exudates in the eyes and nares, and mental lethargy. Nonseptate hyphae are found invading the tissues. Rhinocerebral *Mucor* infection (zygomycosis) is diagnosed. What is the most likely underlying condition?

(A) C5–C8 deficiencies
(B) Epstein-Barr virus infection
(C) Hepatitis A infection
(D) Hepatitis B infection
(E) Ketoacidotic diabetes
(F) Severe neutropenia

11. Which of the following cell surface markers are associated with T helper cells?

(A) $CD2^- \ CD3^- \ CD4^- \ CD8^- \ TCR^-$ cell
(B) $CD2^+ \ CD3^+ \ CD4^- \ CD8^- \ TCR^+$ cell
(C) $CD2^+ \ CD3^+ \ CD4^+ \ CD8^- \ TCR^+$ cell
(D) $CD2^+ \ CD3^+ \ CD4^- \ CD8^+ \ TCR^+$ cell
(E) $CD2^+ \ CD3^+ \ CD4^+ \ CD8^+ \ TCR^+$ cell

12. Which of the following is found only in gram-positive bacteria?

(A) Capsule
(B) Lipopolysaccharide
(C) Outer membrane
(D) Peptidoglycan
(E) Teichoic acid

13. Which of the following has the highest association with hepatocellular carcinoma?

(A) Acute hepatitis A infection
(B) Acute hepatitis B infection
(C) Chronic hepatitis B infection
(D) Epstein-Barr virus infection
(E) Hepatitis B infection with hepatitis D superinfection
(F) Hepatitis E infection

14. Which of the following factors is associated with the virulence of *Yersinia pestis*?

(A) Adhesins
(B) Exotoxin that inhibits protein synthesis by blocking elongation factor 2
(C) Exotoxin that causes an increase in cyclic adenosine monophosphate
(D) Exotoxin that inhibits protein synthesis by binding to the 60S ribosomal subunit
(E) V and W antigens
(F) X and V factors

15. A neonate develops meningitis at 7 days of age. Her mother is 16 years of age, is single, has had multiple sexual partners without barrier protection, and lives in the United States. The baby was born 23 hours after the mother's amniotic sac ruptured. What is the most likely causative agent?

(A) *Escherichia coli*
(B) *Haemophilus influenzae*
(C) *Listeria monocytogenes*
(D) *Neisseria meningitidis*
(E) *Streptococcus agalactiae*

16. Which of the following viruses is a double-stranded RNA virus?

(A) Calicivirus
(B) Flavivirus
(C) Paramyxovirus
(D) Reovirus

17. Which of the following statements characterizes neonatal thymectomy?

(A) It depletes the periarteriolar region of the spleen.
(B) It eliminates germinal center formation.
(C) It enhances graft rejection.
(D) It results in autoimmunity.

18. A 19-year-old college freshman has a sore throat, sore and enlarging cervical lymph nodes, and a fever and is greatly fatigued. A diagnosis of infectious mononucleosis is made. Which of the following factors is present?

(A) Delta hemagglutinin
(B) E1A protein
(C) Large T antigen
(D) TAT protein
(E) VCA protein
(F) Matrix protein

19. Repeated *Neisseria meningitidis* septicemias in an individual should raise physician awareness of what underlying condition?

(A) C5–C8 deficiencies
(B) Chronic hepatitis B infection
(C) Ketosis-prone diabetes
(D) Multiple myeloma
(E) Severe neutropenia

20. In traveler's diarrhea caused by *Escherichia coli,* what is responsible for the fluid and electrolyte disruption?

(A) Adherence causing palisade layers of the bacterium on the surface of the small intestine
(B) Capsule
(C) Invasion of the intestinal lining
(D) Exotoxin that inhibits protein synthesis by blocking elongation factor 2
(E) Exotoxin that causes an increase in cyclic adenosine monophosphate
(F) Exotoxin that inhibits protein synthesis by binding to the 60S ribosomal subunit

21. Which of the following components is a potent neutrophil chemotactic agent?

(A) C1
(B) C2
(C) C5a
(D) C789 complex

22. A formerly vigorous 3-month-old child has developed upper body weakness manifested by droopy eyes and head, poor feeding, and a weak cry. Changes starting with constipation were first noticed 2 days ago. The baby is afebrile and there is no sign of rash. What is the most likely causative agent and where is the infection?

(A) *Bacteroides* species; gastrointestinal (GI) tract overgrowth
(B) *Clostridium botulinum;* GI tract infection
(C) *Clostridium difficile;* GI tract overgrowth
(D) *Clostridium tetani;* tissue infection
(E) *Neisseria meningitidis;* central nervous system infection

23. Which of the following antibiotics has a β-lactam ring in its structure?
> Cephalosporin & Penicillin

(A) Tetracycline
(B) Cephalosporin
(C) Streptomycin
(D) Erythromycin
(E) Griseofulvin
(F) Bacitracin

24. A woman develops cervical carcinoma. What viral protein played a role in the development of the carcinoma?

(A) Large T antigen
(B) E1A protein
(C) E6 protein
(D) TAX protein

25. What bacterial gene transfer process would be inhibited by free extracellular exonucleases?

(A) Conjugation
(B) Generalized transduction
(C) Specialized transduction
(D) Transformation
(E) Transposition

26. An alcoholic presents complaining of chest pain, fever, shaking chills, cough, and myalgia. She was very cold 2 nights ago and says she has felt "poorly" ever since. Her cough is producing rust-colored, odorless, mucoid sputum. Her temperature on admission is 40°C. Her white blood cell count is 16,000 cells/mm^3 and is predominantly neutrophils with an overall left shift. An α-hemolytic, lancet-shaped, gram-positive diplococcus is isolated on blood agar. What is the most likely causative agent?

(A) *Legionella pneumophila*
(B) *Klebsiella pneumoniae*
(C) *Mycoplasma pneumoniae*
(D) *Neisseria meningitidis*
(E) *Streptococcus pneumoniae* → rusty colored mucoid sp

27. A deficiency in nicotinamide adenine dinucleotide (NADH) or nicotinamide adenine dinucleotide phosphate (NADPH) oxidase and an increased susceptibility to organisms of low virulence are characteristic of

(A) chronic granulomatous disease.
(B) angioneurotic edema.
(C) chronic active hepatitis.
(D) Graves' disease.

28. A 10-month-old child presents with a temperature of 39.8°C and lethargy. Brudzinski's and Kernig's signs are both present. What part of the routine health care could have prevented this disease?

(A) A trivalent killed viral vaccine
(B) A polysaccharide vaccine with 23 different antigens
(C) A covalently linked protein–polyribitol vaccine
(D) A viral surface antigen vaccine
(E) A quadrivalent capsular vaccine

29. Which of the following is a nonnucleoside analogue that inhibits herpesvirus DNA?

(A) Acyclovir
(B) Amantadine
(C) Cytarabine
(D) Foscarnet
(E) Interferon

30. Which of the following complement components is most closely related to anaphylatoxin?

(A) C5b
(B) C5a
(C) C1qrs
(D) C4b2a
(E) C2b

31. A Mexican fruit picker has developed subcutaneous nodular lesions along the lymphatics from the initial site of trauma caused by a plum thorn puncture. What is the nature of the most likely causative agent?

(A) Acid-fast organism
(B) Dimorphic fungus
(C) Filamentous fungus
(D) Gram-positive coccus
(E) Gram-negative rod
(F) Helminth

32. Assuming that the route and concentration of the inocula are equivalent, which one of the following inocula would be most antigenic in a normal immunocompetent host?

(A) Homologous red blood cells
(B) Homologous serum protein
(C) Heterologous carbohydrate
(D) Heterologous serum protein
(E) 2,4 Dinitrobenzene

33. Which of the following proteins is associated with the *v-src* oncogene of Rous sarcoma virus?

(A) Protein kinase
(B) Growth factor
(C) DNA-binding protein
(D) G protein

34. A compromised patient is admitted in respiratory distress. She had signs of focal central nervous system (CNS) lesions early in the day and is now in a comatose state. The CNS and pulmonary biopsies show dichotomously branching septate hyphae. What is the most likely underlying condition?

(A) CD4⁺ cell count < 200
(B) Ketoacidotic diabetes
(C) Multiple myeloma
(D) Severe neutropenia
(E) Sickle cell disease

35. Latent infection of neurons occurs with

(A) cytomegalovirus.
(B) herpes simplex virus.
(C) measles virus.
(D) poliomyelitis virus.
(E) rabies virus.

36. In June, an 18-year-old man develops a sore throat with a fever and a nonproductive cough that develops into pneumonia with a severe, prolonged hacking cough but little sputum production. Cryoagglutinins are present. He is treated appropriately and successfully with azithromycin. What is the nature of the most likely causative agent?

(A) Acid-fast organism
(B) Gram-negative coccus
(C) DNA virus
(D) Gram-negative rod
(E) Gram-positive coccus
(F) *Mycoplasma*

37. African sleeping sickness is transmitted by

(A) tsetse fly bite.
(B) invasion of skin in water.
(C) respiratory droplets and direct mucosal contact.
(D) mosquito bite.
(E) reduviid bug bite.
(F) sandfly bite.

38. Which of the following cells actively secretes a specific idiotype of antibody?

(A) CD4⁺ cell
(B) CD8⁺ cell
(C) Mature B cell
(D) Plasma cell
(E) Natural killer (NK) cell
(F) Monocyte–macrophage

39. Vascular inflammation and glomerulonephritis induced by autoantibodies are characteristic of

(A) Arthus reaction.
(B) angioneurotic edema.
(C) systemic lupus erythematosus.
(D) hemolytic anemia.

40. The most frequent cause of the common cold is

(A) coronavirus.
(B) parainfluenza virus.
(C) reovirus.
(D) rhinovirus.

41. In which of the following phases of growth is a gram-positive bacterium most susceptible to the action of penicillin?

(A) Lag
(B) Exponential
(C) Stationary
(D) Decline
(E) Death

42. Which of the following contains O antigen?

(A) Capsule
(B) Lipopolysaccharide
(C) Lipoprotein
(D) Mesosome
(E) Peptidoglycan
(F) Teichoic acid

43. CD8 is a surface membrane protein on T cells and has which of the following characteristics?

(A) It recognizes class I human leukocyte antigens (HLA).
(B) It recognizes class II HLA.
(C) It characterizes T helper cells.
(D) It is strongly chemotactic.

44. Which of the following viruses does NOT use a reverse transcriptase during replication?

(A) Mouse mammary tumor virus
(B) Rous sarcoma virus
(C) Polyoma virus
(D) Human T lymphotrophic virus
(E) Hepatitis B virus

45. Which of the following molecules is genetically encoded on only one chromosome?

(A) Immunoglobulin (Ig) G
(B) IgM
(C) T-cell receptor
(D) Human leukocyte antigen (HLA)-B
(E) HLA-DR

46. Which of the following statements about the prevention of clostridial infections is correct?

(A) The low incidence of spores in the environment makes prevention difficult.
(B) The tetanus vaccine should not be given to pregnant women.
(C) In developing countries, the incidence of neonatal tetanus can be minimized by ensuring the cleanliness of the umbilical stump.
(D) The botulism vaccine should be given routinely to newborns to prevent infant botulism.
(E) Botulism is spread through inhalation of spores.

47. Antivirals that inhibit viral proteases are available for

(A) hepatitis B virus.
(B) herpes simplex virus.
(C) human immunodeficiency virus.
(D) influenza A virus.

48. Which one of the following characteristics describes interleukin-1?

(A) Inhibition of T cells
(B) Initiation of the acute phase reactants
(C) Synthesis restricted to mononuclear phagocytes
(D) Suppression of tumor necrosis factor

49. Which of the following statements about the treatment of cholera is correct?

(A) Ciprofloxacin is critical along with fluids for recovery; clinical response is slow and the patient will remain sick for a few weeks.
(B) Replacement of fluid and electrolytes is most important and will lead to a dramatic improvement; antibiotics will decrease the length of disease and the period of infectivity.
(C) Ciprofloxacin will not alter the course; replacement of fluids and electrolytes will lead to gradual clinical improvement.
(D) Replacement of fluid and electrolytes is most important and will lead to a dramatic improvement; antibiotics are contraindicated.
(E) Antitoxin along with fluid and electrolytes is critical to a rapid clinical response.

50. Which of the following statements concerning $\gamma_2\kappa_2$ antibody is true?

(A) It contains a J chain.
(B) It contains a secretory piece.
(C) It contains a hypervariable region.
(D) It is the initial antibody synthesized after antigen.

51. The initial host defense mechanism that occurs at the first site of primary virus infection is

(A) inflammation.
(B) immunoglobulin M antibody production.
(C) sensitized T-cell production.
(D) interferon production.

52. A noncompliant human immunodeficiency virus (HIV)-positive patient with a CD4$^+$ cell count of 40/mm^3 has a pulmonary infection caused by an organism that requires 4 weeks to grow on Lowenstein-Jensen medium. What is the nature of the most likely causative agent?

(A) Acid-fast organism
(B) Dimorphic fungus
(C) Filamentous fungus
(D) Gram-positive coccus
(E) Gram-negative coccus
(F) Gram-negative rod

53. What characteristic of the influenza A virus allows genetic reassortment?

(A) Poor editing by the RNA-dependent RNA polymerase
(B) Presence of the A-*rec* gene product
(C) Defective chaperone proteins
(D) Poor editing function of the reverse transcriptase
(E) Segmented genome

54. Which of the following conditions is an inflammatory response caused by antibodies reacting with parietal cells of gastric mucosa that results in depressed acid secretion and atrophic gastritis?

(A) Serum sickness
(B) Amyloidosis
(C) Pernicious anemia
(D) Ulcerative colitis

55. What is transferred when an F$^+$ cell is crossed with an F$^-$ cell?

(A) Only some bacterial chromosomal genes
(B) Generally the whole bacterial chromosome
(C) Only the fertility factor DNA
(D) Both the plasmid and chromosomal genes
(E) No genes

56. There is an outbreak of watery diarrhea in 6 members of a party of 20 who ate at a Chinese restaurant the day before. Fried rice is implicated. What is the most likely causative agent?

(A) *Bacillus cereus*
(B) *Giardia lamblia*
(C) Norwalk agent
(D) Rotavirus
(E) *Salmonella enteritidis*
(F) *Staphylococcus aureus*

57. Which of the following cell surface markers are associated with pre–T cells?

(A) CD2$^-$ CD3$^-$ CD4$^-$ CD8$^-$ TCR$^-$ cell
(B) CD2$^+$ CD3$^+$ CD4$^-$ CD8$^-$ TCR$^+$ cell
(C) CD2$^+$ CD3$^+$ CD4$^+$ CD8$^-$ TCR$^+$ cell
(D) CD2$^+$ CD3$^+$ CD4$^-$ CD8$^+$ TCR$^+$ cell
(E) CD2$^+$ CD3$^+$ CD4$^+$ CD8$^+$ TCR$^+$ cell

58. Which of the following phrases best describes a prophage?

(A) Phage that lacks receptors
(B) Phage attached to the cell wall that has released its DNA
(C) Newly assembled intracellular phage particle
(D) Intracellular temperate phage DNA

59. Hookworm infections can be prevented by

(A) not swimming in contaminated water.
(B) not using human excrement as vegetable fertilizer.
(C) heating all canned foods to 60°C for 10 minutes.
(D) avoiding cat litter or taking proper care when changing litter.
(E) wearing shoes outside in endemic regions.

60. Anti-A isohemagglutinins are present in persons with which one of the following blood types?

(A) Type A
(B) Type B
(C) Type AB

61. Which of the following terms best describes bacteria that can use fermentation pathways and contain superoxide dismutase?

(A) Obligate aerobe
(B) Obligate anaerobe
(C) Facultative anaerobe
(D) Aerobic heterotroph

62. Which of the following is the most sensitive type of serologic test?

(A) Virus neutralization
(B) Enzyme-linked immunosorbent assay
(C) Nucleic acid hybridization
(D) Hemadsorption

63. Division and differentiation of B cells leading to production of plasma cells both require

(A) CD4 and CD8.
(B) interleukin (IL)-1 and IL-3.
(C) IL-1 only.
(D) IL-4 and IL-6.

64. Which of the following contains *N*-acetyl-muramic acid?

(A) Lipopolysaccharide
(B) Lipoprotein
(C) Outer membrane
(D) Peptidoglycan
(E) Teichoic acid

65. How is primary amebic meningoencephalitis most likely acquired?

(A) Intravenous drug abuse
(B) Diving or swimming in contaminated water
(C) Using human excrement as vegetable fertilizer
(D) Eating raw fish or seafood
(E) Handling cat litter

66. Which of the following is the most common organism in the human gastrointestinal tract?

(A) *Bacteroides* species
(B) *Clostridium botulinum*
(C) *Clostridium difficile*
(D) *Clostridium perfringens*
(E) *Clostridium tetani*
(F) *Escherichia coli*

67. A Peace Corp volunteer recently returned to rural Africa develops symptoms of liver damage and a blocked bile duct after general anesthesia. What is the nature of the most likely causative agent?

(A) Cestode
(B) Dimorphic fungus
(C) Filamentous fungus
(D) Fluke
(E) Nematode
(F) Protozoa

68. A bacterial growth medium that contains penicillin is a

(A) minimal medium.
(B) differential medium.
(C) selective medium.
(D) complex medium.

69. Which of the following statements concerning *Chlamydia trachomatis* is correct?

(A) It is the most common bacterial sexually transmitted disease among college populations.
(B) It is an intracellular-dwelling virus.
(C) It rarely induces the carrier state.
(D) It is a motile, single-cell animal parasite.

70. Which of the following is also called an endotoxin?

(A) Capsule
(B) Lipopolysaccharide
(C) Lipoprotein
(D) Mesosome
(E) Outer membrane
(F) Peptidoglycan

71. Which of the following regions contains the greatest number of antigenic epitopes in gram-negative bacteria?

(A) Mucopeptide
(B) Lipid A
(C) Teichoic acids
(D) O side chains

72. After extensive oral surgery, a patient who had rheumatic fever as a child did not take the prescribed perioperative prophylactic antibiotics and subsequently developed subacute infective endocarditis. Which of the following is the most likely causative agent?

(A) *Enterococcus faecalis*
(B) *Staphylococcus aureus*
(C) Viridans streptococci
(D) *Streptococcus agalactiae*
(E) *Streptococcus pneumoniae*
(F) *Streptococcus pyogenes*

73. The number of live bacteria in a sample is best determined by

(A) turbidity measurement.
(B) viable count.
(C) dry weight.
(D) protein measurement.

74. Which of the following maternal infections may cause congenital disease?

(A) Infectious hepatitis
(B) Measles
(C) Serum hepatitis
(D) Infectious mononucleosis
(E) Shingles
(F) German measles

75. Which of the following statements characterizes idiotypic determinants?

(A) They are found in the crystallizable fragment of immunoglobulins.
(B) They are found on protein antigens.
(C) They can be antigenic.
(D) They are responsible for rejection of transplants.

76. Which of the following would be found in the urine of a patient with multiple myeloma?

(A) Bence Jones proteins
(B) Complement components
(C) Heavy chains
(D) Crystallizable fragments

77. The presence of delta antigen in a patient's serum indicates

(A) dengue virus infection.
(B) influenza B virus infection.
(C) hepatitis D virus infection.
(D) varicella-zoster virus infection.

78. Which of the following viruses causes croup?

(A) Respiratory syncytial virus
(B) Parvovirus
(C) Reovirus
(D) Parainfluenza virus
(E) Bunyavirus
(F) Arenavirus

79. Which of the following medications blocks virus penetration and uncoating of influenza A virus?

(A) Acyclovir
(B) Amantadine
(C) Cytarabine
(D) Foscarnet
(E) Interferon
(F) Ribavirin

80. Which of the following virulence factors is produced by several genera of bacteria that are notable mucosal colonizers?

(A) Elastase
(B) Hemagglutinin
(C) Immunoglobulin A protease
(D) Mucinase

81. Which of the following is NOT a differential medium?

(A) Eosin-methylene blue agar
(B) MacConkey agar
(C) Mueller-Hinton agar
(D) Tellurite agar

82. Which of the following latent infections is most likely to be activated during immunosuppression?

(A) Infectious hepatitis
(B) Measles
(C) Serum hepatitis
(D) Infectious mononucleosis
(E) Shingles
(F) German measles

83. Which of the following is an infection that produces heterophil antibodies?

(A) Cytomegalovirus
(B) Epstein-Barr virus
(C) Human immunodeficiency virus
(D) St. Louis encephalitis virus

84. Which of the following cells is involved in recognition of antigen in the context of class II histocompatibility antigens?

(A) CD4$^+$ cell
(B) CD8$^+$ cell
(C) Mature B cell
(D) Plasma cell
(E) Natural killer (NK) cell
(F) Null (K) cell

85. Plague is transmitted by

(A) rodent feces.
(B) respiratory droplets.
(C) tick bite.
(D) animal bite, most commonly small rodents.

86. Loose bacterial surface polysaccharide plays a critical role in

(A) gonorrhea.
(B) meningitis with no underlying trauma.
(C) *Mycoplasma* pneumonia.
(D) pyelonephritis.
(E) urinary tract infection.

87. The neuraminidase of the influenza B virus is inhibited by

(A) ganciclovir.
(B) ribavirin.
(C) ritonavir.
(D) zanamivir.

88. Intracellular survival and replication are the major virulence factors rather than exotoxin production for which of the following organisms?

(A) Cholera
(B) Diphtheria
(C) Gastroenteritis caused by enterotoxigenic *Escherichia coli*
(D) Pertussis
(E) Plague

89. All of the following are properties of interferon-γ EXCEPT

(A) induction of 2′,5′-adenyl synthetase.
(B) host cell–specific gene product.
(C) direct inactivation of eIF-2 (eukaryotic initiation factor-2).
(D) toxic side effects when used clinically.

90. Assuming that route and concentration of inocula are appropriate, an immune response is expected to all of the following EXCEPT

(A) 2,4 dinitrobenzene.
(B) heterologous red blood cells.
(C) heterologous carbohydrates.
(D) heterologous enzymes.
(E) heterologous immunoglobulins.

91. Six 18-year-old women return from a recent Canadian camping trip with abdominal cramping, gas, pain, and diarrhea that is pale, greasy, and malodorous. They drank untreated stream water on the last 2 days of the trip after losing their water filter. What is the most likely causative agent?

(A) *Baylisascaris procyonis*
(B) *Entamoeba histolytica*
(C) *Giardia lamblia*
(D) Norwalk agent
(E) *Salmonella enteritidis*
(F) *Vibrio parahaemolyticus*

92. One advantage of a live, attenuated vaccine is

(A) it does not produce persistent infections.
(B) the viral strain does not revert to virulant forms.
(C) it has an unlimited shelf life.
(D) it induces a wide spectrum of antibodies.

93. Which of the following is an RNA tumor virus associated with the neurologic disease topical spastic paraparesis?

(A) AKR leukemia virus
(B) Human immunodeficiency virus
(C) Human T lymphotrophic virus type 1
(D) Rous sarcoma virus

94. All of the following molecules are within the immunoglobulin superfamily EXCEPT

(A) T-cell receptor.
(B) immunoglobulin E.
(C) human leukocyte antigen (HLA)-A and other class I histocompatibility antigens.
(D) HLA-DR and other class II histocompatibility antigens.
(E) C4 and other class III histocompatibility antigens.

95. All of the following statements about exotoxins are true EXCEPT

(A) they are heat stable at 100°C.
(B) they are produced by both gram-positive and gram-negative bacteria.
(C) they may be neutralized by antitoxins.
(D) they are proteins.

96. The role of macrophages in the immune response includes all of the following functions EXCEPT

(A) antigen engulfment.
(B) production of interleukin (IL)-1.
(C) production of IL-2.
(D) production of endogenous pyrogen.
(E) presentation of antigen in context of class II histocompatibility antigens.

97. CD4 cells are involved in all of the following processes EXCEPT

(A) acting as a "helper function" for B cells.
(B) processing and presenting antigens.
(C) producing and releasing interleukin-2.
(D) regulating intensity of natural killer cell and null cell activity.
(E) producing and releasing interferon-γ.

98. B cells can be involved in all of the following processes EXCEPT

(A) capping and internalization of antigen bound by surface immunoglobulin receptors.
(B) antigen processing and presentation.
(C) production and release of interferon-γ.
(D) maturation to plasma cells.
(E) expression of class II histocompatibility antigens on the cell surface.

99. What major trait does *Neisseria meningitidis* have that is NOT found in *Neisseria gonorrhoeae*?

(A) β-Lactamase resistance
(B) Capsular polysaccharide
(C) Inability to metabolize glucose
(D) Inability to metabolize maltose
(E) Oxidase production

100. Viral transcription

(A) occurs in a specific temporal pattern for most RNA and DNA viruses.
(B) involves a virion transcriptase for negative-sense, enveloped RNA virus.
(C) occurs in the nucleus for poxviruses.
(D) may be inhibited by amantadine hydrochloride.

101. Which of the following statements about children who have survived infant botulism is true?

(A) Elevated cerebrospinal fluid pressure occurs in over half of the children, resulting in some permanent neurologic defects.
(B) Almost all of the children have some permanent neurologic defects.
(C) There is some permanent muscle weakness following recovery that, like polio, may worsen late in life.
(D) Recovery is expected to be complete in all children who survive.

102. All of the following compounds are mitogens that stimulate human T cells to proliferate EXCEPT

(A) lipopolysaccharide.
(B) concanavalin A.
(C) pokeweed mitogen.
(D) phytohemagglutinin.

103. In addition to the "bull neck" appearance and the pseudomembrane, symptoms of diphtheria involve the

(A) skin (cutaneous diphtheria).
(B) kidneys.
(C) heart and nerves.
(D) liver and kidneys.
(E) ears and sinuses.

104. All of the following substances are T-independent antigens EXCEPT

(A) endotoxin.
(B) lipopolysaccharide.
(C) polymerized flagellin.
(D) phytohemagglutinin.
(E) Epstein-Barr virus.

105. Subacute spongiform encephalopathy describes degenerative central nervous system diseases caused by

(A) arbovirus.
(B) BK virus.
(C) JC virus.
(D) prions.

106. All of the following substances are mediators of immediate (type I) hypersensitivity EXCEPT

(A) histamine.
(B) anaphylatoxins.
(C) slow-reacting substance of anaphylaxis.
(D) eosinophilic chemotactic factor of anaphylaxis.
(E) kinins.

107. A typical antibody molecule has all of the following characteristics EXCEPT

(A) it consists of at least two identical heavy and two identical light chains.
(B) it has at least two antigen-binding sites.
(C) it has only one specificity for antigen.
(D) it is a glycosylated molecule.
(E) it has two constant domains on each of the heavy chains.

108. In the following pairs of organisms, which two are easiest to distinguish from each other by Gram stain?

(A) *Bacillus* and *Clostridium*
(B) *Salmonella* and *Shigella*
(C) *Haemophilus* and *Escherichia*
(D) *Corynebacterium* and *Lactobacillus*
(E) *Listeria* and *Proteus*

109. A neonate with very low Apgar scores dies 2 hours after birth. Autopsy reveals disseminated granulomatous lesions throughout; some are caseating, but they are not calcified. During her pregnancy, the mother most likely had a septicemia caused by

(A) *Escherichia coli.*
(B) group B streptococci.
(C) *Listeria monocytogenes.*
(D) parvovirus B19.
(E) *Toxoplasma gondii.*

110. Which of the following cells interacts directly with antigen-presenting cells?

(A) CD4$^+$ cell
(B) CD8$^+$ cell
(C) Mature B cell
(D) Plasma cell
(E) Monocyte–macrophage
(F) Null (K) cell

111. The virulence of *Francisella tularensis* is most highly associated with

(A) adherence.
(B) the capsule.
(C) intracellular replication.
(D) an exotoxin that inhibits protein synthesis by blocking elongation factor 2.
(E) a Shiga-like toxin.

112. A 15-month-old child living in a religious community that does not vaccinate their children develops meningitis. A gram-negative rod is seen in the cerebrospinal fluid. What is the most likely causative agent?

(A) An enterovirus
(B) *Escherichia coli*
(C) *Haemophilus influenzae*
(D) *Neisseria meningitidis*
(E) *Streptococcus agalactiae*

113. Following several tick bites while hiking through a wilderness park in the southeastern United States, a 19-year-old man develops fever, sore throat, malaise, headache, nausea, and a rash on the lower parts of both his arms and legs. When he starts feeling worse and his wrists and ankles begin to swell, his companions take him to an emergency department. The man's temperature is 38.9°C. Which of the following should be at the top of the differential diagnosis list?

(A) Epidemic typhus
(B) Lyme disease
(C) Q fever
(D) Rocky Mountain spotted fever
(E) Streptococcal pharyngitis

114. Which of the following is a characteristic of streptococci?

(A) Gram-negative cocci usually strung in diplococci or chains
(B) Endotoxin
(C) Fimbriae
(D) Coagulase
(E) Catalase

115. A patient with *Pseudomonas aeruginosa* septicemia develops shock, which is triggered by

(A) catalase.
(B) lipid A.
(C) flagella from gram-negative bacteria.
(D) O-specific polysaccharide side chain of endotoxin.
(E) teichoic acid-peptidoglycan fragments.

116. A burn patient has an infected area with odiferous, blue-green pus. What is the most likely causative agent?

(A) *Aspergillus fumigatus*
(B) *Pseudomonas aeruginosa*
(C) *Staphylococcus aureus*
(D) *Streptococcus pyogenes*
(E) *Vibrio vulnificus*

117. Which of the following viruses induces characteristic giant, multinucleated cells?

(A) Respiratory syncytial virus
(B) Parvovirus
(C) Reovirus
(D) Parainfluenza virus
(E) Bunyavirus
(F) Arenavirus

118. Which of the following is a nucleoside analogue that inhibits reverse transcriptase?

(A) Acyclovir
(B) Amantadine
(C) Cytarabine
(D) Zidovudine
(E) Interferon
(F) Ribavirin

119. Infection with which of the following organisms is more often noted for the production of a lymphocytosis rather than a mononucleosis?

(A) Epstein-Barr virus
(B) *Bordetella pertussis*
(C) Human immunodeficiency virus
(D) *Listeria monocytogenes*

120. In which one of the following fungal scalp infections is hair loss most likely to be permanent?

(A) Anthropophilic tinea capitis
(B) Black-dot tinea capitis of adults
(C) Favus (tinea favosa)
(D) Zoophilic tinea capitis

121. A child presents with impetigo with bullae. A gram-positive, β-hemolytic, catalase-positive, coagulase-positive coccus is isolated. Which of the following is the most likely organism?

(A) Group A streptococcus
(B) Group B streptococcus
(C) *Staphylococcus aureus*
(D) *Staphylococcus epidermidis*

122. A woman who is an intravenous drug abuser and who has worked as a prostitute for the last 20 years now has an aortitis. She has no mucosal ulcerations or exanthems. Her VDRL (Venereal Disease Research Laboratory) test is negative and her fluorescent treponemal antibody absorption test is positive. What is the most likely diagnosis?

(A) Early primary syphilis
(B) Lyme disease
(C) Secondary syphilis
(D) Latent syphilis
(E) Tertiary syphilis

123. Which of the following infections is known to increase susceptibility to pneumonia caused by *Streptococcus pneumoniae*?

(A) Epstein-Barr virus infection
(B) *Haemophilus influenzae* type b or d infection
(C) Influenza virus infection
(D) *Mycobacterium tuberculosis* infection
(E) *Mycoplasma pneumoniae* infection

124. Which strain of *Corynebacterium diphtheriae* is pathogenic?

(A) Those producing the blackest colonies on tellurite medium.
(B) Those with a plasmid with *tox*⁺ genes.
(C) Those with chromosomal *inv*⁺ genes.
(D) Those lysogenized by corynebacteriophage-β

125. What is the vector for Chagas disease?

(A) Lice—genus *Pediculus*
(B) Mites
(C) Mosquitoes—genus *Aedes*
(D) Mosquitoes—genus *Anopheles*
(E) Reduviid bugs
(F) Sandflies

126. The T-cell antigen receptor is associated with which of the following characteristics?

(A) It is a monomeric immunoglobulin M.
(B) It requires free antigen for triggering.
(C) It is associated with CD4 or CD8.
(D) It is nonspecific.

127. Which of the following cell surface markers are associated with T lymphocytes immediately before differentiation into T helper cells and cytotoxic T cells?

(A) CD2⁻ CD3⁻ CD4⁻ CD8⁻ TCR⁻ cell
(B) CD2⁺ CD3⁺ CD4⁻ CD8⁻ TCR⁺ cell
(C) CD2⁺ CD3⁺ CD4⁺ CD8⁻ TCR⁺ cell
(D) CD2⁺ CD3⁺ CD4⁻ CD8⁺ TCR⁺ cell
(E) CD2⁺ CD3⁺ CD4⁺ CD8⁺ TCR⁺ cell

128. Which of the following cells is capable of attacking a certain tumor cell spontaneously (i.e., without prior sensitization)?

(A) Monocyte–macrophage
(B) CD8⁺ cell
(C) Mature B cell
(D) Plasma cell
(E) Natural killer (NK) cell
(F) Null (K) cell

129. A patient has a catheter infection. A biofilm is present on the catheter. What is the most likely causative agent?

(A) *Enterococcus faecalis*
(B) *Staphylococcus aureus*
(C) *Staphylococcus epidermidis*
(D) *Streptococcus agalactiae*
(E) *Streptococcus pneumoniae*
(F) *Streptococcus viridans*

130. How does *Mycoplasma pneumoniae* differ from *Rickettsia prowazekii*?

(A) It is a prokaryote.
(B) It is dimorphic.
(C) It lacks a cell wall.
(D) It has a single chromosome.
(E) It is intracellular.

131. Which of the following drugs induces 2,5A synthetase?

(A) Acyclovir
(B) Amantadine
(C) Cytarabine
(D) Foscarnet
(E) Interferon
(F) Ribavirin

132. Bacteria are protected from phagocytosis by

(A) the capsule.
(B) lipopolysaccharide.
(C) lipoprotein.
(D) the mesosome.
(E) the outer membrane.
(F) peptidoglycan.

133. Stimulation of the T helper subset 1 (T_H1) cell population with processed antigen and interleukin (IL)-1 can reciprocally activate macrophages if it releases

(A) complement components.
(B) IL-2.
(C) IL-6.
(D) interferon-γ.

134. Which of the following viruses has a segmented, ambisense genome?

(A) Respiratory syncytial virus
(B) Parvovirus
(C) Reovirus
(D) Parainfluenza virus
(E) Bunyavirus
(F) Arenavirus

135. A patient with sickle cell anemia is most likely to have repeated septicemias with

(A) *Candida albicans.*
(B) nontypeable *Haemophilus influenzae.*
(C) *Mycobacterium avium-intracellulare.*
(D) *Salmonella enteritidis.*
(E) *Staphylococcus aureus.*

136. Which of the following complement components attaches to the crystallizable fragment of immunoglobulin M?

(A) C5b
(B) C5a
(C) C1qrs
(D) C4b2a
(E) C2b

137. What is the current state of epidemiology for whooping cough?

(A) Like diphtheria, pertussis has nearly been eradicated by vaccination except for 4–7 imported cases/year.
(B) There are hundreds of pertussis cases/year, but only imported or in partially vaccinated or unvaccinated babies.
(C) There are thousands of pertussis cases/year, but only imported or in partially vaccinated or unvaccinated babies.
(D) There are thousands of pertussis cases/year, some imported, some in partially vaccinated or unvaccinated babies, and some in junior high children, and adults whose immunity has waned.

138. Why does *Clostridium difficile* cause diarrhea?

(A) *C difficile* invades, surviving and causing disease in a mechanism similar to that of *Listeria*.
(B) *C difficile* invades, secreting two surface toxins inside the cells.
(C) *C difficile* stacks itself on the colonic surface to cause maladsorption and the appearance of a pseudomembrane.
(D) *C difficile* exotoxins damage the cells, causing a disruption in transport and attracting polymorphonuclear cells to cause the appearance of a pseudomembrane.

139. What does a zone of induration greater than 15 mm mean in interpreting a tuberculin skin test?

(A) Active infection with *Mycobacterium tuberculosis*
(B) Active infection with any of the nontuberculous mycobacteria
(C) Anergy
(D) Antibody titer to *M tuberculosis*
(E) Previous infection with *M tuberculosis*
(F) Vaccination with bacillus Calmette-Guérin (BCG) vaccine only

140. Which of the following is most likely to cause urinary tract infections?

(A) *Bacteroides* species
(B) *Clostridium botulinum*
(C) *Clostridium difficile*
(D) *Clostridium perfringens*
(E) *Clostridium tetani*
(F) *Escherichia coli*

141. Which of the following is the most appropriate and effective method for reducing the transmission of toxoplasmosis?

(A) Avoid intravenous drug abuse.
(B) Avoid swimming in contaminated water.
(C) Avoid using human excrement as vegetable fertilizer.
(D) Cook fish and seafood thoroughly.
(E) Heat all canned foods to 60°C for 10 minutes.
(F) Avoid cat litter or take proper care in changing litter.

142. Which of the following statements about endogenous type C viruses is correct?

(A) They are defective viruses.
(B) They are pathogenic for their hosts.
(C) They cause tumors in their hosts.
(D) They have a provirus form.

143. Which of the following diseases is caused by a virus that uses a reverse transcriptase during replication?

(A) Infectious hepatitis
(B) Measles
(C) Serum hepatitis
(D) Infectious mononucleosis
(E) Shingles
(F) German measles

144. Which of the following statements regarding the clinical manifestations and consequences of *Neisseria gonorrhoeae* infection is true?

(A) Pharyngeal infection is always mild and mimics viral sore throat.
(B) Dermatitis involves rash over the trunk and extremities.
(C) Ophthalmia neonatorum is always mild.
(D) Both men and women can be asymptomatic.
(E) Urethral symptoms are painless.

145. How is drug resistance transferred in most gram-negative bacteria?

(A) Unidirectional transfer of DNA by conjugation
(B) Conjugal exchange of the DNA from both participants in the cross (drug resistance is generally dominant)
(C) Transformation
(D) Generalized transduction

146. An 18-year-old Iowan dirt bike racer, who recently raced for the first time in the desert south west, presents in September with cough, malaise, low-grade fever, myalgias, and chest pain. Rales are heard and respiratory infiltrates are noted on radiograph. Sputum stained with calcofluor white and viewed on an ultraviolet microscope shows large blue-white fluorescing spherical structures with round cells inside. What is the most likely causative agent?

(A) *Candida albicans*
(B) *Coccidioides immitis*
(C) *Histoplasma capsulatum*
(D) Influenza virus type A
(E) *Mycoplasma pneumoniae*
(F) *Streptococcus pneumoniae*

147. Which of the following cells is involved in antigen processing and presentation?

(A) CD4$^+$ cell
(B) CD8$^+$ cell
(C) Mature B cell
(D) Monocyte–macrophage
(E) Plasma cell
(F) Null (K) cell

148. A patient presents with explosive, watery, noninflammatory diarrhea along with headache, abdominal cramps, nausea, vomiting, and fever. Symptoms began the day after eating raw oysters in August. What is the most likely causative agent?

(A) *Giardia lamblia*
(B) Norwalk agent
(C) Rotavirus
(D) *Salmonella enteritidis*
(E) *Staphylococcus aureus*
(F) *Vibrio parahaemolyticus*

149. A tuberculosis patient who is also human immunodeficiency virus (HIV) positive has a CD4$^+$ count of 60 because he is inconsistent in taking any medication. He also has small sites of dissemination throughout his body. What was the most likely route of dissemination?

(A) Blood stream
(B) Nerves
(C) Contiguous spread through the tissues
(D) Lymphatics

150. A 28-year-old homosexual man is seen with a solitary indurated penile ulcer with fairly clean margins, no obvious raised granulomatous areas, and no discoloration. He reports that it began as a hard nodule and that it is not painful. Regional lymphadenopathy is noted. What is the most likely causative agent?

(A) *Haemophilus ducreyi*
(B) Herpes simplex virus type 2
(C) *Histoplasma capsulatum*
(D) Human papillomavirus, serotype 11
(E) *Neisseria gonorrhoeae*
(F) *Streptococcus pyogenes*
(G) *Treponema pallidum*

151. A 3-year-old girl presents with a temperature of 38.2°C, a sore throat, difficulty swallowing, and vomiting. Examination reveals that the soft palate and posterior oral cavity are reddened with vesicular lesions. No tonsillar abscess or exudate is seen. The epiglottis is not swollen. She is fully vaccinated. The test for cell-wall carbohydrate is negative. Blood and Thayer-Martin agar cultures have been set up. What is the most likely causative agent?

(A) Coxsackievirus type A
(B) *Haemophilus influenzae*
(C) *Mycoplasma pneumoniae*
(D) *Neisseria meningitidis*
(E) *Streptococcus pyogenes*

152. A 7-year-old boy is seen with malaise, fever, sore throat, and swelling of both ankles and wrists. He has a macular rash that began on his hands and feet (including his palms and soles) and is progressing inward. A wood tick (*Dermacentor*) was removed 6 days earlier after his return from scout camp in Tennessee. What is the most likely causative agent?

(A) *Borrelia burgdorferi*
(B) Coxsackievirus type A
(C) *Francisella tularensis*
(D) *Streptococcus pyogenes*
(E) *Rickettsia prowazekii*
(F) *Rickettsia rickettsii*

153. Which of the following diseases is associated with the delta agent?

(A) Infectious hepatitis
(B) Measles
(C) Serum hepatitis
(D) Infectious mononucleosis
(E) Shingles
(F) German measles

154. Which of the following is a regulatory gene of human T-cell lymphotropic virus I (HTLV-I) that transactivates transcription?

(A) Delta hemagglutinin
(B) E1A protein
(C) Large T antigen
(D) TAT protein
(E) VCA protein
(F) TAX protein

155. Which of the following viruses has an oncogene that codes for a guanine-nucleotide–binding protein?

(A) Mouse mammary tumor virus
(B) Rous sarcoma virus
(C) Polyomavirus
(D) Human T lymphotrophic virus
(E) Hepatitis B virus
(F) Harvey sarcoma virus

156. β-Lactamase production is a major problem in which one of the following organisms?

(A) *Corynebacterium diphtheriae*
(B) *Neisseria meningitidis*
(C) Methicillin-sensitive *Staphylococcus aureus*
(D) *Treponema pallidum*

157. Which of the following viruses lacks a functional virogene?

(A) Mouse mammary tumor virus
(B) Rous sarcoma virus
(C) Polyomavirus
(D) Human T lymphotrophic virus
(E) Hepatitis B virus
(F) Harvey sarcoma virus

158. Which of the following complement components is most closely related to C3 convertase?

(A) C5b
(B) C5a
(C) C1qrs
(D) C4b2a
(E) C2b

159. How can you reduce your chances of acquiring *Vibrio parahaemolyticus* illness?

(A) Avoid intravenous drug abuse.
(B) Avoid swimming in contaminated water.
(C) Avoid using human excrement as vegetable fertilizer.
(D) Cook fish and seafood thoroughly.
(E) Heat all canned foods to 60°C for 10 minutes.
(F) Wear shoes outside in endemic regions.

160. Which of the following cells has surface immunoglobulin M and surface immunoglobulin D?

(A) CD4$^+$ cell
(B) CD8$^+$ cell
(C) Mature B cell
(D) Plasma cell
(E) Natural killer (NK) cell
(F) Null (K) cell

161. Which of the following viruses is a type B RNA tumor virus?

(A) Mouse mammary tumor virus
(B) Rous sarcoma virus
(C) Polyomavirus
(D) Human T lymphotrophic virus
(E) Hepatitis B virus
(F) Harvey sarcoma virus

162. Which of the following antibiotics causes misreading of mRNA?

(A) Tetracycline
(B) Cephalosporin
(C) Streptomycin
(D) Erythromycin
(E) Griseofulvin
(F) Bacitracin

163. Which of the following antifungal drugs is fungicidal and appropriate for systemic use?

(A) Amphotericin B
(B) Chloramphenicol
(C) Econazole
(D) Griseofulvin
(E) Itraconazole
(F) Nystatin

164. What is the mechanism of action of the aminoglycosides?

(A) Damage to the membrane
(B) Inhibition of DNA gyrase
(C) Inhibition of mycolic acid synthesis
(D) Binding to 30S ribosome
(E) Binding to 50S ribosome

165. How is *Borrelia burgdorferi* transmitted?

(A) Lice—genus *Pediculus*
(B) Mites
(C) Mosquitoes—genus *Aedes*
(D) Mosquitoes—genus *Anopheles*
(E) Ticks—genus *Dermacentor*
(F) Ticks—genus *Ixodes*

166. Which of the following infections is a co-factor in Burkitt's lymphoma?

(A) Cytomegalovirus infection
(B) Hepatitis A virus infection
(C) Hepatitis B virus infection
(D) Influenza virus type A infection
(E) *Mycoplasma pneumoniae* infection
(F) Epstein-Barr virus infection

167. After a trip to Peru to adopt a 6-month-old baby, a 32-year-old woman and her new baby both develop profuse, watery diarrhea with flecks of mucus. Both are hospitalized because of the severity and rapidity of the dehydration, but neither one is febrile. What is the most likely causative agent?

(A) *Campylobacter jejuni*
(B) *Escherichia coli* O157
(C) *Salmonella typhi*
(D) *Vibrio cholerae*
(E) *Vibrio parahaemolyticus*

168. What is the nonvertebrate host for the plasmodia?

(A) Lice—genus *Pediculus*
(B) Mites
(C) Mosquitoes—genus *Aedes*
(D) Mosquitoes—genus *Anopheles*
(E) Tsetse fly
(F) Sandflies

169. A 45-year-old man has mental degeneration after a prolonged but inapparent infection. At autopsy, a subacute spongiform encephalopathy is found. What is the nature of the most likely causative agent?

(A) Acid-fast organism
(B) Dimorphic fungus
(C) DNA virus
(D) Viroid
(E) Prion

170. Which of the following genetic mechanisms is responsible for the conversion of non-toxigenic strains of *Corynebacterium diphtheriae* to toxigenic strains?

(A) Lysogenic phage conversion
(B) In vivo transformation
(C) Reciprocal genetic recombination
(D) Conjugation

171. Which of the following cell surface markers are associated with cytotoxic T cells?

(A) $CD2^-$ $CD3^-$ $CD4^-$ $CD8^-$ TCR^- cell
(B) $CD2^+$ $CD3^+$ $CD4^-$ $CD8^-$ TCR^+ cell
(C) $CD2^+$ $CD3^+$ $CD4^+$ $CD8^-$ TCR^+ cell
(D) $CD2^+$ $CD3^+$ $CD4^-$ $CD8^+$ TCR^+ cell
(E) $CD2^+$ $CD3^+$ $CD4^+$ $CD8^+$ TCR^+ cell

172. Which of the following agents oxidizes proteins?

(A) Alcohols
(B) Chloroform
(C) Detergents
(D) Ethylene oxide
(E) Iodine

173. What is the first event in a patient who ultimately develops *Neisseria meningitidis* meningitis?

(A) Crossing the blood–brain barrier
(B) Meningococcemia
(C) Skin lesions
(D) Upper respiratory colonization
(E) Waterhouse-Friderichsen syndrome
(F) Traumatic implantation directly into the brain

174. In a high-frequency recombination (Hfr) cross with an F^- bacterial cell, each having a single DNA molecule, what is the most likely outcome?

(A) Bacterial genes will be transferred from the Hfr cell to the F^- cell, but there will be no change in the "sex" of either cell.
(B) Some genes will be transferred and the recipient cell will become Hfr.
(C) Only plasmid genes will be transferred.
(D) Each cell may acquire genes from the other.

175. A patient with acquired immunodeficiency syndrome has severe, nonresolving diarrhea. Acid-fast oocysts are seen in the stools, which are not gray and greasy. What is the most likely causative agent?

(A) *Cryptococcus*
(B) *Cryptosporidium*
(C) Enterotoxic *Escherichia coli*
(D) *Giardia*
(E) *Salmonella*
(F) Enterohemorrhagic *E coli*

176. Which of the following cells is involved in the recognition of antigen in the context of class I histocompatibility antigens?

(A) $CD4^+$ cell
(B) $CD8^+$ cell
(C) Mature B cell
(D) Plasma cell
(E) Natural killer (NK) cell
(F) Null (K) cell

177. At their proper levels, which of the following agents would be most effective in inactivating a naked capsid virus on a surface (e.g., a countertop) or for surface disinfection of a stethoscope?

(A) Chlorine
(B) Chloroform
(C) Detergents
(D) Ethylene oxide

178. Cellulitis develops in a 26-year-old man after he is bitten by his girlfriend's unvaccinated cat. What is the most likely dominant organism involved in the infection?

(A) *Bartonella (Rochalimaea) henselae*
(B) *Calymmatobacterium granulomatis*
(C) *Pasteurella multocida*
(D) *Toxoplasma gondii*

Answers and Explanations

1–F. The null (K) cell is the predominant cell involved in antibody-dependent cell-mediated cytotoxicity.

2–B. *Cryptococcus* is the only medically important yeast with a capsule. The capsule consists of polysaccharide, which is antigenic and diffuses away from the cell in cerebrospinal fluid. Antigenic tests used to detect capsular polysaccharide are twice as sensitive in rapid diagnosis of cryptococcal meningitis as microscopic examination using India ink. Antibodies are never used because it takes too long for them to form.

3–B. The childhood disease roseola is caused by human herpesvirus 6. Parvovirus B19 causes erythema infectiosum (fifth disease), another childhood disease characterized by a rash.

4–E. The California and La Crosse viruses, which have mosquito vectors, are both bunyaviruses.

5–D. This patient has a fungal infection requiring an oral antifungal, such as an imidazole, griseofulvin, or terbinafine.

6–C. The question refers to generalized transduction, in which an error at the packaging stage creates a transducing virus. In contrast, specialized transduction can only be carried out by temperate phages that can integrate their DNA into the bacterial DNA. Temperate phages insert their DNA into a specific integration region of the bacterial DNA. When the repressor, which maintains the integrated prophage state (lysogeny), is damaged, excision is induced. If the excision process is not perfect, a bacterial gene on either side of the integration site can be excised out, replicated with the phage DNA, and integrated into the phage progeny. The progeny, having lost some of their own genes and having picked up one bacterial gene from one side of the integration site, are transducing; however, they can only transduce genes on either side of the prophage integration site, and thus the term "specialized" transduction.

7–D. The patient's age and symptoms (and the viral clue) indicate that rotavirus is the primary suspect.

8–F. *Streptococcus pyogenes* is a group A streptococci that has an M protein on its outer cell walls that interferes with phagocytosis in the immunologically naive individual. M12 strains are often nephritogenic.

9–B. Diptheria toxin and *Pseudomonas* exotoxin A are both adenosine diphosphate–ribosylating toxins that irreversibly inactivate elongation factor 2 and inhibit protein synthesis. Although they have similar modes of action, they differ in their cellular targets and antigenicity.

10–E. Ketoacidotic diabetes is a major predisposing condition for zygomycosis, although lymphoma and leukemia also predispose the patient to zygomycosis.

11–C. A T helper cell would have all of the listed markers except for CD8.

12–E. Teichoic and teichuronic acids, which are polymers containing ribitol or glycerol, are found in the cell walls or cell-wall membranes of gram-positive bacteria.

13–C. Individuals with chronic hepatitis B infection have an increased risk of hepatocellular carcinoma. Persons with superinfections involving hepatitis B with D rarely survive long enough to develop carcinoma. Because hepatitis A and E are naked viruses and do not set up long-term chronic infection, they are rarely associated with hepatocellular carcinoma. Epstein-Barr virus also has no association with hepatocellular carcinoma.

14–E. The pathogenicity factors important in plague are calcium dependency, V and W antigens, outer membrane proteins, the F1 envelope antigen, pesticin, coagulase, and fibrinolysin.

15–E. *Streptococcus agalactiae* (group B streptococci) is the most common cause of neonatal meningitis. It is most prevalent in young women with multiple partners and is most likely to infect the baby during a protracted delivery. *Escherichia coli* is the second most common cause of neonatal meningitis. *Listeria* is a less frequent cause of neonatal meningitis and other severe diseases in newborns. *Haemophilus influenzae* and *Neisseria meningitidis* rarely cause neonatal meningitis.

16–D. Reoviruses are the only double-stranded RNA viruses.

17–A. A thymic-dependent area of the spleen is the periarteriolar region, whereas the germinal center contains predominantly B lymphocytes. Removal of the thymus aids in graft retention because it results in the absence of effector T cells. Thymectomy does not result in autoimmunity.

18–E. The VCA protein, or viral capsid antigen, is the main component of the Epstein-Barr virus (EBV) capsid. EBV is the causative agent of infectious mononucleosis.

19–A. The killing of *Neisseria meningitidis* organisms is primarily dependent on complement-mediated cell lysis. Patients with genetic deficiencies in C5–C8 cannot carry out complement-mediated lysis of bacterial cells and have repeated septicemias with *N meningitidis*.

20–E. Traveler's diarrhea is most frequently caused by enterotoxigenic strains of *Escherichia coli* that produce the heat-labile (LT) and heat-stable (ST) toxin. LT is an exotoxin that causes an increase in cyclic adenosine monophosphate.

21–C. The complement component C5a promotes chemotaxis. The complement components C1, C2, and the C789 complex do not promote chemotaxis.

22–B. The child most likely has infant botulism, which is caused by ingestion of the spores (not the toxin) of the anaerobe *Clostridium botulinum*. The immature intestinal flora allow germination of the spores and the subsequent vegetative growth with in vivo production of the toxin.

23–B. Cephalosporin drugs have the β-lactam ring as do the penicillins. They also inhibit cell-wall biosynthesis and are inactivated by some β-lactamases.

24–C. Cervical carcinoma is caused by oncogenic strains of human papillomavirus (most commonly 16, 18, and 31). The early protein E6 is associated with the oncogenic potential of human papillomavirus.

25–D. In transformation, the DNA is extracellular before it is picked up by the competent cells; during this period, the DNA is subject to the extracellular exonucleases. Because the DNA in generalized and specialized transductions is protected extracellularly by the virus capsid, it is not subject to extracellular exonucleases. In conjugation, the DNA is never outside of a cell. Transposition is a mechanism of inserting a transposon into another molecule of DNA and has no extracellular transport mechanism associated with it.

26–E. *Streptococcus pneumoniae* is the most common causative agent of pneumonia in alcoholics. *Klebsiella pneumoniae* is less common but even more deadly because of the high incidence of abscesses. (Almost all of the patients who have pneumonia caused by *K pneumoniae* suffer from chronic lung disease or alcoholism.) If foul-smelling sputum had been present, then anaerobes would most likely be involved. *Legionella* and *Klebsiella* are both gram-negative rods. *Neisseria meningitidis* is a gram-negative diplococcus. Neither *Legionella* nor *Mycoplasma* would have grown on blood agar.

27–A. Only patients with chronic granulomatous disease exhibit a deficiency in nicotinamide adenine dinucleotide (NADH) or nicotinamide adenine dinucleotide phosphate (NADPH) oxidase and increased susceptibility to organisms of low virulence. Chronic granulomatous disease is an inherited condition.

28–C. Based on the description of the disease, the child has bacterial meningitis. The only listed and routinely administered childhood vaccine that prevents meningitis is the *Haemophilus influenza* vaccine, which is a conjugate polysaccharide protein vaccine as described in choice C. The polysaccharide vaccines are not routinely administered to babies because of poor immunological response. The new heptavalent polysaccharide-protein conjugate vaccine for *Streptococcus pneumoniae,* approved in 200 but not listed in the question would also be a possible corrected answer.

29–D. Foscarnet inhibits herpesvirus DNA polymerase directly.

30–B. C5a (anaphylatoxin II) is analogous to C3a (anaphylatoxin I). C5a binds to a specific receptor on the mast cell and causes histamine release during complement activation.

31–B. *Sporothrix schenckii,* a dimorphic fungus, is found in the environment on various plant materials. Subcutaneous infections begin with traumatic implantation of contaminated plant material such as mine timber slivers, thorns, or the combination of wires and sphagnum moss (used by floral designers). The resulting sporotrichosis is characterized by a fixed nodular subcutaneous lesion or lesions along the lymphatics from the initial trauma site. When found in tissues, the fungus grows as an oval to cigar-shaped yeast. It grows as sporulating filaments in the environment and has a worldwide distribution. Cases are most common in tropical regions because people are less likely to wear protective clothing (e.g., long pants, long-sleeved shirts).

32–D. Heterologous serum protein would have the greatest antigenicity of the structures listed. It is "foreign," is usually of appropriate weight, and has a very well-defined tertiary and quaternary structure.

33–A. The *v-src* oncogene associated with the Rous sarcoma virus codes for a tyrosine protein kinase with a biologic activity that results in cellular transformation.

34–D. Invasive aspergillosis is found primarily in patients with neutrophil counts less than $500/mm^3$. Patients with cystic fibrosis or chronic granulomatous disease may also have invasive aspergillosis.

35–B. Herpes simplex viruses have the ability to become latent in neurons and reactivate (replicate) under certain conditions that are not well understood.

36–F. *Mycoplasma* is a common cause of pneumonia in teenagers and young adults. During the course of the infection, some autoagglutinating antibodies (cold agglutinins) are formed against red blood cells. The antibodies are inactive at normal body temperature, but agglutinate red blood cells at 4°C.

37–A. African trypanosomiasis (African sleeping sickness) is transmitted by tsetse flies.

38–D. The plasma cell, with its well-developed rough endoplasmic reticulum, is the producer of specific, secreted antibody.

39–C. Glomerulonephritis is a hallmark of patients with systemic lupus erythematosus, which is a vascular inflammation induced by autoantibodies produced by a variety of cellular antigens.

40–D. Although many viruses, including coronaviruses and parainfluenza viruses, cause upper respiratory tract disease, rhinoviruses are the most frequent cause of the common cold.

41–B. Gram-positive bacteria would be most susceptible to penicillin in the exponential phase, because this is the phase in which cell-wall synthesis is greatest.

42–B. O antigen or O-specific side chains are major surface antigens in the polysaccharide component of lipopolysaccharide.

43–A. CD8 recognizes class I human leukocyte antigens selectively. It is found on suppressor and cytotoxic T cells. CD4 characterizes T helper cells.

44–C. Although hepatitis B virus is a DNA virus, it needs a reverse transcriptase to replicate. Therefore, only polyoma virus is not dependent on this enzyme activity for replication.

45–E. Of the molecules listed, only the class II histocompatibility antigens, which include HLA-DR, HLA-DQ, and HLA-DS, are totally encoded on one chromosome (chromosome 6). Immunoglobulin (Ig) G and IgM are encoded on the H chain of chromosome 14 and the kappa chain of chromosome 2 or the lambda chain of chromosome 22. The T-cell receptor is encoded on the alpha chain of chromosome 7 and the beta chain of chromosome 14. The class I histocompatibility antigens are encoded on the alpha chain of chromosome 6 and on the β_2-microglobulin of chromosome 2.

46–C. In developing countries, the incidence of neonatal tetanus can be minimized by ensuring the cleanliness of the umbilical stump. The high incidence of clostridial spores in the environment makes prevention extremely difficult. Tetanus vaccine should be given to pregnant women to boost maternal antibodies. A botulism vaccine that seems to be somewhat effective is available for laboratory workers investigating *Clostridium botulinum,* but not for other populations. Botulism is spread in infants by the ingestion of spores and in adults by the ingestion of contaminated food containing the exotoxin.

47–C. Human immunodeficiency virus is the only virus that can be treated with antivirals whose mechanism of action is the inactivation of a viral protease.

48–B. Interleukin-1 aids in the initiation of the acute phase response to bacterial invasion. It is synthesized by many cell types, it activates T cells, and it can act synergistically with tumor necrosis factor.

49–B. Fluid and electrolyte replacement is most important in the treatment of cholera. Antibiotics alone will not work but antibiotics with the water and electrolytes will most often be successful and will reduce carriage.

50–C. All antibodies contain a hypervariable region at which antigen is bound. Immunoglobulin (Ig) G does not contain a J chain because it is a singular entity. It is preceded in synthesis by IgM. Only IgA contains a secretory piece because it needs to be transported across mucosal surfaces.

51–D. Because interferon is produced in the first cell infected by the virus, it is the first host defense mechanism that occurs in response to a primary virus infection.

52–A. *Mycobacterium avium-intracellulare* or *Mycobacterium tuberculosis,* both acid-fast organisms, are the most likely causes of this pulmonary infection in a patient with acquired immunodeficiency syndrome. *Pneumocystis carinii* cannot be cultured yet.

53–E. Influenza A virus, which causes a localized respiratory infection, has a segmented genome composed of eight pieces of negative-sense, single-stranded RNA, which can "reassort" when two different strains infect the same cell.

54–C. This syndrome is exhibited by patients with pernicious anemia and is not characteristic of the other diseases.

55–C. An F$^+$ cell contains the fertility factor in the free plasmid state. In the cross between an F$^+$ cell and an F$^-$ cell, chromosomal genes are not transferred because they are not covalently linked to the plasmid. Only the plasmid genes are transferred.

56–A. *Bacillus cereus,* found in rice, is not killed by steaming. The addition of eggs and other ingredients to make fried rice encourages growth if the fried rice is not held at a high temperature. Onset of watery diarrhea may occur within 2 hours or as long as 18 hours after consumption and is in response to the presence of toxin.

57–A. A pre–T cell is a lymphocyte with no discernible T-cell markers.

58–D. The integrated intracellular form of the DNA of a temperate phage is called a prophage.

59–E. Hookworm filariform larvae may grow in the soil in endemic regions and can penetrate skin. Wearing shoes has been shown to greatly reduce the transmission of hookworm.

60–B. The isohemagglutinins (anti-A and anti-B) are found only in individuals who do not possess the homologous antigenic determinant.

61–C. Facultative anaerobes grow in the presence or absence of oxygen; a respiratory mode is used when oxygen is present, and fermentation occurs when it is not. Facultative anaerobes contain the enzyme superoxide dismutase, which aids aerobic growth by preventing the accumulation of the superoxide ion. Obligate aerobes do not have fermentative pathways and require oxygen for growth; obligate anaerobes lack superoxide dismutase. The heterotrophs require preformed organic compounds for growth.

62–B. Enzyme-linked immunosorbent assays are approximately 1000-fold more sensitive than the other serologic tests listed. Nucleic acid hybridization is not a type of serologic test.

63–D. Amplification of pre–B cells along the pathway leading to the terminal plasma cell requires interleukin (IL)-4 and IL-6. IL-1 is involved mainly in T-cell activation. CD4 and CD8 function during interaction of the T cell with antigen-presenting cells.

64–D. Peptidoglycan (mucopeptide and murein) is a complex cell-wall polymer containing *N*-acetylglucosamine and *N*-acetylmuramic acid and associated peptides.

65–B. Swimming in contaminated waters may cause infection with *Acanthamoeba* or *Naegleria,* which may develop into meningoencephalitis.

66–A. *Bacteroides* is the most common organism in the human gastrointestinal tract, greatly outnumbering *Escherichia coli, Clostridium perfringens,* and *Clostridium difficile,* which are also part of the normal flora of the gastrointestinal tract.

67–E. Adult *Ascaris lumbricoides* is a roundworm that maintains its position in the gastrointestinal tract by continual movement "upstream," not by attaching. It is noted for migration into the bile duct, gallbladder, and liver, producing severe tissue damage. This process is often exacerbated by fever, antibiotics, and anesthetics.

68–C. A selective medium permits growth in the presence of agents that inhibit other bacteria. A minimal medium contains the minimum quantity and number of nutrients capable of sustaining growth of the organism. A differential medium differentiates among organisms on the basis of color due to different fermentation or pH.

69–A. Of the bacteria causing sexually transmitted diseases, the bacterium found most prevalently in college-age students is *Chlamydia trachomatis.* It is a small, intracellular-dwelling bacterium that often induces the carrier state. *Trichomonas vaginalis* is a motile, single-cell parasite.

70–B. Endotoxin activity is associated with the lipid A component of lipopolysaccharide found in the outer membrane of gram-negative bacteria.

71–D. O side chains contain the greatest number of antigenic epitopes in gram-negative bacteria. The mucopeptide, lipid A, and teichoic acids are poorly antigenic because they have few antigenic epitopes. Teichoic acids are not found in gram-negative bacteria.

72–C. Viridans streptococci, which are part of the normal oral flora in humans, are noted for their ability to attach to damaged heart valves when they enter the circulation after oral surgery.

73–B. Turbidity, dry weight, and protein are all indirect indices of the true number of bacteria in a sample. Even viable counts, which measure live bacteria, do not always give a true count because bacteria may clump and aggregate, thus appearing as a single entity.

74–F. The rubella virus, which causes German measles, can cause a congenital rubella syndrome if the fetus is infected during the first 10 weeks of pregnancy.

75–C. Because idiotypic determinants on antibodies contain amino acid sequences in the $(Fab')_2$ variable regions that are unique to the respondent, they can be antigenic.

76–A. The Bence Jones proteins are dimers of free light chains found in the urine of some patients with multiple myeloma (plasma cell tumors).

77–C. The delta antigen is a phosphoprotein involved in the replication process of hepatitis D virus.

78–D. Croup, an early childhood upper respiratory tract infection, is caused by type 2 parainfluenza viruses.

79–B. Amantadine blocks the penetration and uncoating of influenza A viruses and may be used prophylactically.

80–C. Colonization of mucous membranes often involves immunoglobulin A proteases.

81–C. Mueller-Hinton agar is widely used for drug susceptibility testing because a wide range of organisms grow on it; however, it is not a differential medium. A differential medium allows differentiation of two different kinds of bacteria, whereas an enrichment medium contains added growth factors to encourage the growth of certain bacteria. A selective medium may have inhibitors to prevent the growth of certain bacteria. Tellurite, eosin-methylene blue, and MacConkey media are all differential media.

82–E. Immunosuppression can cause the reactivation of varicella-zoster virus from neurons, which results in shingles.

83–B. Heterophil antibodies (which react with sheep erythrocytes and are the basis for the "mono" spot test) are produced during most Epstein-Barr virus infections.

84–A. $CD4^+$ cells, or T helper cells, recognize antigen in the context of class II histocompatibility antigens on the surface of macrophages and other antigen-presenting cells. The natural ligand for CD4 is the class II molecule.

85–B. Plague is generally transmitted in one of two ways: either by flea bite or by respiratory droplets from an untreated person with the pulmonary form of plague.

86–B. For all major causative agents of meningitis that are extracellular (and these are the major ones), the capsule (polysaccharide) is important for successful hematogenous spread to the central nervous system; examples include *Cryptococcus,* meningitis-causing strains of *Haemophilus influenzae* (type b capsule), *Neisseria meningitidis,* and *Streptococcus pneumoniae.* All of these causative agents have polysaccharide capsules that allow survival in the blood stream in an immunologically naive individual so they can reach the blood–brain barrier. The major virulence factors in urinary tract and ascending urinary tract infections are pili or adhesions that attach to the uroepithelium. *Mycoplasma* does not have a capsule.

87–D. Zanamivir is used for prophylaxis and treatment of influenza A and B virus infections. It inhibits the neuraminidase of the virus, thereby preventing release of the virus from the cell.

88–E. The virulence of *Yersinia pestis* does not depend on exotoxins. Instead, it depends on a variety of other factors, the most important of which is its ability to proliferate intracellularly. Associated with this ability and virulence are Ca^{2+} dependence; V and W antigens; *Yersinia* outer membrane proteins; F1 envelope antigen; coagulase, pesticin, and fibrinolysin production; and pigment absorption.

89–C. Interferon-γ does not directly inactivate eIF-2 but induces a protein kinase that phosphorylates it, thus rendering it inactive.

90–A. All heterologous compounds may elicit some antibody response. Dinitrobenzene is a hapten by definition and, under normal circumstances, should not elicit an immune response.

91–C. Pale, greasy, malodorous stools with malabsorption after drinking untreated stream or lake water strongly suggests a *Giardia lamblia* infection. The organisms can be detected most reliably by a fecal antigen test because they attach to the intestinal mucosa.

92–D. An advantage of live, attenuated vaccines is that they induce a wide spectrum of antibodies. Disadvantages include the possible production of persistent infections, reversion to highly virulent strains, and a limited shelf life.

93–C. Human T lymphotrophic virus type 1 causes adult acute T-cell leukemia, but is also associated with tropical spastic paraparesis, a slowly progressive (10 or more years) neurologic disease endemic in some areas of the Caribbean.

94–E. Of the molecules listed, only the complement components are outside the basic structure of the immunoglobulin superfamily.

95–A. Exotoxins are heat-labile proteins that are released or secreted by certain gram-positive and gram-negative bacteria. Antitoxins are antibodies that neutralize toxins.

96–C. Macrophages have all of the functions listed except interleukin-2 (IL-2) production. IL-2 is produced by activated T cells.

97–B. CD4 cells, or T cells, have all of the functions listed except for processing and presenting antigens.

98–C. B cells are not known to produce interferon-γ.

99–B. *Neisseria meningitidis* generally makes a capsule, which gonococcus (*Neisseria gonorrhoeae*) does not. Both strains use glucose and produce oxidase. Meningococcus (*N meningitidis*) does ferment maltose.

100–B. A unique feature of negative-sense RNA virus replication is the presence of an RNA-dependent RNA polymerase (transcriptase), which synthesizes mRNA from the viral genome.

101–D. The neurotoxin involved in infant botulism, unlike bacterial meningitis, does not cause elevated cerebrospinal fluid pressure, so recovery should be complete.

102–A. All of the listed compounds are T-cell mitogens except lipopolysaccharide, which is a B-cell mitogen.

103–C. *Corynebacterium diphtheriae* does not invade tissues; rather, the exotoxin enters the blood stream and affects tissues, primarily the heart and nerves.

104–D. All of the listed compounds are both T-independent antigens and B-cell mitogens except for phytohemagglutinin, which is a T-cell mitogen.

105–D. Prion diseases cause a brain pathology described as a subacute spongiform encephalopathy that occurs in the gray matter of the brain due to vacuolation of cells and processes and astroglial hypertrophy and proliferation.

106–B. Complement is not directly involved in the type I anaphylactic reaction, and the anaphylatoxins C3a and C5a would not be mediators. Both C3a and C5a, however, do cause mast cells to release many of the mediators important in anaphylaxis.

107–E. There are at least three constant domains on the heavy chains of an immunoglobulin (or antibody) molecule, and there may be as many as four (as in immunoglobulins E and M).

108–E. *Listeria* is a gram-positive rod, whereas *Proteus* is a gram-negative rod. *Clostridium*, *Lactobacillus*, *Corynebacterium*, and *Bacillus* are all gram-positive rods, whereas *Haemophilus*, *Escherichia*, *Salmonella*, and *Shigella* are all gram-negative rods.

109–C. *Listeria* may cause in utero infections or may infect the baby during delivery. In utero *Listeria* infections are generally severe and are characterized by caseating, granulomatous lesions. Except for *Toxoplasma* and parvovirus, the other organisms listed cause infections acquired during birth. *Toxoplasma* usually manifests with calcified central nervous system lesions in the baby. Parvovirus B19 can cause anemia and hydrops fetalis when it crosses the placenta.

110–A. CD4$^+$ cells directly interact with antigen-presenting cells.

111–C. The ability of *Francisella tularensis* to survive intracellular killing and to replicate intracellularly are the most important known virulence factors.

112–C. The only gram-negative rods are *E. coli* and *H. influenzae*. The causative agent is more likely to be *Haemophilus influenzae* in this age child.

113–D. The rash associated with *Rickettsia rickettsii* originates on the ankles or wrists and spreads to all parts of the body.

114–C. Streptococci are gram-positive organisms, so they do not possess an endotoxin. They attach to endothelial cells via their fimbriae and associated lipoteichoic acids. They are nonmotile. They are distinguished from staphylococci because they are catalase negative. Of the medically important bacteria, only *Staphylococcus aureus* and *Yersinia pestis* are coagulase positive.

115–B. *Pseudomonas* is a gram-negative organism; therefore, the patient has a gram-negative septicemia. Endotoxic activity is associated with lipid A. No toxicity is associated with the O polysaccharides, the flagella from gram-negative bacteria, or catalase. Teichoic acid-peptidoglycan fragments trigger gram-positive shock.

116–B. Some strains of *Pseudomonas aeruginosa* produce a blue-green pigment, which is clinically notable in burn wounds infected with *Pseudomonas*.

117–A. Respiratory syncytial virus causes the formation of characteristic giant cells that can be observed in nasal secretions.

118–D. Zidovudine is an analogue of thymidine, which, when converted to a triphosphate form by cellular enzymes, inhibits reverse transcriptase in human immunodeficiency virus.

119–B. *Bordetella pertussis* is unusual among bacterial infections in that it causes a lymphocytosis. A mononucleosis-like presentation may occur during the first year of human immunodeficiency virus infection.

120–C. Scarring and permanent hair loss are most likely to occur with favus (tinea favosa).

121–C. Although groups A and B streptococci and *Staphylococcus aureus* are β-hemolytic, only the streptococci are catalase negative. Only *S. aureus* is both β-hemolytic and coagulase positive.

122–E. The fluorescent treponemal antibody absorption (FTA-abs) test detects specific antibody and is positive slightly earlier than the Venereal Disease Research Laboratory (VDRL) test (about 1 week earlier); it remains positive with or without antibiotic therapy. The VDRL test detects less specific reaginic antibodies, which sometimes decline without treatment in tertiary syphilis. Therefore, based on the serologic data, this patient could have very early primary syphilis or untreated tertiary syphilis. With primary syphilis one would expect some mucosal lesions instead of aortitis. Thus, the symptoms are consistent with tertiary syphilis.

123–C. Pneumococcal pneumonia is most frequent in patients with some damage to mucociliary elevators in the upper respiratory tracts. Antecedent measles, influenza virus infections, and alcoholism predispose patients to pneumococcal pneumonia.

124–D. Only toxin-producing strains of *Corynebacterium diphtheriae* cause diphtheria. The genes directing the production of the toxin are located on molecules of corynebacteriophage-β DNA, which may infect and lysogenize *C diphtheriae* causing production of the toxin. Neither plasmids nor the chromosome contain the genes to direct the synthesis of the toxin. Repressor molecules for the *tox*$^+$ gene are on the chromosome, however. Both toxigenic and nontoxigenic strains of *C diphtheriae* will be gray to black on tellurite medium.

125–E. Chagas disease (South American trypanosomiasis) is transmitted by reduviid bugs that defecate as they bite. The trypanosome is actually in the feces, which is scratched into the bite site. Reduviid bugs are also called kissing, assassin, or cone-nosed bugs.

126–C. The T-cell antigen receptor is specific for antigen bound to an antigen-presenting cell. It is a multicomponent molecule associated with CD3. Transmission of the signal also involves association with major histocompatibility complex (MHC) class II molecules via CD4 and with MHC class I molecules via CD8.

127–E. Maturing T cells have both CD4 and CD8 markers before differentiation into T helper cells (CD4$^+$) and cytotoxic T cells (CD8$^+$).

128–E. The natural killer (NK) cell is capable of spontaneously attacking and destroying certain tumor cells.

129–C. *Staphylococcus epidermidis* is noted for its ability to secrete biofilms and adhere to intravenous lines. *Streptococcus mutans* (a viridans streptococci) is also noted for the production of a dextran biofilm that adheres these organisms to dental surfaces and causes dental plaque.

130–C. Both *Mycoplasma pneumoniae* and *Rickettsia prowazekii* are prokaryotic microorganisms. However, *M pneumoniae* lacks a cell wall; it is extracellular.

131–E. Interferon, a host-encoded glycoprotein that is produced in response to virus infection, induces the synthesis of several antiviral proteins, including 2,5A synthetase.

132–A. The capsule is a well-defined structure usually composed of polysaccharide that is external to the cell wall and protects the bacteria from phagocytosis, prior to opsonization.

133–D. Of those listed, Interferon-γ is the only potent activator of the macrophages.

134–F. The short genome RNA molecule of arenavirus is ambisense—that is, the 3′ half has negative sense and the 5′ half has positive sense.

135–D. Sickle cell anemia patients have problems with septicemias with encapsulated organisms, such as pneumococcus and *Klebsiella*. Of those listed, only *Salmonella enteritidis* has a prominent capsule and so is noted for causing repeated infections in sickle cell carriers. *Staphylococcus aureus* only rarely is encapsulated.

136–C. C1qrs is the functional link between antibody on a cell surface and activation of the classic complement cascade.

137–D. Pertussis is badly underreported. Babies are born with little immunity and so are very susceptible before complete vaccination; disease is more severe the younger the baby. Babies are infected by older children and adults who acquire pertussis when their immunity wanes, which happens 5 years or longer after vaccination. Partial immunity generally prevents neurologic consequences and death. Twelve to twenty percent of afebrile coughs in adults are pertussis.

138–D. *Clostridium difficile* causes the production of exotoxins, which cause diarrhea and production of the pseudomembrane.

139–E. The tuberculin test indicates previous infection with *Mycobacterium tuberculosis* or *Mycobacterium bovis* from between several weeks to 5 years. It does not provide proof of current active infection with *M tuberculosis*. The tuberculin test detects cell-mediated immunity and not antibody. If a person is infected with a nontuberculous strain of mycobacteria, usually the skin test is smaller. Specific skin tests for some of these nontuberculous strains of mycobacteria are available. Vaccination with bacillus Calmette-Guérin (BCG) vaccine should not result in this large a zone of induration.

140–F. *Escherichia coli* is a common causative agent of urinary tract infection. The strict anaerobes do not cause urinary tract infections.

141–F. One route of spread of toxoplasmosis is through contaminated cat litter. The other is through the ingestion of undercooked meat.

142–D. Endogenous type C viruses are retroviruses that are not pathogenic for their hosts and often replicate when cells harboring them are placed in culture. Their genetic material exists in a provirus form in host cells.

143–C. The hepatitis B virus, the hepadnavirus that causes serum hepatitis, uses a virus-encoded reverse transcriptase during replication.

144–D. Both men and women with *Neisseria gonorrhoeae* infection can be asymptomatic, thus facilitating the spread of gonorrhea. Pharyngeal infection can be severe with manifestations similar to those of a streptococcal sore throat. Dermatitis usually occurs as a simple pustule over the inflamed joint. Ophthalmia neonatorum is rapidly destructive, causing blindness if untreated.

145–A. The DNA in bacterial conjugation (a single strand) goes only from the donor parent to the recipient and not vice versa. Conjugation requires a series of genes (e.g., conjugal DNA metabolism, sex pili) and is the major mechanism of transfer in gram-negative bacteria. Transduction is a major mechanism in the transfer of *Staphylococcus aureus* drug resistance.

146–B. The causative agent can only be *Coccidioides immitis* from the description of the spherules and endospores in the sputum along with the huge potential for exposure in a person new to the endemic area. Without the results of the microscopic examination it possibly could have been *Histoplasma capsulatum* pneumonia since he is from Iowa, but it is unlikely and no exposure was given for bird or bat guano. The patient is the right age-group for *Mycoplasma* pneumonia, but again the microscopic exam points instead to *Coccidioides.*

147–D. The monocyte–macrophage is the classic example of an antigen-presenting cell (APC). Other macrophage-like cells (e.g., Kupffer's cells, Langerhans' cells of the skin) probably share this APC function.

148–F. *Vibrio parahaemolyticus* is the most likely causative agent. It is found in raw oysters from contaminated oyster beds, usually in late summer.

149–A. The description fits miliary tuberculosis, which results from hematogenous spread of *Mycobacterium tuberculosis.*

150–G. Only *Treponema pallidum* and *Haemophilus ducreyi* produce nodular penile lesions that ulcerate. Major clues leading to the diagnosis of *T pallidum* are the hard nodule or chancre and the lack of pain. *H ducreyi* produces soft, painful chancres. *Histoplasma capsulatum* produces mucous membrane ulcerations, generally in compromised patients who have disseminated infections. Human papillomavirus produces warts that do not ulcerate. Herpes simplex virus type 2 would have nerve pain associated with it. *Neisseria gonorrhoeae* generally causes urethritis with an exudate. Group A streptococci cause impetigo, which is not nodular.

151–A. Symptoms of coxsackievirus herpangina include sore throat, such as that caused by *Streptococcus;* however, vesicular lesions are present on the soft palate, and tonsillar abscesses are not seen. Generally, the patient's temperature is lower in herpangina, and no left shift is noted in a white blood cell count. Epiglottitis caused by *Haemophilus influenzae* is not likely in a vaccinated child. *Mycoplasma* does cause sore throat but is not associated with vomiting or difficulty swallowing and would not manifest as vesicular lesions. *Neisseria meningitidis* also is less likely because of the vesicles.

152–F. Several organisms produce exanthems. The tick, the locale (southeastern United States), the wrist and ankle swelling, the macular nature of the rash, and the progression of the rash are most suggestive of Rocky Mountain spotted fever caused by *Rickettsia rickettsii. Borrelia* is generally spread by the *Ixodes* tick; vasculitis is not prominent and the rash spreads in a somewhat circular pattern. *Francisella* may be spread by ticks, but generally results in an ulcer at the tick site and is not associated with a rash.

153–C. The delta agent, a defective virus, causes a more severe form of serum hepatitis than that observed with hepatitis B virus alone.

154–F. TAX protein is a human T-cell lymphotropic virus I (HTLV-I) transcriptional activator thought to be involved in cellular transformation.

155–F. The *ras* gene of the Harvey sarcoma virus codes for a guanine-nucleotide–binding protein, which has biologic activity that causes cellular transformation.

156–C. Production of β-lactamases had become a major problem in *Staphylococcus aureus,* so nafcillin and methicillin were developed. Now, due to the mutation of penicillin-binding proteins, many methicillin-sensitive *S. aureus* have become resistant to those compounds. Because there is little β-lactam resistance of any kind, penicillin G and erythromycin are the accepted drugs of choice (along with antitoxin) for *Corynebacterium diphtheriae* infections. Penicillin G is the drug of choice for both *Treponema pallidum* and *Neisseria meningitidis,* but rare resistant strains of *N. meningitidis* are beginning to appear.

157–F. Harvey sarcoma virus, like most viruses with high oncogenic potential, is a defective virus that lacks at least one functional virogene.

158–D. The C4b2a moiety, formed sequentially after the attachment of C1 to antibody, will cleave C3 and is thus called C3 convertase.

159–D. *Vibrio parahaemolyticus* is a marine organism that is transmitted through ingestion of raw or undercooked seafood.

160–C. Possession of multiple classes of surface immunoglobulin is a hallmark of the mature B cell. This cell can be driven to plasma cell formation and subsequent antibody secretion by exposure to the appropriate antigen.

161–A. Mouse mammary tumor virus (the Bittner virus) is a type B RNA tumor virus.

162–C. Streptomycin binds to the 30S ribosomal subunit, thereby causing misreading of mRNA.

163–A. Both amphotericin B and nystatin are fungicidal, but nystatin is not used for systemic infections.

164–D. Aminoglycosides are bactericidal for many aerobic gram-negative bacteria.

165–F. *Borrelia burgdorferi* causes Lyme disease. The reservoirs are deer and white-footed mice. The vector carrying the bacterium to humans and dogs is the *Ixodes* tick.

166–F. Antecedent Epstein-Barr virus infection in a malarial region is associated with Burkitt's lymphoma.

167–D. The mention of Peru should raise suspicion of cholera. (Rotavirus would have to be ruled out for the baby, but it is not one of the choices.) The loss of fluids and electrolytes is rapid and most severe with *Vibrio cholerae.* The lack of fever and lack of pus and blood in the stools suggests that the causative agent is not *Campylobacter* or *Salmonella.* The lack of blood also decreases the chance of *Escherichia coli* O157. If untreated, cholera may lead to dehydration, hemoconcentration, and hypovolemic shock.

168–D. Malaria is spread by the *Anopheles* mosquito, which is also the definitive host.

169–E. Creutzfeldt-Jakob disease is an unconventional slow virus, or prion disease.

170–A. A toxigenic strain of *Corynebacterium diphtheriae* is produced as a result of lysogenic phage conversion after a temperate bacteriophage infects a nontoxigenic strain of the organism.

171–D. A cytotoxic T cell would have all of the listed markers except for CD4.

172–E. The organic solvents and detergents primarily disrupt the membrane; detergents also physically remove microorganisms. Ethylene oxide alkylates proteins while iodine is an oxidizing agent (as is chlorine).

173–D. *Neisseria meningitidis* is an immunoglobulin A protease producer with a capsule; these virulence factors play a role in the upper respiratory colonization that is followed by invasion of the blood stream and that precedes meningitis. Skin lesions develop from overproduction of outer membrane, which is excreted without being incorporated causing endotoxin shock and petechiae which progress to frank purpura. Waterhouse-Friderichsen syndrome is late and occurs when the adrenal glands are involved.

174–A. The donor cell, which transfers part of one of the two strands of its DNA, will duplicate any areas of single-stranded DNA and so will not change genotype, including its "maleness." Only a portion of the integrated fertility factor and some bacterial genes on that strand of DNA will be transferred, so the recipient cell may pick up some new bacterial genes. But because the last thing to be transferred in would be the rest of the fertility factor, the cell almost never becomes Hfr.

175–B. Acid-fast oocysts are seen in infections with *Cryptosporidium,* a protozoan that causes severe, nonresolving diarrhea in patients with acquired immunodeficiency syndrome. In general, the bacterial causative agents are more responsive to treatment.

176–B. CD8⁺ cells, or cytotoxic T cells, recognize antigen in the context of class I histocompatibility antigens on the surface of all nucleated cells. The natural ligand for CD8 is the class I molecule.

177–A. The organic solvents will not be effective in this situation. Ethylene oxide as a toxic explosive gas is not used for open surface contamination. Diluted household chlorine (1:5) is effective.

178–C. Cat bites are most commonly a mixed infection with *Pasteurella multocida* as the dominant organism. *Bartonella (Rochalimaea) henselae* is involved in cat scratch fever.

Index

References in *italics* indicate figures; those followed by "t" denote tables